Somatic Exercises

by Kristin McGee

for dummies®
A Wiley Brand

Somatic Exercises For Dummies®

Published by: **John Wiley & Sons, Inc.**, 111 River Street, Hoboken, NJ 07030-5774, www.wiley.com

For general information on our other products and services, please contact our Customer Care Department within the U.S. at 877-762-2974, outside the U.S. at 317-572-3993, or fax 317-572-4002. For technical support, please visit https://hub.wiley.com/community/support/dummies.

Wiley publishes in a variety of print and electronic formats and by print-on-demand. Some material included with standard print versions of this book may not be included in e-books or in print-on-demand. If this book refers to media that is not included in the version you purchased, you may download this material at http://booksupport.wiley.com. For more information about Wiley products, visit www.wiley.com.

Library of Congress Control Number: 2025933268

ISBN 978-1-394-29821-1 (pbk); ISBN 978-1-394-29822-8 (ebk); ISBN 978-1-394-29823-5 (ebk)

Contents at a Glance

Table of Contents

Ten Tips for Enhancing Your Somatic Experience

Introduction

Hi! I'm excited to share with you the basics of somatic exercise. *Soma* is the Greek word for body. Somatic exercise is about getting to know your body and what you can learn from it as you get to know it better. There are many different forms of somatic movements, ranging from breathwork to Pilates. This book covers somatic exercises and give you a brief overview on how somatic movement can benefit you on many levels.

The beauty of somatic exercise is that you don't have to judge yourself. You're the observer noticing what you discover as you move your body or practice. You'll learn how to slow down and allow things to come up. It's like running your hands through a pile of sand at the beach and seeing what shells appear. You can look at each shell and see if it's been chipped or is still in one piece, if it's shiny or has lost some of its sheen. You're sifting through the loose granular substance and examining parts of it that have been shaped through many years of experiences or waves washing over them. Our emotions and experiences are like the waves and each area of our body is like a shell. To examine things closer, we need to slow down and do a little digging.

About Somatics

Somatic movement explores many different ranges of motion. Somatic exercise starts with slowing down and listening to your breath and body before you begin to move. Somatic exercise provides a way to chip away at the armor, let the sand fall, and discover the various shapes underneath. You can improve on what you find; or you can work to repattern or reprogram ways that you move so you have more freedom in your body, which in turn can open more space in your mind.

You may see many exercises in this book that seem familiar or are performed in different environments or in other exercise modalities. The main thing to remember is that when you approach exercise "somatically," you shift your focus entirely inward, tuning into the sensations of your body as you move, rather than worrying about external goals like building muscle or burning calories. This creates a more mindful, gentle practice, where the emphasis is on noticing and releasing subtle tension throughout the movement.

Here's what makes somatic exercise unique:

>> **Deep focus on internal sensations:** Instead of just going through the motions, you tune in to how your body feels with each movement — paying attention to any tightness or discomfort and allowing it to melt away.

>> **Slow, intentional movements:** Somatic exercises tend to be slower, giving you the time to check in with your body's response. It's all about being present and aware with each step and each stretch.

>> **Movement for the sake of movement:** There's no pressure to hit specific targets, like lifting heavy weights or pushing yourself to the max. The goal is simply to move and connect with your body in a meaningful way.

>> **Mind-body connection:** Somatic practices are about bringing your mind and body into harmony, directing your awareness to your body's sensations, and truly feeling each moment as you move.

For example, consider a regular arm stretch — you might normally reach as far as you can. But in a somatic stretch, you extend your arm slowly and notice how your shoulder and upper arm feel, gently releasing any tightness as you move deeper into the stretch. It's all about the experience, not the result.

This approach can apply to every movement you learn in this book!

About This Book

In this book, you become familiar with the various types of somatic exercise, including how you can learn them and incorporate them into your daily life. Some may resonate more than others, and this is the beauty of the book. You can experiment with and experience many kinds of somatic exercises.

This book guides you slowly, step by step, into the treasure house of somatics. You find out how to strengthen your mind and enlist it to unlock your body's extraordinary potential. A sound body requires a sound mind, and I show you how to improve or regain the health and wholeness of both.

I know you're busy, so I've organized this book in the easy-access way the *Dummies* series is known for. You may choose to read the book from cover to cover, or you may read any section or chapter as it calls to you. Whether you're interested in becoming more flexible, more fit, less stressed, or more peaceful and joyful, this book contains all the good advice and practical exercises you need to get started.

I've endeavored to make this book relevant to busy people like you. Not all somatic movement needs to be therapeutic — you may just love to discover how good it feels to move just for the sake of moving. You don't have to measure your progress by any external compass. You just get to grow at your own pace and in your own time and for no reason other than to get to know yourself better.

Foolish Assumptions

I know you're no dummy! But if you're a newbie to somatic exercises, I know you'll appreciate starting with the basics. You don't need prior knowledge of somatics to benefit from this book. You don't need to be trained in anything to start. You can be any level and any age. You just need a willingness to be open to what's been stored in your body.

If you do have some experience with somatics and want to understand the fundamentals more deeply, this book will also serve you well. For you, I provide detail and a fair amount of depth across the spectrum, but always in a clear and direct manner.

Icons Used in This Book

Throughout the book, you'll notice little pictures in the margins. These icons point you to information that you may not want to forget or, in some cases, you may decide to skip over.

These tips point you toward helpful information that can make your somatic journey a little smoother.

When I point to information for you to remember, that means I think it's worthwhile for you to pause and make a mental note of the information; it can help you down the road in your understanding and practice.

Please take note of all warnings. Somatics is safe, but injuries can and do happen, and I don't want that to be your experience.

Beyond the Book

In addition to the book content, you can find valuable free material online. I provide you with a Cheat Sheet that addresses questions that may be first and foremost in your mind. Check out this book's online Cheat Sheet by searching www.dummies.com for **Somatic Exercises for Dummies Cheat Sheet**.

You can also check out video clips online of many of the poses you learn in this book at www.kristinmcgee.com.

Where to Go from Here

Somatic Exercises For Dummies is both an introduction and a beginner's reference. You can read the chapters one after the other and practice along, or you can dip into the book here and there, reading up on the subjects that currently interest you.

If you're a newcomer to somatics, I recommend that you spend some time with the table of contents and leaf through the book to get a general sense of how I have structured and approached the material. You probably want to begin your reading with the first two chapters, which give you a picture of the somatics landscape.

If you aren't new to somatics and you want a refresher course, you can also use this book as a reliable guide in answering your questions. Perusing the table of contents is a good starting point for you as well. You may find yourself gravitating to later chapters that zero in on specific categories of postures, or exercises and routines for specific needs, or ways to custom-design a personal practice. And of course, the index is always useful to locate specific information on any topic of interest.

Whether you're completely new to this practice or already familiar with its benefits, you're in the right place. This book guides you through each aspect of somatics exercises so you can confidently design flows that nurture your body, refresh your mind, and support your well-being.

Okay, then, are you ready to change your relationship to your body? Let's get started!

1

Getting Acquainted with Somatic Basics

IN THIS PART . . .

Learning all about somatic exercises.

Understanding the benefits of somatic exercises.

Guiding your somatic practice to fit your personal needs.

Chapter **1**

Somatic Movement in a Nutshell

We all hold many amazing memories in our bodies. We also hold on to traumatic events and experiences that may be holding us back from living our best lives. Through somatic movement, you can unlock things that are stored and start to process events that you may not realize are creating unhealthy patterns and thoughts.

Somatic exercise is a form of exercise that uses the mind-body connection to discover things about ourselves and release physical and emotional tension. I like to think of somatic exercise as a "work in" as opposed to a workout. Somatic exercise is movement for the sake of movement, not for an external result. With somatic exercise, you are not concerned with an outcome or a result. You are instead looking to connect with your body in a way that makes it safe to process things that may be stored inside.

TIP

Soma refers to the living body, as indicated by Thomas Hannah, a pioneer in the somatic field.

Somatic movement requires a certain kind of patience and focus. The goal is to be fully in touch with your body, mind, and breath as you practice somatic exercises.

Understanding the Mind-Body Connection

Our bodies and minds are connected. When something happens to us mentally or emotionally, it's often stored physically. We may not even realize it at the time and then may create movement patterns based around the trauma.

Have you ever been thinking about something and notice that your shoulders are up to your ears? Or have you ever been moving your body and the next thing you know you've completely spaced out? So often in life we are thinking or moving, but not in the moment. I see people at the gym on the treadmill, watching television or listening to music; or some are on a stationary bike reading a book or magazine. It's impossible to be fully connected to what your body is doing when you are multitasking.

Somatic movement is the opposite of multitasking. Instead, you connect your mind and your body and pay attention to how the two are united in the same task. When we are mindful of what we are doing and present in the moment, it's miraculous how time moves differently. Many call it a *flow state*. You are so all in on what you are doing that you lose sense of anything else. You are in the flow, and nothing gets in your way.

REMEMBER

Finding that mind-body connection can tune you into all aspects of your life. It takes practice and somatic movement can help you get better and stay in that zone more often.

Exercising the Somatic Way

The concept behind somatic exercise isn't too complex. As human beings, though, we are programmed to be "doing" as opposed to "being." Because of this, learning to slow down and listen intently to our bodies can be challenging.

There isn't an external goal when it comes to somatic movement. Yes, you will notice the benefits. Maybe you'll be stressed or you'll lose a little weight, or reduce pain, or feel better. But you're not doing somatic exercises for that reason. You're moving your body in a way that feels good and helps you understand yourself better. Focusing on the mind-body connection is the ultimate goal of somatic movement. Through this process, you will experience some incredible breakthroughs and results. The first goal isn't the result, but you will inevitably see changes as you put in the work to get to know yourself better.

Somatic exercise is a body-based practice that involves noticing what you are sensing. As you start using your senses as you move, you'll start to release tension. You'll find ways of freeing up space. You'll connect to your breath. The goal, if there is one, is to become at home in your body.

You can practice somatic exercises on your own or with a trained somatic therapist. You can work on body awareness and connection using titration, pendulation, breathwork, and grounding exercises:

>> *Titration* involves gradually and carefully exploring traumatic experiences by working with small pieces at a time to avoid getting overwhelmed.

>> *Pendulation* involves moving between two sensations — safety and discomfort, or expansion and contraction — so that you can slowly release these in a balanced way.

>> *Breathwork* combines conscious breathing techniques with body awareness. The goal is to enable physical, mental, and emotional well-being. You learn to use your breath as a powerful tool to release tension, promote self-awareness, and foster a deep connection with oneself.

>> *Grounding exercises* root you in the present moment, helping to deregulate the central nervous system. When you focus on your body's contact with the floor or with the Earth, you are able to be in the moment and calm yourself.

HOW SOMATICS HELPED ME

I struggled for many years to feel at home in my body. I remember in my early teen years I was uncomfortable with the signals my body was giving me as I entered puberty. I started controlling what I was eating and lost quite a bit of weight. I was borderline anorexic, and my parents were unfamiliar with what was happening. I went to a counselor and surprisingly she gave me a workout VHS tape to bring home and start moving my body. She wanted me to start eating healthier and gain an appreciation for how my body moved and supported me at the same time. I wasn't doing the at-home workouts for an external result; rather she wanted me to feel myself from the inside and appreciate my body for how it could move and breathe and nourish itself. Eating disorders of any kind involve losing a valuable connection between the conscious mind and the physical self. Somatic movement and exercise help foster the mind/body connection.

(continued)

(continued)

This was my first experience with somatic movement. Thank goodness I realized how important it was to eat healthy, and I got back to a normal weight. I was also a dancer and in dance we'd look in the mirror and compare ourselves. When I went to college, I fell back briefly into the trap of punishing my body by restricting and then overeating. I lost track of feeling myself from the inside and cherishing what my body could do for me.

At this point, I discovered yoga, and it honestly changed my life. I started going to the local yoga studio near me in the East Village every day. I started to feel more connected to myself than ever before. I cried often in *Savasana* (the final relaxation posture at the end of a yoga class to soak in the effects of the practice) as I let go of my harsh inner critic. I learned to listed to my natural hunger cues and trust that my body knew what it needed. I tapped into my breath and found healthier ways to cope and manage my anxiety. Yoga helped me activate my parasympathetic nervous system so I could get out of flight or fight mode and relax. Somatic movement like yoga saved my life. This may sound dramatic, but I honestly think had I not discovered yoga (which then opened up the door to many other forms of somatic exercises), I wouldn't be the person I am today. See Figure 1-1.

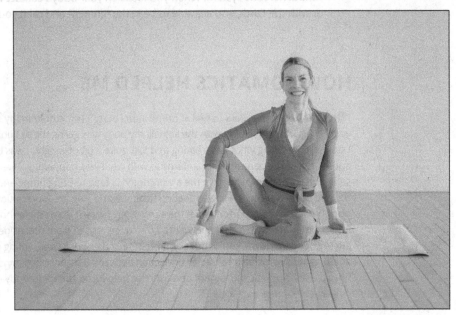

FIGURE 1-1:
The author feeling lighter after a somatic movement session.

Photograph by Guen Egan

Calming vs activating the nervous system

Somatic movement has a calming effect on the nervous system. The stress of many people's daily lives has led them to be more reactive and living in fight-or-flight mode constantly. This can lead to illness and disease. It's important to find things that can help you tap into a heightened state. Somatic exercise activates the parasympathetic (rest and digest) nervous system. When you move in a mindful way and incorporate deep breathing, you allow your body to settle down. It's not easy to constantly be on high alert. Many people need a way to relax and release.

Yoga, meditation, Pilates, walking in nature, Tai Chi, and dance are all forms of somatic movement. They allow you to connect with yourself and your senses.

Differentiating somatic work from other exercises and treatments

There are, of course, other ways to calm the nervous system, such as listening to classical music, talking to a friend, or reading a good book. The difference between somatic movement and other treatments is that you use your body to process your emotions first, instead of your mind. People often try to "think" their way out of a stressed state or an anxious mood. *Soma* means "of the body" and, in somatics, you start with your body and let it guide you to a better state. You move with purpose and connectedness. As you connect your mind and body, you can start to unravel what's putting you on high alert.

Psychotherapy

Talk therapy is the basis of psychotherapy, but in somatic therapy, the body is the starting point. Instead of talking through your issues, you become aware of bodily sensations and learn to feel safe in your body so you can achieve healing. You can explore your thoughts, emotions, and memories more easily when your body is aware and you're tapping into the areas where you've held tension and tightness due to certain experiences. Somatic exercise can certainly be a nice complement to talk therapy, but they are not the same thing.

Massage

Somatic massage focuses on the mind-body connection to help improve overall well-being. It can help you become more in tune with your body and understand how and where you store difficult memories or experiences. In addition, it can relieve tension, pain, and stress and can improve circulation. A somatic massage may include effleurage (long gliding strokes), petrissage (kneading movements), tapotement (percussive tapping), and friction (pressure applied to certain areas), deep touch, light touch compression, light shaking, and assisted stretching. During a session you may feel yourself yawning, shaking, laughing, crying or letting go of stored trauma.

A regular massage is where you go in and have your sore muscles rubbed. Although it can also be very beneficial, it is much different than a somatic massage.

Working out

When you're working out, you usually have an external goal you want to accomplish. You may want to build muscle, lose weight, or train for a specific sport or event. Somatic exercises, on the other hand, focus on the body's internal sensations, perceptions, and experiences. You can perform any workout or sport with a somatic approach as long as you're emphasizing the connection between the physical sensations and your emotional and mental state. Most workouts focus on the physical. Somatic movements have you "working in" as much as you're "working out."

Exploring the History of Somatic Exercises

Somatic exercises can be traced back to ancient Eastern practices as well as the work of philosophers and teachers in the late 19th and 20th centuries. Many somatic practices draw from Eastern healing practices such as Tai Chi, yoga, meditation, and breathwork. These ancient techniques were used as teachers developed practices that used a body-based approach to learning.

Ancient yogis were always using their bodies as tools to explore and refine their minds. They used breathwork and postures to gain a deeper understanding of and access to their consciousness. The yoga philosophy views the mind and body as interconnected, not separate. Yoga *asanas* (postures) and breathwork are used to cultivate awareness of sensations that can help quiet the mind and focus attention inward. In the late 19th and 20th centuries, philosophers and teachers developed practices that use a body-based approach to learning.

Thomas Hanna, a philosopher and educator, coined the term *somatics* in the 1970s. His belief was that many ailments were caused by a disconnect between the mind and the body. He found that focusing on the body movement, education and mindfulness could improve physical and mental health. He called his work *Hanna Somatic Education* and said that many negative health effects could be due to sensory-motor amnesia.

Other pioneers in the world of somatic movement include:

>> **Frederick Matthias Alexander** was an actor who created the Alexander Technique after losing his voice and linking it to poor posture and bad habits. His technique helps people release tension in their muscles and change harmful habits.

>> **Dr. Moshé Feldenkrais** developed the Feldenkrais Method, which is a somatic system of movement he developed after combining his martial arts and relaxation techniques. He believed that thoughts, feelings, and movement are related and can influence each other.

>> **Ida Pauline Rolf** received her PhD in biochemistry and later went on to do more research in organic chemistry. Her drive came from trying to find solutions to her own health problems and discovered that proper alignment, physiologic function, and anatomical structure are the basis of many healing methods. She created a system of hands-on deep work (called "Rolfing") on the fascia and the muscles to rebalance the body.

>> **Dr. Milton Trager** developed the Trager Approach, which is a somatic movement technique that uses gentle touch and movement to improve joint mobility and release physical and mental patterns. *Mentastics* is the term for his active movements that the client does after they have work done to them by a practitioner on a table. His approach is based on his idea that a physical change can follow a change in mindset.

>> **Bonnie Bainbridge Cohen** created body-mind centering, which explores movement and consciousness through a combination of movement, anatomy and touch.

From the ancient yogis to the dancers, actors, PhDs, and more, somatic movement has been developed by many people and practices. It all comes from the same place — a union of the mind and body.

Recognizing Why Somatic Exercise Is Useful

By now you realize that somatic exercise can help you become more aware of your body and mind and the connection between the two. Somatic exercise can help you physically and mentally. It has myriad benefits, including these:

>> Somatic movement relieves stress by helping you focus on how your thoughts affect you and what sensations are happening in your body. You can

understand what you need and manage your response to stress so you become more responsive and less reactive.

>> Somatic movement can help with pain relief through gentle movement and mindful awareness.

>> Somatic movement can help improve posture and strengthen and realign muscles.

>> Somatic movement can help you achieve better balance, mobility, and flexibility.

>> Somatic movement can help you process stuck tension and memories and help you learn more efficient and effective ways of moving. You can also become more aware and in touch with your body, so you have a better sense of your emotions.

>> Somatic movement can lead to pain reduction, increased mobility, and stress management and relief. You'll find you have reduced stress and less anxiety, depression, and other mental health issues as you develop a better relationship with yourself and connect your mind and body. You can also work on healing deep-seated trauma by releasing muscular tension and issues you have stored in your body.

>> Somatic movement helps you tune into your body's wisdom. You'll cultivate awareness of physical sensations and your emotional state. You'll learn to listen and understand what your body is telling you.

>> Somatic movement can help support personal growth and enhance your emotional well-being. As you discover what your body is telling you, you also recognize what it does for you. You can work with your body and mind to grow to new levels.

The bottom line is that you can find a deeper connection to your body. This is what helped me heal so much when I had an eating disorder and especially when I would slip back into unhealthy eating patterns. You'll begin to get a better understanding of your physical needs, and you'll listen to your body on a deeper level. You'll recognize its true hunger cues, rest cures, when you're pushing too far outside of your comfort zone, and when you may need to give yourself a bit more motivation.

Looking at Current Trends

Somatic practices have become increasingly popular in the Western world over the last 50 years. They are taught in many programs and used by professionals (including medical and physical therapists) to help with pain relief and trauma recovery.

Somatic yoga has become increasingly popular. Somatic yoga differs from regular yoga in that it focuses on the internal experience of the body and less on external alignment. Somatic yoga takes a more intuitive approach; it helps you move with the flow of energy in your body. Somatic yoga has no end result or peak pose to achieve. It can help you connect with your emotions and release trauma. People turn more to somatic yoga because of its deeper benefits.

Somatic healing modalities are also on the rise. People want to take care of themselves and move in a way that does not add more stress to their lives. Some people who are very active are turning to somatic movement for recovery. Others who are inactive find somatic movement as a great entry point to move in a mindful way that promotes health and balance. They use somatic movement to stay injury-free and carry it into anything else they choose to do.

Some other cool new trends include using virtual reality and biofeedback to improve the outcomes of somatic therapy. Neuroimaging and biomarkers can lead to more personalized somatic intervention. Generative somatics integrates trauma healing at the individual and systemic levels.

Somatic dance has also become quite popular. Group dance gatherings are becoming a popular wellness practice in many arenas. I think with the rising trend of sober outings, somatic dance is a wonderful outlet for people to come together. Somatic dance is also great on your own and is a way to unwind at the end of the day, instead of grabbing a drink.

Combining somatic movement with other workouts is also becoming popular. If you're focusing on mobility, body awareness, and alignment, somatic exercise is great before a workout. It can enhance movement efficiency and help reduce your risk of injury. After a workout, somatic movement can help you recover and release tension and return to a state of calm and awareness. It's like having a *Savasana* at the end of every workout.

Somatic exercises will continue to gain popularity because they are effective tools for holistic well-being. It isn't expensive to start and you only need your mind and body and a willingness to get to know yourself better. You can choose from many styles of yoga and Pilates, go to a Feldenkrais practitioner, try the Alexander Technique, practice Tai Chi, or start with a book like this one!

IN THIS CHAPTER

» **Building proprioception**

» **Becoming aware of your inner emotional wellness**

» **Releasing anxiety and staying in the present**

» **Expressing anger healthily**

» **Staying mobile and fit as you age**

Chapter 2

Appreciating the Benefits of Somatic Exercises

S omatic exercises can have such a profound effect on your life because they enhance how your mind and body connects. *Soma* is the Greek term for body. Your body stores everything you've experienced, and you can't find out what it's storing until you do a deep dive physically into your body. That's where somatic exercises come in. They can help you uncover tension and unhealed experiences your body is holding, and then release trauma on an internal level.

Sometimes, simply just becoming conscious of what you're keeping in can be challenging. Only when you start to move and breathe in a way that gets you into your body and out of your head, can you actually be aware of how and where you harbor tension. You feel better because you aren't walking around unaware of what's weighing you down.

In this chapter, I show you how somatic exercises can help in so many ways. When you participate in somatic exercises, you deepen your emotional balance, ease your anxiety, manage stress, and release your anger. Practicing somatic exercises on a regular basis can also help you manage your relationship with food, alleviate chronic pain, increase flexibility and mobility, foster relaxation, and heal trauma.

Our inner worlds are so rich and wonderful, it's time we start to explore them more!

TIP

Before diving into any of these practices, consider checking with your doctor. Creating a safe, supportive space allows you to move freely and feel prepared for any physical or emotional release that may arise as you explore deeper layers of your somatic journey.

Enhancing Self-Awareness

How often do you walk around thinking about how you're holding your head? How often do you sit and think about your posture? On most days, you probably go about your activities without being aware of how you move or hold yourself. On the surface, lack of body awareness may not seem like a big deal, but it is. Knowing where your body is in space is called *proprioception*. Proprioception also closely ties into how your body stores trauma.

When you experience trauma — whether physical, emotional, or psychological — your body sometimes creates areas of tension or disconnection to protect you from the pain. A big benefit of somatic exercises is that they can help you improve your proprioception and help you bring these unconscious patterns to the surface, allowing you to release stored trauma and regain a sense of presence and ease in your body. Somatic exercises such as yoga, dance, and breathwork are naturally proprioceptive and can help you become more aware of what may be debilitating you.

WARNING

Proprioception worsens as we age. Over time, we lose awareness of areas of tension and how we hold ourselves, leading to restricted or imbalanced movement patterns and possible injuries. However, practicing somatics can slow this decline.

Many people aren't concerned with proprioception unless they engage in physical activities that require them to focus on where their bodies are in space. For example, some professional athletes work to improve their proprioception because their performance depends on it. Professional gymnast Simone Biles had a temporary case of "twisties" (a phenomenon where gymnasts suddenly lose their proprioception), which prevented her from competing in the 2021 Olympics. Her coach said in order to overcome the twisties and improve her well-being and performance, she had to know herself better and set boundaries. She listened to him, worked with him and others to heal and train, and regained her proprioception and — eventually — her ability to compete. This turned out to be a career and life-saving decision; she went on to win four medals in the 2024 Olympics.

Whether you're going for the gold or just trying to cope with daily life, it's smart to become more aware of where your body is in space and how you can move it. It's really quite fun to explore how our bodies move in space and to become more self-aware of how we move in our daily lives.

Try this exercise to improve your proprioception:

1. **Stand with your feet hip-width distance apart and place your hands on your hips.**

2. **Shift your weight onto your right foot and lift your left foot off the ground a few inches.**

3. **Hold this position for up to 30 seconds and then switch sides.**

4. **Repeat this process two to three times.**

TIP

Tai Chi is a form of somatic exercise that is incredible for proprioception because of its continuous, slow circular movements while weight shifting. For more about Tai Chi, check out *T'ai Chi For Dummies* by Therese Iknoian.

BEING MINDFUL IS POWERFUL

When you listen to your body, it gives you information and insight that you would never tap into otherwise. At the gym, I often see people running on a treadmill while watching television or riding a bike while reading a book or magazine. They do get some benefit from raising their heart rates and breaking a sweat, but afterwards I can't imagine they gained much insight about themselves. Of course, it is okay to want to tune out the world or distract yourself from what your body is feeling on occasion, but in the long run, mindful somatic movement will empower you to connect on a deeper level. You may end up finding yourself running to no music and just listening to your breath. Or taking your bike ride outdoors in nature to feel the fresh air on your skin and take in the view. With mindfulness comes power.

Deepening Emotional Balance

Pro tip: No one ever calms down after someone tells them to calm down. To learn how to calm and self soothe, you need to get in touch with your emotions and connect with how they make you feel physically and mentally. A great benefit of somatic exercise is that it can help you do just that. Somatic exercise deepens your emotional balance by teaching you how to cope with difficult feelings — some of which you may not even be aware. Have you ever noticed that when you're walking around with chronic discomfort or pain, like a sore back or tense shoulders, you're extra crabby or have less patience? That stored trauma becomes physical tension, which then affects your mental state. It's a cycle — but luckily, somatic exercise can help you break it.

TIP

As you learn to identify where you tend to hold tension and then release that physical stress by using somatic exercise, you can feel more emotionally balanced.

For example, I often clench my jaw. I've had to wear a nightguard for years because I have so much tightness in my jaw and mouth. However, once I started doing more somatic breathwork, I found I clenched my jaw and grinded my teeth less at night.

The more you practice somatic exercises, the better you become at maintaining your emotional balance. You can see your emotions for what they are and not get carried away by them. One of my favorite Pema Chodron quotes is, "You are the sky. Everything else is just the weather."

REMEMBER

Often times, people aren't present enough to their experiences. Somatic exercise helps you fully experience your life and emotions instead of pushing them away. Taking time each day to connect with yourself through somatic work can really benefit your emotional state.

Easing Anxiety

Somatic movement promotes mind-body awareness, which is a powerful tool for reducing anxiety. Anxiety often stems from worrying about the future or fixating on things beyond your control. When you feel anxious, your body tenses up, and your mind races to try and manage things that may not even be happening yet.

One of the biggest benefits of somatic exercise is its ability to ground you in the present moment. By focusing on what's happening *right now* — like how your body moves and how you're breathing — you can shift your focus away from anxious thoughts about the future. Personally, I've found when I ground myself in the present through somatic exercise like yoga, that I can let go of what I can't control and focus on the here and now. Once I do that, I feel my body relax.

When you practice somatic exercise, you also train your nervous system to release tension instead of wind up. The more often you practice *breathwork* or other somatic techniques, the easier it is to tap into deep breathing and relaxation when things feel out of control. By focusing inward, you also allow yourself time and space to figure out what causes you anxiety, which is different for everyone. This helps you discover what causes you stress and how you can manage or avoid those triggers.

REMEMBER

Breathwork is a collection of breathing practices that can help you manage your mental, emotional, or physical state. It can be used to improve your health and well-being, and can be practiced anywhere, anytime.

Everyone is different, and not all somatic exercises work the same for all. Find your jam! Not everyone loves yoga. You may prefer Tai Chi or breathwork, or you may enjoy Pilates. Or maybe you like casual movements you can fit into your everyday routine, like turning walking into a somatic exercise by paying attention to your footfalls and your breath.

As you get to know yourself better through somatic exercise, you'll discover an entire arsenal of tools that can help you stay mindful and present. In the present moment, you'll no longer be anxious about the future or ruminating about events from the past. Somatic exercises provide a way to tap into your body's innate ability to relax and let go.

A simple way to release anxiety quickly is through a somatic exercise called *progressive muscle relaxation*:

1. Find a comfortable sitting or standing position.

2. Tense your feet as you inhale, then release the tension as you exhale.

3. Work your way up your body, tensing and releasing all parts until you end at your head. Be sure to take slow, deep breaths as you inhale.

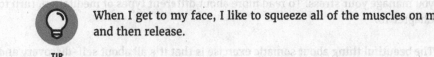

TIP

When I get to my face, I like to squeeze all of the muscles on my face all at once, and then release.

Managing Stress

Let's face it: We live in a very stressful world. All people are fighting their own inner battles while dealing with the stress of trying to make ends meet, taking care of themselves (and loved ones possibly), and getting blasted with news from social media and television that can be very upsetting. It's up to you to find ways to bring more peace and calm into your life.

I personally have a mantra meditation I often use where I repeat in my mind, "Peace Begins with Me" while tapping each of my fingers consecutively to my thumb starting with the pointer finger. And yep, you guessed it — that's somatic technique at work!

REMEMBER

Much like managing anxiety, somatic exercise can help you manage stress by getting you to pay attention to your body and internal sensations during movement. When you develop a connection between your mind and body, you improve your ability to regulate emotions and manage stressful situations in everyday life. I often say I practice yoga not for what it helps me with while I'm on my mat, but for what it does for me off of my mat. The meditation sets me up to manage stress, and since stress is cumulative, a daily practice (or twice daily) helps me remove my stress as it builds.

I think of it like a washing machine. If you make the mistake of setting it straight to the spin cycle without washing your clothes first, you'll just be wringing out dirty clothes. It's the same with self-care: You can't skip the process of cleaning out the stress and tension. You need to wash, rinse, spin, and repeat. And just like how clothes keep getting dirty, life keeps throwing challenges your way, so regular maintenance is key. If you stop too soon — like opening the washing machine before the cycle finishes — you won't get the full benefit.

REMEMBER

It's imperative to give yourself enough time to connect and reset. I always notice when I've skipped a few of my daily meditations.

I personally do a *Vedic* style of meditation twice a day for 20 minutes. Meditation is much like yoga in the fact that you may need to try a few different styles or teachers before you find something that gels with you. You may also find you need a moving type of meditation or going for a mindful hike a few times a week helps you manage your stress. To read more about different types of meditation, turn to Chapter 10.

The beautiful thing about somatic exercise is that it's all about self-discovery and connecting to your body; in return, you learn more about your mind and can manage your stress and emotions. All somatic exercises can help with stress management; but I particularly love breathing exercises. When people get stressed, they tend to hold their breath, which raises their blood pressure and elevates cortisol levels. Breathwork can help you calm down immediately by bringing awareness to your breath. Take deep, slow breaths to soothe your *parasympathetic nervous system* and get out of fight-or-flight mode. Head over to Chapter 4 if you want to learn more about how your parasympathetic nervous system works.

When you learn to manage your stress, you create a ripple effect of calmness around you. It's easier said than done but with a little bit of practice and daily somatic exercises, you can alleviate the pressure that builds up.

Expressing Anger

Somatic exercises, which help increase body awareness, can help you manage your anger. Managing your anger is important because when you suppress it, it can turn into depression. Women especially struggle with this because society often discourages them from expressing their anger. However, men aren't off the hook either. Although men are typically allowed to show anger more so than women, they are more depressed as well. The world is very complicated, and we can't save it through somatic exercises (well not entirely, anyway), but I do think if each person did their part to get to know themselves better and learn how to manage anger in a healthy way, we'd all be better off.

In yoga practice, there's a posture called Lion's Pose that's fantastic for doing just this:

1. **Start with your knees on the floor.**

2. **Breathe in, and as you do, lift your buttocks up off of your heels while rounding your spine in and pulling your fists toward your stomach (see Figure 2-1a).**

3. **Exhale while you extend your spine and shoot your arms out, releasing your palms. Stick your tongue out and make a very large "ROAR" sound, just like a lion (see Figure 2-1b).**

The Lion's Pose can feel really silly at first, but it's beyond therapeutic for letting go of anger. Look, there are many times when we all just want to shout or scream or punch something. I'm a single mom of three boys and teaching them to manage their anger is one of the hardest but also most rewarding jobs.

REMEMBER

Anger in and of itself isn't bad. In fact, there are no bad or good emotions. Emotions are just feedback and our natural reactions to situations.

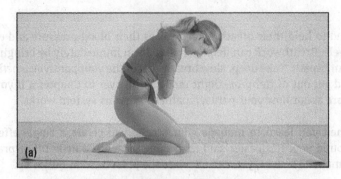

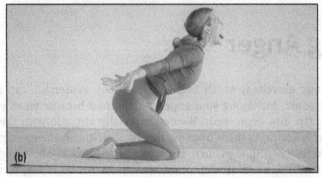

Photograph by Guen Egan

FIGURE 2-1:
Preparing for the
Lion's Pose (a)
and roaring like
a lion (b) can help
release anger.

It's okay to get angry, but it's even better to figure out how to channel the anger in a healthy way. You certainly don't want to lash out at anyone or do anyone (including yourself) harm, but if you don't let your anger out in some way, you end up bottling it up and eventually — like a pressure cooker — you just explode. Letting out a mighty lion's roar every now and then can be a very beneficial way to control your anger.

Even though communicating about your feelings is important, you have to be mindful of whether you're being productive. The thing about anger is that some-times only talking things through can escalate your anger if you're solely focused on trying to prove a point or win an argument.

TIP

When you feel the conversation going nowhere or starting to ramp up, it's better to take a timeout and do something physical to release the pent-up anger.

Have you ever noticed how much better you feel after exercising? You may be angry at your spouse or friend, and after a long run, you come back and might even almost forget what bothered you so much.

Or what about this trick that I got from a meditation teacher friend: When you're arguing with someone, hold their hand and see if that helps. Being in physical contact and aware of that connection is somatic in nature. It can be very calming.

TIP

One of my favorite nonviolent ways to release anger is called the "anger release shake." Stand with your feet hip-width apart and shake your hands vigorously. Let the shaking spread throughout your body. You can even make sounds like the lion's roar or a growling noise. Try for one to two minutes or once you feel a release. Then stop and take some deep full breaths and notice how you feel.

It's funny, without even realizing it, my first-born son and I did this often when things were upsetting in our household. We'd literally turn on Taylor Swift's "Shake It Off" and dance and shake like crazy. It was very therapeutic somatic anger management exercise!

REMEMBER

Don't judge yourself if you feel silly. Allow yourself to just shake it off!

Supporting a Healthy Relationship with Food

Weight loss isn't one size fits all, nor is somatic movement. While somatic exercise in and of itself won't lead to direct weight loss, it can help on many related levels. Because somatic movement connects your mind and body, it helps you become conscious of and honor what your body tells you it needs, including food.

Additionally, somatic exercises can lower cortisol levels. Cortisol is often called the "stress hormone," and when your cortisol levels are elevated, you're more prone to storing fat, particularly in the abdomen. This is why somatic exercises — with their emphasis on slower movements, deeper breaths, and nurturing your mind-body connection — can be so effective in managing stress and weight loss. Speaking of stress, it can lead to emotional eating or binge eating, which can lead to weight gain. When you use somatic exercises to reduce your overall stress, you may find that your emotional eating decreases as well.

WARNING

However, I think you have to be really careful with weight loss, especially in the beginning of your journey. In fact, I would challenge you to possibly let go of losing weight as a goal for now and just aim to use somatic exercise to get to know yourself better. Use it to be observant without being judgmental and listen to what your body is telling you. You are unique, and you deserve to freely find the path that works for you.

HOW YOGA SAVED ME

I often say that yoga (which is a form of somatic movement) saved my life. I had a lot of anxiety as a child and at one point, I harnessed it by becoming overly obsessed with the number of calories I ate. Looking back on this time, I didn't really have a healthy outlet. Although I loved to sing and dance, with all of my school work, I didn't have much time for it. I also played tennis, but it was a competitive sport and the goal was on the outcome, not on turning inward. I got too thin and it wasn't healthy. Thank goodness my father is a doctor and he noticed quickly and took me to the hospital where they explained to me if I didn't start eating more, I could actually die. I started therapy at the time, but it wasn't very helpful. I did start eating more but it wasn't in a very balanced way. I wasn't in touch with my hunger cues and I was still counting calories in my head. When I discovered yoga in college, I finally felt like I was getting in touch with myself. I finally started listening to my body and eating intuitively. I stopped obsessing over calories and I ate healthy foods in portions that felt good for me.

I am forever grateful for my yoga, Pilates, meditation, and breathwork practice. I discover something new about myself every time I get on my mat. In a world where so much is judged from the outside, it's a beautiful experience to get more in touch with what's on the inside.

For example, when I was restricting my food intake in unhealthy ways in high school, somatic exercise — yoga specifically — helped me get in touch with my body and listen to my true hunger cues, versus what my head was telling me to eat (or not eat). I talk more about my personal experience in the sidebar entitled, "How Yoga Saved Me."

Look at young babies — they eat when they are hungry and stop when they are full. They don't have the desire to overeat because that would make them uncomfortable, and they only seek comfort. Many adults are different, though. They often decide to accept the discomfort that comes along with eating too much. Think about when the desserts come after dinner: You eat them because they taste too good to resist, even though you might be full. The reverse is true, too — as it was with me in high school — where people deny themselves food they may really need because they want to lose weight or control their lives for unhealthy reasons, or simply because they aren't aware of what their bodies need.

I'm also guilty of multitasking during lunch. I often type up emails and do other work while I scarf down a salad, but because I'm not being mindful of my meal, the food never really registers with my body and brain, and later, I end up wanting something sweet or filling, which is not the greatest choice for my body. I've now made it a goal during meals to use somatic exercises to stay conscious. I stop everything else I'm doing to focus on and really enjoy my food, which helps me choose foods that work best for my body and digest it better.

TIP

When you foster your mind-body connection through somatic exercise, that connection can trickle down into you discovering more about the food your body actually needs and what works for you.

Although somatic exercises may not feel like a huge workout at first, they help you gain flexibility, coordination, and strength. As a result, you may experience less pain and be more likely to move more in your daily life, indirectly leading to weight loss. It's a big circle: You're likely to feel better when you use somatic movement to stay active because it connects your mind and body, and keeping your mind connected to your body usually inspires you to move more. More movement also means more energy. The more energy you have, the more you move. It's a great boomerang effect.

Pilates is another form of somatic movement that hits two targets with one arrow. Not only does it lower your cortisol level, it strengthens your core. Pilates focuses on building your core from the inside out (or the deepest layer of abdominals) while also strengthening other muscles, and it's very beneficial for many people. I personally relied heavily on my Pilates practice after carrying my twin boys to term, delivering them via c-section, and feeling like I had completely lost connection to my core. Somatic exercises like Pilates helped me reunite and reconnect to the deep abdominals and also heal my *diastasis recti* (a split of the *Linea alba*, the connective tissue that connects the two sides of the rectus abdominis).

NEAT BENEFITS

NEAT, or Non-Exercise Activity Thermogenesis, refers to the calories you burn through daily activities that aren't considered structured exercise. These movements include things like walking around the house, taking the stairs, cleaning, or even fidgeting. While it's not the same as somatic exercise, NEAT plays a significant role in overall health because it keeps your body in motion throughout the day.

The benefits of NEAT are substantial when it comes to weight management and energy expenditure. Research shows that small, frequent movements like standing instead of sitting or walking to the store instead of driving can add up over time, helping you burn more calories. By integrating more NEAT into your life, you stay more active without the need for intense workouts.

While NEAT isn't a mindful, body-aware practice like somatic exercises, both encourage regular movement and help reduce the amount of time spent sitting or being sedentary. This can lead to better overall health, improved mobility, and an easier time managing your weight. By increasing NEAT alongside your somatic practice, you can maximize your body's natural energy output.

Alleviating Chronic Pain

Somatic exercise is perfect for pain management in the very fact that it works on both the physical level and the emotional level. Somatic movement can also help us become more aware of repetitive movements that can exacerbate certain painful conditions. Think of someone who types all day long. Overtime they may end up with carpal tunnel syndrome. Or someone who is on their feet all day long and always shifts to one side who eventually has pain in one leg or their lower back. Tennis players can end up with tennis elbow and so can carpenters, from overusing their hammer hand. While most people can't change their profession or career, they can find ways to manage how they move.

Somatic exercise can also help you manage chronic pain by teaching you to listen to your body's signals and differentiate between pain and discomfort. I often teach my students about distinguishing between pain and discomfort when they're in a yoga pose, reminding them that feeling discomfort is okay — and even good.

REMEMBER

As a matter of fact, if you never felt discomfort in life, you wouldn't grow. Discomfort teaches you to manage your breath and "grow through what you go through." When you can breathe during, say, an intense yoga posture, you can breathe in other intense situations in your life.

When discomfort creeps in during a yoga pose in the form of a little warming sensation in the stomach or a muscle, or you experience a bit of an opening feeling, you can take deep breaths and see if you can manage and stay with the discomfort. Of course, when it gets too intense, you should back off of the pose and find a position that feels manageable to breathe through. This whole somatic process teaches you that you can live (and grow) through some discomfort. It makes you resilient and reminds you that you can do hard things!

WARNING

Pain is completely different. You do not want to feel pain in any yoga pose. The old days of "no pain, no gain" are long gone, and that philosophy is the exact opposite of what you try to achieve when you practice somatic exercises. Pain can be direct like a sharp shooting sensation, or you may hear a pop then some pain, or it can be blunt force like too much pressure on your knee. Avoid pain at all costs.

Chronic pain is a different story. Often, people live with chronic pain due to lack of mobility, deterioration of joints, or having excess stress on their joints. Students often complain to me about how much their back hurts. Yoga poses can help open up tight areas around your back, but more often than not, it's the deep breathing and stress management from yoga and other somatic movement that starts to alleviate your pain.

You can use somatic exercises to find out what's causing the pain and then work on finding exercises to correct the movement pattern and strengthen or stretch other muscles surrounding the painful area, bringing you back into balance.

TIP

Use *body-scan meditation* to breathe into painful areas in your body and work on releasing what you can (turn to Chapter 5 for the step-by-step process). Sometimes the root of your pain is purely physical, and other times, it's emotional. As your work through your body, you start to connect the dots and figure out how to alleviate your pain.

Increasing Flexibility and Mobility

My favorite topic is flexibility and mobility! Mobility is so important. It allows you to move freely without pain and live a healthy life. Having more range of motion can even help you relax and create more space for your breath. When you can breathe deeper and move freely, you tend to be happier than you are if you're constricted. Having good mobility can help you

>> Avoid injury

>> Improve athletic performance

>> Increase balance

>> Increase range of motion

>> Prevent health complications

Somatic exercises increase your flexibility and mobility while deepening your connection to your breath and body. Often people don't even realize how tight or stiff they are until they start to work on opening their muscles and bodies up.

For athletes, mobility is especially crucial. You can't swing a tennis racquet through its full range of motion if your shoulders are tight. A football player can't get into certain positions without mobility in their hips. When I was training for my marathon, I realized how important it was to keep my mobility so I could find a full range of motion in my stride. And golfers need good range of motion to swing a golf club. I have taught many golfers how to do somatic exercises, and their golf games improved dramatically. I think it's due to the increase of mobility and flexibility, but also their ability to stay calm under pressure.

REMEMBER

Athlete or not, everyone's flexibility and mobility benefits from somatic exercise! One of the reasons I fell in love with yoga is that it made stretching fun (in my opinion, anyway). Stretching is one of those things that most people tend to save for last or never get around to doing. Unfortunately, it's really not good to skip stretching.

Even deep diaphragmatic breathing can help you create more mobility in your rib cage (flip to Chapter 4 for the how-to on diaphragmatic breathing). Everything is connected, just like that old song reminds: "The hip bone's connected to the thigh bone." Everything in your body works in unison. When you unlock one area, you may find you need to then open another area. It's actually quite fun to discover how and where you need to create more space in your body. When you have more space, you feel more spacious and less constricted. Walking around stiff all day long isn't very pleasant.

You can even do somatic exercises in a chair. Chair yoga is a wonderful place to start for many beginners. Mindful yoga practices that are slow and use lots of props can also be helpful. Certain yoga postures are really good for alleviating tightness in the hips, shoulders, and upper and lower back. Yoga can even create more mobility and flexibility in the ankles and feet, which is key. As an old Chinese proverb says, "You die from the feet up." Once you lose mobility in your feet, you have issues with balance and stability. You want your "wheels" to be on straight and to have a full range of motion, and you want your feet to be balanced and have the ability to move freely.

TIP

Start as slowly as you want to, building your practice by incorporating a few new moves a day. The beauty again of somatic movement is that it's your practice. No expectations, no judgment. You're just getting to know yourself better and freeing up space so you can move with ease.

Fostering Relaxation

If one thing's for certain, it's that everyone could benefit from even just a little rest and relaxation. I lived in New York City for 30 years. I loved the energy of the city and constantly being on the go, but I never realized how draining it could be until I left for more open air.

Here's a story that perfectly illustrates what I mean. At the end of every yoga class (including the ones I taught or took in NYC), students take *savasana* or Corpse Pose. In the Corpse Pose, you do absolutely nothing. You don't fall asleep; you just completely let go. I've had some of my most relaxing moments ever in savasana. Savasana somehow just takes you away to a very mellow serene place where there's no place to go, nothing to do, and no one to be. The best part of the practice, in my opinion, is this final relaxation, yet so often, I'd see busy New Yorkers rush out of class and skip savasana. The problem is if you don't recharge your batteries, they eventually die. It reminds me of the Anne Lamott saying, "Almost everything will work again if you unplug it for a few minutes, including you."

TIP

By tuning in to yourself and your inner peace, you allow your nervous system to relax. If you stay in fight-or-flight mode, you end up running on adrenaline, but it eventually runs out. Then you might grab a cup of coffee to keep going. Later, you end up crashing and feeling worse.

Taking time to rest and reset can help you lead a more balanced and effective life. It's impossible to be like the Energizer Bunny and go, go, go all the time. I personally think some people keep themselves busy so they don't have to deal with their emotions. Somatic exercises encourage you to slow down and take a much-needed break.

REMEMBER

Somatic movement gives you a steady state of healthy energy. Your breath is really what gives you the most lasting fuel. When you take in plenty of oxygen, your metabolism works efficiently, your head feels clear, and you have stamina.

Almost all somatic exercises incorporate breath awareness in some way. Your breath is your life force and directly linked to your emotional state. When you breathe rapidly, you feel more tense. When you breathe slowly, you feel more at ease. Just stopping to take a few slow deep breaths throughout the day can help tremendously with fostering relaxation.

In addition to breathwork, somatic exercises usually incorporate slow, gentle movements, which help release tension. They also help you become more aware of your thoughts, feelings, and what your body is telling you in a nonjudgmental way. When you are more at peace with your emotions, you feel calmer. When you practice somatic exercises, you're also respecting your limitations. You aren't pushing yourself to finish the last heavy rep or run an extra mile, even when you're exhausted. You can find a balance and honor where your body's at in any given moment or on any given day. Just giving yourself grace when you move is relaxing and less stressful on your nervous system.

For example, I roll out my yoga mat almost every day, but I listen to my body and move according to what its needs are for that particular moment or day. I don't set any time limits or force myself to do anything. I just listen to my breath and find a nice flow and connection with my body. And when I practice Pilates, I start from a place of rest before jumping into the harder core exercises. I check in with my body and see where it's at.

REMEMBER

As an ex-New Yorker, believe me when I say it's okay to slow down. It is okay to relax. You deserve to feel at home and at peace with yourself. You deserve a long savasana at the end of a practice. Let everything soak in, because that is the time when your body is reaping the benefits of the movement you just practiced.

Healing Trauma

You hold trauma in your body. You will never think or talk therapy your way out of trauma. It is true, it is impossible to just talk your way through all of your experiences. "Our issues are in our tissues," I often say. When I was a young girl, I had a horrible appendicitis. I woke up and told my mom my side hurt. She thought I was constipated and sent me to school. I ended up in the hospital a few hours later and luckily got there just in time before my appendix burst. After having my surgery, I would often feel phantom pain in my right side. I was completely healed and fine, but my nervous system hadn't quite processed it. This is just a small example of how bodies harbor trauma. My trauma was physical. People often hold emotional trauma in their bodies, which can be even harder to unlock.

The stress I carry in my jaw when I grind my teeth at night could be from anxiety. It could also be from having a very difficult time speaking up for myself. I definitely avoid conflict at all costs. I really have a hard time when it comes to managing expectations and being able to hold my ground. I often just want to please people. People-pleasing has its downside, though. You have to find a happy medium between taking care of your own needs and being aware of the needs of others.

Life is fun and complicated and scary and sad and full of its ups and downs. There are times when you feel amazing, and there are times when you don't feel so great. All of your joy, grief, pain, elation is carried in your body. When you are present to experience your emotions, your mind and body process them and you move on in a healthy way. After a very traumatic experience, like being rushed to the hospital as a fourth grader because my appendix was about to rupture, people's nervous systems can get stuck in "freeze" mode. Symptoms of trauma then start to manifest physically. Somatic exercise is a bottom-up approach and focuses on how the body is storing trauma as opposed to trying to talk through a traumatic experience.

TIP

You can use somatic exercises to release trauma because they connect the mind and body. They bring your focus to body awareness to help process and release tension. Mindful movement and tense-and-release exercises can also help certain muscles get out of being stuck in a state of stress. In order to release the trauma, you need to process it. Somatic exercises allow you to have a safe space to do a deep dive into your body and slowly work on letting go of traumatic after-effects in a negative way.

I am reminded of when an animal is rescued from an abusive owner. It takes them quite a while to feel safe again to even be pet or held by someone else, even if they are safe. The pet's nervous system has been wrecked and you see this trauma manifesting in their physical state. They may shake, cringe, shy away, or even lash out and bite. I wonder if the animal is going through somatic movements instinctually to process their trauma.

REMEMBER

Your basic needs include not only water, food, air, and shelter, but also exercise and rest. I'd even include hugs or some sort of physical connection. Somatic exercise is a way to meet your needs while also releasing what is holding you back. When you live with built-up trauma, you are like the rescue pet constantly on high alert. You need to create a safe space within yourself to feel okay and engage with the world around you. A healthy inner world leads to a healthier life and healthier relationships.

Practicing somatic exercises not only benefits you, it benefits those around you. I am a much better mother when I am consistent with my meditation and yoga practice. I am able to constantly process micro traumas that occur on a regular basis as well as examine deeper traumas that have been stored for years.

WARNING

Sometimes your trauma is too much to face alone. If you feel like you need extra support, be sure to enlist professional help from a counselor or psychologist as well. See Chapter 4 for more on somatic therapists.

Somatic exercise is more than just moving your body. The soma, or body, is like a giant sponge that absorbs everything from emotions to experiences to injuries to life events. All of these shape you into who you are as a unique being. Everyone comes from different backgrounds, upbringings, cultures, and environments. People's history, personal battles, jobs, and health conditions mold them into who they are. You can't compare yourself to others; we are all special in our own way.

IN THIS CHAPTER

» **Exploring whether somatic exercise fits your personal needs**

» **Guiding your practice with solid goals**

» **Choosing the right time and place to enhance your somatic experience**

» **Deciding what equipment you need, if any**

» **Staying safe while you practice**

Chapter **3**

Preparing for Your Somatic Journey

Preparing for your somatic journey is important because — just like anything new on which you embark — laying the groundwork ahead of time helps you manage your expectations, declare goals, and set yourself up for success. And taking notes in a journal or an app on your phone can help you keep track of what you learn on this journey. But I'm getting a little ahead of myself here. Before you launch into this experience, do a little exploration so you can figure out whether somatic exercise is a fit for you. In this chapter, I walk you through that self-discovery process for deciding whether somatic exercise is a good fit for you.

I start by showing you the ins and outs of researching, personal reflecting, and goal-setting. Once you know your personal motivation for practicing somatic exercises (I call that "your why"), I help you consider which types of somatic exercise will help you meet your goals. Then I share with you all sorts of tools and equipment you'll need based on which type of somatic exercises you gravitate toward. The tool and toys can be a big factor in determining which path you take with somatics — at the end of the day, we all still have budgets to contend with, am I right?

I also go over how to select *where* to practice (you might even find the perfect spot right in your home that inspires you) and to create a schedule and choose the time of day that makes the most sense for you, making commitment much more likely.

This chapter also features tips for taking accountability and being proactive in your practice, ensuring that you know how to keep yourself safe if your somatic movement brings up trapped emotions or trauma (and how to find professional help if you want it).

Deciding Whether Somatic Exercise Is For You

Pop quiz:

>> Do you want to increase your mobility and flexibility?

>> Do you want to improve emotional regulation?

>> Do you want to experience a deeper mind/body connection?

>> Do you want to find a way to process triggers?

>> Do you feel stuck in your life?

>> Do you want to feel better in the way you move throughout your day?

If you answered "yes" to any of these questions, there's a good chance somatic exercise might be just what you're looking for. To dig deeper, start by doing a little research online or at the library or bookstore (you're already off to a great start with this book, which is a top-tier resource, if I do say so myself). Also, ask around! Even if they've never mentioned it before, your friends, coworkers, or family members might have experience with somatic movement. Bring it up and see what happens — they may have valuable insight to share!

As you collect research, tune into what resonates for you. Do you feel like you need an emotional release? Maybe you work in a high-pressured job, or maybe you have a lot of stress to manage at home. You may have possibly gone through a recent break up or moved to a new city. There are many times in your life when you may feel extra tension and really need to find a way to cope with it. Since somatic exercises can help you tap into how your emotions influence how you feel physically, they can be very beneficial in helping you process and move through stressful times in your life.

Stress is inevitable, and different somatic movements are an incredible way to manage it. You can use somatic breathwork to home into where you're feeling anxious in your body. You can use yoga to open up tight areas that you never realized were storing so much physical tension. You can use Tai Chi to move your energy and notice how it feels when you're doing things in a slow and controlled way. To learn more about how to do these movements, turn to Chapters 5 and 7.

TIP

Somatic movement might also help improve chronic pain. Somatic practices can ease your pain by helping you bring mindful awareness to tender areas and breathing or moving through the pain. Somatic exercises can help restore a sense of peace and harmony in your body. Movement in general is good pain management. Somatic movement takes basic movement a step further by allowing you to acknowledge where the pain is coming from and guiding you in how to manage it better.

You can also take up somatic exercise to help you alleviate stress. The same way somatic movement helps you pinpoint your painful areas in your body, it also helps you become aware of your reactions to stress. When you can learn to focus on your thoughts and become aware of your bodily sensations, you have more sense of control. Bringing awareness to your body and its sensations can be very therapeutic and can help bring a sense of relaxation and stress relief.

One of the most important aspects of somatic movement (in my opinion), is that it helps you cope with trauma. Even though nearly everyone experiences traumatic circumstances, many are unaware of just how much they've been through. Somatic movement helps you slow down and listen to what your body is telling you.

REMEMBER

When you slow down and listen to your body, you can start to cope with any heavy emotions stored in your body and find ways to let them go so that you can relax your nervous system and live a healthier life. For more on how somatic movement can help you process and heal, turn to Chapter 2.

As you take stock of different stressors, physical and emotional pain, and other factors that influence your well-being, you don't have to rush to judgment simply because you want relief. Consider whether somatic exercise is truly in alignment with your needs and is something you can commit to fully. To be successful with somatic exercises, you need time and space to practice and the dedication to continue with your practice so that you can feel and witness the profound effects it will have on your mind and body over time.

Setting Goals

Clear goals are the starting point for all successful endeavors, including somatic exercise. They help you stay accountable and celebrate your progress!

Think about what you're looking to get out of somatic exercise. As you think, keep in mind that somatic exercise isn't about physical results as much as it is about lifestyle changes and feeling balanced and peaceful in your day-to-day life. These thoughts are the earliest form of your goals. Record them as they come to you. Don't worry about being perfect. You can make changes to this list any time you want.

Your goals can be anything you want, such as

>> Increasing awareness of your bodily sensations, positions, posture, and movements.

>> Relieving body tension, discomfort, and pain.

>> Improving your movement efficiency, fluidity, and grace.

>> Deepening or developing a mind-body connection.

>> Releasing trauma.

>> Learning to regulate your emotions.

REMEMBER

Choose goals that are less externally-oriented (for example, weight loss or muscle gain) and more about how you want to feel internally (for example, feel calm or be fully present).

After you identify your somatic exercise goals, I recommend that you create a strategic plan that includes steps you can implement on the way to your big goals. Breaking up your goals into little bite-sized pieces prevents you from getting overwhelmed and giving up.

My boys are in school, and they all have weekly lessons, monthly goals, and yearly calendars. You can do the same thing for yourself. Write out your daily goals, weekly ideas, monthly plans, and yearlong forecast. It's really cool to look back each week and give yourself a high five for doing what you set out to accomplish. In a year from now, you'll have transformed in ways you never thought possible.

Taking the first step

TIP

Make your goals and steps reasonable and doable for you. Don't set out to do too much in the beginning. Slow and steady always works best. You've been living your life for years already; you can't expect it all to change overnight. Adopting somatic exercise into your life takes practice!

If you don't practice, you won't evolve (in your somatic exercises or life in general). The beauty of somatic exercise is that, once you start, you'll notice how much better you feel. The better you feel because of somatic exercise, the more you'll want to incorporate it into your life. And the more you incorporate it into your life, the more your practice takes hold.

"But will it always be this wonderfully easy self-sustaining cycle, Kristin?" you may be asking. "Are you saying all I have to do is start and the rest takes care of itself?" Well, no. Sorry to be so blunt, but that's truth. Look, you and I both know that even with the best, most doable goals, life gets in the way sometimes and finding the time (or the space or the motivation. . .) to practice isn't always easy. Having goals and those little steps along the way can make a huge difference in your ability to stay the course. You never have to accomplish everything today; just try to focus on one step.

REMEMBER

Setting somatic goals isn't a one-and-done experience. Since somatic exercises can help increase awareness of your body's responses, the more you practice, the better you become at noticing how different movements affect you, and you can adjust your goals based on what you learn along the way. You may start out wanting to improve your mind-body connection and the next thing you know, you're setting goals for a regular meditation practice. Or you may want to increase your flexibility, and soon enough, you're rolling out your yoga mat a few times a week.

When you're just starting out with somatic exercise, feeling hectic and overwhelmed is very normal, but feeling that way also makes sticking with a practice very difficult. Press on, though, my friend. As somatic movement helps you release built-up emotions and calm your nervous system, you get clearer and calmer in your mind. Your goals evolve and align as you shift. When you're in a relaxed state more often, you'll be pleasantly surprised by how easy it is to make that commitment to show up for yourself.

TIP

As you practice (especially in the beginning), I suggest recording your progress so you not only stay accountable, but can also easily see your accomplishments. Go old school and write everything down in a notebook or daily planner, or use an electronic device like a smart watch or fitness tracker. You can also keep note on your phone or a computer log. Find out what works best for you and be diligent about taking notes and adjusting as you need to. Listen to your body and recognize when you need to stop or take a break.

I know if I don't write something down, I rarely do it. I always schedule my somatic movement routines into my calendar on my phone and I won't book a meeting over them or let other commitments get in the way. I take my somatic practice seriously because I know that everything else falls into place when I'm in a better place mentally and physically.

For more on setting goals and staying motivated, see Chapter 15.

Discovering your why

Your "why" is the deeper motivation or purpose that drives your actions and decisions, shaping how you engage with life and what you ultimately strive for. Once you know your why, it's much easier to stick to your somatic exercise goals. You can continue to return to your why on the days you don't feel like moving or you think you're too busy to do some breathwork.

Discovering your why starts with self-awareness. What is it that makes you tick? What gets you out of bed in the morning? What makes you excited? What are your values? How do you want to feel? There are many things you can ask yourself daily to help you identify why you do the things you do. Why did you choose to read this book?

In order to get the most out of your experience, you must have some curiosity around getting to know yourself better through somatic movement. You don't have to have all of the answers right away. Even if you did, your why may change or evolve over time. I know when I first started practicing yoga, my why was "to figure myself out." Over time, my why has evolved to "learning how to be the best version of myself that I can be." Your why may change at different stages of your life, too.

My why is much more important to me now because if I can be the best version of me, my kids are getting the best mom version of me, my clients are getting the best teacher version of me, and my friends and family have the best version of me-me. If I don't show up for myself and work on the issues that are inside me first, I can't show up fully for others.

To find your why for starting a somatic journey, try

>> Writing down your thoughts, feelings, and actions every day

>> Challenging your assumptions so you can start to see new perspectives

>> Taking notice of your recurring thoughts and look for common themes

>> Thinking about your core values, what fulfills you, and what leaves you wanting more

>> Making a list of everything you value and then narrowing it down to determine your five most deeply held values

>> Thinking about the subjects, activities, and passions that engage your curiosity

>> Taking note of what you naturally excel at

>> Looking at your skill set and think about what you're good at

>> Believing in yourself and imagining the life you want to live

>> Working with a coach or a mentor to help you dig deeper

After you find your why, you can better focus on choosing somatic exercises to match it.

Choosing exercises to meet your goals

With somatic movement, you have so many options, you can tailor the exercises to meet your why and your goals.

TIP

If you want to find more space in your body, you can focus on yoga and mindful stretching. If you are looking to calm your mind, you may focus more on breathwork and meditation. Maybe you want to get more movement into your routine; you can do Pilates or mindful walking or hiking. Or maybe Tai Chi is the perfect form of movement for you to find more focus, balance, and ease in your life.

There are so many options, and you don't have to pick just one, because many complement each other. For example, I love how my yoga practice and Pilates complement each other so well. My meditation routine pairs well with breathwork and yoga.

Also be honest about where you are in your fitness journey. Don't look to achieve an outside goal. Choosing your exercises is about you finding movement that meets you where you are and helps you go deeper inside of yourself to create meaningful changes and develop a closer connection to yourself. Be realistic about what it is you want to work on and find the exercises that pair best with your goals.

REMEMBER

You have the freedom to experiment with what works for you. You can always choose something different if you find you're not achieving what you want.

I recommend you try each form of exercise for at least three weeks. You may want to give up sooner, but stick with it. You need at least 21 days to really see if you're enjoying a practice and can implement it into your life. Because it can be challenging and you're going deeper into yourself, you may have the urge to resist it or stop too soon. For anything to become a habit, you need to give it at least three weeks.

You may also find that you like certain exercises, but you just need a little help in tailoring them so that they can meet your goals. In that case, you may want to consult with an expert in the somatic movement you're interested in. (To learn how to find someone to help you, see the sidebar in this chapter called "How to choose professional guidance.") You can also enlist a friend or find classes that inspire you. Look into local somatic yoga classes or join a mindful walking group.

The sky's the limit and as you start to meet your goals, keep creating new ones. It's really cool to see how limitless somatic practice is. You keep discovering new things about yourself and inherently want to set new milestones to reach. Your journey is yours to go at your own pace. Your goals are your own. You can let people in on them or keep them private. Some people do better when they let others in on their progress. Others like to keep it closer to their chest. You'll find out along the way what suits you.

Knowing Where and When to Practice

Pick where and when you practice so it's more likely you'll stick with it. I personally love to do my practice first thing in the morning. This way, I know nothing can get in the way later in the day. If you are not a morning person, you might dread the thought of having to do your exercises first thing, so schedule your practice for midday or early evening. Tailor your exercise to fit your needs throughout the day. If you have more energy in the morning, you can do something a bit vigorous. Or maybe you like a gentle to start your day and have more energy midafternoon. Perhaps you like to end the day on a calm note. There is no one way or right or wrong way when it comes to what time of day you practice. It's your practice! You get to decide.

TIP

Unlike other types of physical exercise, many somatic exercises can help you wind down and relax from the day, so don't worry about practicing them in the evening.

Once you start practicing these exercises, you'll probably find that you move more intuitively throughout your day. There are some days when I miss my morning practice, but after sitting for too long, I naturally start to do some stretches or some chair yoga because somatic movement has been a part of my life for so long. Due to my somatic exercise practice, I find I listen to what my body needs day in and day out. Sometimes I want a more rigorous flow, other days I want a very gentle, yin-style practice.

Where you practice is similar to when you practice. I think having a dedicated space that is distraction-free with enough room to move is ideal. You can set up a great area in your home that is welcoming and useful.

REMEMBER

You can move anywhere and anytime. I've done chair yoga in an airport. I've meditated while waiting for my sons to get out of school. You can tap into your body in any given moment. Breathwork is always available. You don't need a special place to do any of these exercises. Many people practice Tai Chi in the park, enjoying the connection to the outdoors as well as their bodies.

Setting the scene

When you are practicing somatic movement you can set the scene to your liking. You have the opportunity now to see what resonates with you. The best environment is typically a quiet, private space where you can focus on your feelings and movements without distraction. Do you have a room in your home that can serve as a peaceful space?

Keep in mind that everyone is different. Even though most people like a quiet, isolated environment for somatic practice, that doesn't mean everyone does (or has the access to such a space). If you prefer to practice somewhere that's more public (or your space limitations at home necessitate that you do), that's totally okay! The key is tuning into what works for you and working with what you've got. Personally, I love having a clean space that allows me to focus on my movement and uniting with myself, but at the same time, I have a cat who often joins me and I welcome him into my space.

TIP

You don't need a space solely dedicated to your practice. You can use rooms or areas that you don't need to rearrange or set up. For example, I meditate twice a day in my bedroom. I love the back support my headboard gives me and I add a little pillow behind my back as well. I have a set routine and place, which makes it more likely for me to keep up my practice.

Picking the perfect spot

To find your space, try a few different locations and see which one you start to gravitate toward. You may find one place that lends itself to the energy you're looking for when you practice somatic movement.

Tune into what resonates with you to help you unwind and focus:

>> Do you like having natural light, or are lamps more your speed?

>> Does clutter distract you? Do you need a tidy space, or can you block it out?

>> Does the space make your mind feel too busy or anxious, or does it calm you? For example, practicing in your home office may trigger you to think about all the work you need to do. Or if you're too close to your kids' rooms, you may worry about their clutter.

>> Do you want to be behind a closed door, or is an open space okay?

You can even have a few spaces or settings that are welcoming and available. Don't get too rigid because life happens. Have some back-up plans and different areas in your home so you can set the scene wherever you may be. My yoga space varies depending on the time of day and whether my kids are home with me or at school.

REMEMBER

Nothing's going to be perfect (especially at first), but setting up a homey place also reminds you that you can feel at home in your body. Everything is connected.

Once you find an area for your practice, set it up in a simple way and keep it up permanently if you can. If you set out your mat or meditation cushion where you can see them often, you're more likely to use them. Make it a bit sacred. Let your loved ones know that your area is for you to ensure you have that special time for yourself and movement. Even when I was in a very small apartment, I still had a designated corner where I kept my journal, mat, and props. I always sit on my bed for my meditations because it's the perfect spot for me (and my cat Lucky).

When you find the perfect spot or spots, design them to your liking:

>> Plants are great for increasing the oxygen around you, making your breath-work easier.

>> Light tones, sunlight, pleasant smells, and relaxing sounds can all assist you in your practice.

>> If you have a carpeted floor, that may be enough softness to work with. If your floors aren't carpeted, try using a cushioned mat. You may want to see how different textures make you feel. For example, I can't meditate on a hardwood floor even on my meditation cushion because my ankles are quite bony and I'm distracted by the sensation on my legs instead of my mantra or my breath.

REMEMBER

Experiment with your favorite spots and see what resonates with you. Most importantly, have fun with it. You're designing a place to get more in touch with yourself, so the space should bring you joy and happiness. This is just the beginning and an important part of your somatic journey!

Working with the environment you've got

Maybe you don't have to have a pristine studio or even a separate room in which to practice. You can make do with what you have and where you are.

TIP

If you have a tight space or you can only sneak in some movement when you're at work or at the gym, find a place that is as quiet as possible. You may live in a smaller apartment or have a home filled with a lot of stuff. As a mom of three boys, I am familiar with excess games, toys, plushies, and electronics. When we were in a small New York City living space, I found that my bed or comfy couch made sense for meditations. The space next to my bed in front of my full-length mirror was great for yoga or Pilates practice when the kids were home. When they were at school, I could use a little bit more space in the open dining area, which was in front of the big window with lots of light. Sometimes all you need to create space is a meaningful object. For example, light a candle to set the tone or hang a painting or picture with a motivational mantra or phrase to put you in the right mental space.

The words you speak to yourself are very important. Practice replacing negative thoughts with positive ones and you'll be more motivated to do things that make you feel good.

REMEMBER

You have more creative freedom than you realize. It's a matter of being creative and strategic. It's like hiring a professional organizer to redesign your closets. You may even invest in hiring someone to help you create an environment in your home or apartment that can work for you. Or look online to see how others have created welcoming spaces.

TIP

You can also carry a few reminders that help you connect to your mind and body easier, like an essential oil, an eye mask, or a set of headphones that play soothing music. You can turn whatever space you have into a place for somatic movement. You don't have to spend much money if you're on a tight budget. A few items that resonate with you and light your desire to move your body and connect with yourself are all you need.

Establishing a schedule

Everyone needs a routine and some boundaries. I love to give my boys freedom, but if they have too much, they don't get anything done. They like to know their schedule for the week and when their after-school activities are. Most people are similar and thrive in an environment that has consistency.

Set a routine of sorts and write it down. You can write a schedule by the day, week, month, or even year. Add an outline of what you want to do and how you want to feel as a result of your schedule and practice. Commit to showing up at the times you schedule for yourself. Be kind to yourself and give yourself a schedule you can achieve in the beginning. Otherwise, you run the risk of becoming discouraged.

TIP

Prioritize yourself and your practice, but make it manageable. Start with two to three days of somatic exercise per week. Fewer than two days makes it harder to get into a habit, but something is better than nothing. If you can aim for at least two days you're off to a good start.

If you're a morning person who has time at the beginning of the day, try starting with Tuesday and Thursday at 8:00 am. Or maybe you need a weekday and a weekend day. Choose the time and day that you like the best and find a rhythm. Hopefully you'll notice you want to do more, and you can add an extra day or two to your schedule. Eventually, you'll be moving mindfully three or four times a week.

You know you best. I can't tell you when to practice. All I can tell you is to give yourself a routine and stick to it. If you notice the times aren't working, switch them. If you prefer to do a different day, that's fine.

You're going to feel great when you nail down a somatic exercise schedule that works for you. You'll feel even better when you stick to that schedule. You'll be amazed at how much you start to grow and blossom within your routine. You don't have to be so rigid that you get upset when the routine is thrown off for various reasons. Keep an open mind and always a plan B so it's easy to get right back on track. A schedule helps you stay committed even when you're traveling or have big life events (eventually, you may find that you want to be more involved in your movement during these times because they keep you grounded and calm in the midst of chaos).

You are the captain of your ship. Just remind yourself you want to move in the direction of your dreams. Don't let the waves steer you off course. Make your way through the tough patches and you'll find calmer water. Soon it all becomes second nature and you start living the life you've always dreamed of.

Choosing a time of day

TIP

Mornings are generally helpful for waking up your body — your mind may be more alert but your body will be stiffer. In the evening, your body is warmed up but your mind might be more foggy and tired. If you wait to do your practice toward the end of the day, you may be more prone to skip it. On the other hand, a before bed practice can help you unwind and release the day. You just have to be mindful not to do something too active that it keeps you awake.

The bottom line? Do what works best for you and what is going to keep you consistent. Tailor the time of day around the type of somatic movement you're doing. For instance, if you are doing a mindful hike, it might make sense to do it earlier in the morning to start your day with fresh air and sunlight. If you're doing a restorative or Yin yoga practice, you may be more apt to do it later in the day when you need to wind down. You can play around with the time of day and the type of somatic movement you're doing. There is no right or wrong way. This is your journey. Just pick something you enjoy and make the space for it.

You can make it all happen. I know you can.

REMEMBER

You come first. If you prioritize your well-being, you'll be much more available to others too. Don't feel guilty for setting time aside for you.

Adopting proactive and responsive practices

Being proactive about your practice means that you can anticipate changes and address issues before they happen. Set up your space, get your equipment ready, and have a schedule. When you are proactive, you can prevent problems that may occur, which helps you have a positive experience with your somatic journey. My dad used to always say, "proper prior preparation prevents poor performance." You aren't "performing" so to speak, but you should be as prepared mentally and physically as possible when trying somatic exercise. Take away the barriers that could prevent you from getting on your mat or doing your exercise:

>> Set an alarm if you plan to get up early.

>> Set out whatever you need for practice the night before.

>> Designate and set up your space.

>> Create the time that you'll need by not scheduling anything over it.

>> Turn your ringer off or set your phone to airplane mode in advance so you're not tempted to pick up your phone.

WARNING

If you don't spend enough time being proactive, you may end up being reactive when things don't go according as planned. Being reactive often leads to hasty decisions and unnecessary stress, leaving you feeling out of control and unprepared to handle challenges effectively. When you are proactive in setting up your time, place, and schedule, you create circumstances that benefit you. You're also more relaxed and able to respond when things come up unexpectedly.

On the other hand, *responsive practice* involves being able to focus on and take an intelligent approach to your practice, responding in real time to circumstances. When you are moving in a somatic way, you can home in on what your body is telling you and adjust if you need to. For example, if you're involved in a yoga practice a few times a week and you wake up one morning with a runny nose, making downward dog difficult, you can tailor your practice so that you do more standing upright postures or seated upright postures. If you plan to practice Tai Chi outdoors and it's raining, you have a back-up plan for where to practice. If family members are home, give them the heads up you need some quiet time and that you'll tell them the exact time you'll be available. The same goes with work obligations.

TIP

If you're a new parent, it may be challenging to find the time and perfect spot, but you can still sneak in a few moments here and there to give your body and mind what it needs. You can keep the baby monitor on while they sleep and go to your little sanctuary to fit in a bit of somatic movement.

I remember when I was training for my first marathon. I had a very set schedule for my training plan. I had my short runs mapped out for the week and my longer runs set for the weekend. I had my shoes, my water, and my energy gels all ready to go. I had cold weather gear and layers so I could adjust to the weather. I was really on top of it all — or so I thought. See, there were days when I'd just have started my run and then get I'd get a call from the school to come pick up one of my sons who was sick that day. Or I'd be out on a long run and my calf would cramp up so badly I couldn't make it any farther.

Because I have spent years and years practicing somatic yoga, Pilates, breathwork, and meditation, I was able to respond in a way that was appropriate — that was *responsive* and not reactive. I would give up my run immediately to tend to my son. I'd stop running if my body cramped in a way that would make it worse if I tried to push through it. I was aware of the difference between pain and discomfort and always made sure to listen to my body.

When you are setting yourself up for your somatic movement, your goal is to proactively take all of the steps needed to ensure that you stay in tune with yourself during the practice, readily able to respond in ways that make sense in the moment. The last thing you want to do is get injured or distressed and then stop practicing all together.

Ensuring Your Safety

When it comes to practicing safely, there are some things to consider:

>> **Be mindful of your physical safety.** Make sure you have plenty of space clear of any sharp objects or furniture. If you're practicing outside, be aware of dangers and hazards, including other people. You can get lost in your movement and connection with yourself, but it's also important to remain aware of your surroundings.

>> **Ensure that you have the correct equipment if you're using props.** Make sure you have a good mat. For more on the equipment you need, see the section later in this chapter called "Gathering Tools and Equipment."

>> **Check with your physician to make sure you're cleared for exercise.**

>> **Ensure you're comfortable and wearing proper clothing and shoes.** If you are hiking, you need the proper boots or sneakers. If you are walking, invest in good walking shoes. If you are dancing or doing yoga, make sure you're wearing non-restrictive clothing that is also comfortable and supportive.

>> **Ensure you have space and freedom to move.**

>> **Know your limits and don't push past your level of flexibility or strength until you're ready to progress.**

TIP

Before diving into any new regimen, consider checking with your doctor. Creating a safe, supportive space allows you to move freely and feel prepared for any physical or emotional release that may arise as you explore deeper layers of your somatic journey.

How do you know when you're overdoing it? It's important to distinguish between pain and discomfort. Discomfort is necessary for growth. If you don't feel some discomfort, you're probably not testing your potential. If you feel direct pain, though, you need to back off. You're not going for "no pain no gain."

You'll gain a lot more in the long run if you ease into things slowly. Listen to your breath and body and start to nudge yourself into new territory, but do it in a safe way that isn't too extreme or too fast. For example, with my marathon training, if I added on too many miles at once, my body would suffer. I gradually added mileage each week (no more than 10 percent) and increased my speed slowly so that I could maintain good form and progress in a safe way.

It's not worth getting injured or pushing yourself too fast. "Forward" is a perfectly valid pace. You have plenty of time. You don't have to get anywhere. You don't have a set deadline unless you want to give yourself guidelines and benchmarks. Your goal can simply be to keep going and not get injured.

REMEMBER

Since somatic movement is a mind/body exercise, you're not only being mindful of your physical exertion, you also want to be mindful of how you are feeling and any mental strain. You may not realize how emotional it can be to uncover areas in your body that hold a lot of trauma or tension. Be gentle with yourself as you are repatterning old grooves. You've formed these grooves over many years, and it can take some time to create newer, healthier patterns. The goal is to not be a broken record or keep playing the same toxic song over and over again.

You can get stuck in one way of thinking or moving or using old defense mechanisms. I feel like it's taken me 30 years of yoga, meditation, and Pilates to become who I am now and I still have many, many more years to go. Every time I step on my mat, I discover something new. I know I have a lifetime of unlearning and relearning — as well as new learning — ahead of me. You do too!

Somatic movement gives us all the opportunity to heal and move on. It also allows us to create a safe place in our bodies so that our minds have the time to process what we've stored. When you have a good mind-body connection, you can keep finding more unity and harmony within. I share a mantra often with my students, "peace begins with me."

REMEMBER

If you find a peaceful place within you, you'll feel safe enough to keep letting go of what no longer serves you. You'll feel comfortable examining the heartaches you've gone through and instead of shying away from the hurt, you can process it. You can turn your mental pain into power. You're unpacking the emotional baggage through movement. You're creating a less painful physical body, as well as a less-stressed mind.

Gathering Tools and Equipment

The right tools and equipment make your somatic exercise routine accommodating and fun. It's like buying new shoes — you have to try a lot on to see what fits you properly. Your equipment should meet your needs and feel great to use. You can pick your tools depending on what exercises you decide to try.

First off, I highly recommend a mat. You can use a yoga mat for yoga, Pilates, breathwork, mindful stretching, and more. A good yoga mat should last you several years if not more. (I've had the same yoga mat for over 15 years!) There are many types to choose from. Some mats are made of cork and some are made of cotton or PVC. Figure 3-1 shows a few examples. The problem with PVC is that it's not very eco-friendly. Some TPE (thermoplastic elastomer, which is made of plastic and rubber) mats are fully recyclable, yet are generally less durable than PVC mats of the same thickness. You can also choose jute, which is very eco-friendly.

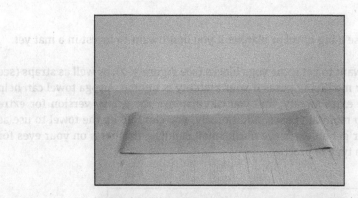

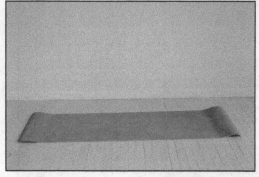

FIGURE 3-1:
Yoga mats come
in a variety of
materials.

Photographs by Guen Egan

Yoga mats can vary in thickness and surface texture. In addition to choosing one that feels good to you, select one that has

>> A grippy underside so the mat doesn't slide around on the floor.

>> A non-slip surface to help keep your hands and feet in position and not sliding around on the mat.

>> Enough padding to be supportive, but not too much that it throws off your balance or creates instability.

>> Easy-to-clean material that can wipe down easily and doesn't absorb sweat. You can also look for one that is naturally antimicrobial, to keep your mat clean and free from odor and perspiration.

Save money by finding a mat that has enough padding to use for yoga and Pilates. Too thin of a mat isn't comfortable when you're lying on your back doing abdominal work. You can always get a thin mat if you need to travel often. Or consider a thinner travel mat and an at-home mat that is a bit heavier and more padded and durable.

You can also use a big towel or blanket if you don't want to invest in a mat yet.

You may also want to get some yoga blocks (see Figure 3-2), as well as straps (see Figure 3-3) for modifying poses if your mobility is limited. A yoga towel can help you if you get extra sweaty, and you can also use the grippy version for extra friction to help maintain poses. Additionally, you can fold up the towel to use as an eye mask or get an extra eye mask/small sandbag that rests on your eyes for any restorative type of practice.

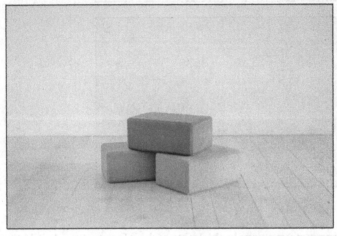

FIGURE 3-2:
Yoga blocks help you modify poses.

Photograph by Guen Egan

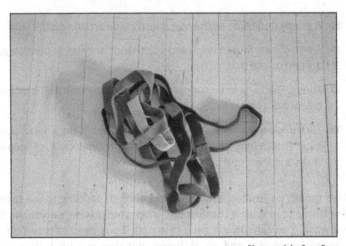

FIGURE 3-3:
Yoga straps also help you modify poses.

Photograph by Guen Egan

You can also get a meditation cushion like you see in Figure 3-4 or blanket to sit on, which can be used for seated poses.

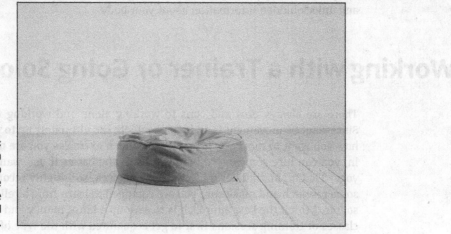

FIGURE 3-4: A meditation cushion can help you feel more comfortable in seated yoga poses.

You may want to invest in some Pilates at-home equipment, like a band or a small ball or a magic circle. These help you gain more insight and keep your practice interesting. All of these Pilates props can help you connect deeper to your core and enhance your mat practice. They can even help you mimic some of the moves you don on the Pilates equipment.

CLEANING YOUR EQUIPMENT

You can clean your mats with a solution of water and a little bit of vinegar and an essential oil such as lemon or lavender. Just a spritz after each practice and wipe it down with a towel. I've also thrown my mat in the wash machine on gentle cycle and hang it to dry, but only once every few months if it really needs it.

I also use the same vinegar spray to wipe down my Pilates equipment. I like to run my yoga towel through the wash after practice. I fold up my blankets nicely and store everything in a clean closet. If you get into the habit of taking care of your props, they'll last longer and stay germ free. My boys even know not to play with my equipment, as fun as it may look!

A good pair of hiking boots or walking shoes is necessary for walks and hikes. Other equipment used for somatic movement might include a tuning board, which is a balancing device that gives you an experience of constant motion and flow. It's portable and can help you connect to your body, connect to the outer world, and unlock hidden information about your body.

Working with a Trainer or Going Solo

There are always pros and cons to working alone and working with a trainer. Since somatic movement is an inside-out job; it's ultimately up to you to discover how you want to move. Once you decide which exercises you are most interested in, you can hire someone to help you learn the basics if you want. Breathwork, yoga, Tai Chi, and Pilates all have their nuances, so I highly recommend you do some research and make sure you are equipped to learn from a reliable, reputable source. I think the best approach is to save up a bit of money and invest in a few classes or training sessions first to get acquainted with the type of somatic exercise you want to do. After that, you can explore more on your own and every now and then check back in with your trainer or teacher.

You may want to hire a private yoga teacher to help you get started, however, private instruction can be expensive. If it's not in your budget, you can find a studio or online resources or learn through books and your own self practice.

If you are doing somatic dance or mindful walking, you don't need someone to tell you how to do it. You just need to be accountable and get out of your own way and do it. You can dance freely in your living room at the end of the day and explore your body in space. You can go on mindful walks and pay attention to your breath as you move. You can even incorporate somatic principles into exercises you already do. You can become more aware of your body, mind, and breath when you're running, for instance. You can even do some meditative breathing while on the golf course.

TIP

You also have to know your favorite learning style and approach. Think about something you enjoyed learning in the past and apply those same principles here. For example, I love working with coaches and mentors to help me gain a deeper understanding of myself, but that's not the only way. Many people prefer to do it all on their own.

Whatever you decide to do, it's also not set in stone. Maybe you start off on your own journey by yourself and then find later that you want some additional work with a trainer. Or perhaps you start out from the beginning with a trainer and then later feel like you can keep going on your own.

I think when it comes to somatic exercise, it's best to eliminate black and white thinking and be comfortable with the gray areas in life. Ideally, you'll find that you don't have to live in the extremes and can keep finding a middle ground. This helps you return to your center and learn to move through life with a sense of ease.

HOW TO CHOOSE PROFESSIONAL GUIDANCE

When you're looking for a trainer or studio to start a somatic practice with, make sure you have vetted them well and feel comfortable with them and their space. Start out by asking friends or family members who are already practicing where they go or who they recommend. Then dig deep. Read reviews online. Ask to see the providers' credentials. Interview them — ask them all kinds of questions about their experience and personality — and see how you feel. Have a conversation. Don't be shy about asking tough questions, either. Remember you're hiring them. You don't have to be afraid to ask all the questions up front.

With studios, you may want to ask if they have a new student special since you are trying to figure out what type of somatic movement resonates with you and would like to sample a few different classes. A new student discount or trial pass allows you to explore without committing long-term to a specific style or teacher until you've found your groove.

Pay attention to the atmosphere of the studio or training environment. Is it welcoming? Are the instructors approachable and responsive? The energy of the space can influence how well you connect with your practice. You want to feel supported, not intimidated. Don't hesitate to visit the studio in person before making a final decision — sometimes the vibe of the space can tell you more than any online review.

I can't even tell you how many different types of yoga I've tried or the number of Pilates studios and teachers I've gone to throughout the years. Keep an open mind. You always learn something new from the experience no matter what. Remember, this is your practice — finding the right fit might take some time, but once you do, it'll be worth the effort.

2

Exploring Fundamental Somatic Practices

IN THIS CHAPTER

» **Understanding somatic breathing and its benefits**

» **Exploring the impact of breathing on the sympathetic and parasympathetic nervous systems**

» **Uncovering somatic breathing techniques to use every day**

» **Connecting your breath to your movement**

» **Working with a somatic therapist**

Chapter **4**

Inhaling and Exhaling: Somatic Breathwork

This chapter covers a person's most important function: Breathing. Let's face it: If you aren't breathing, you aren't alive. Your breath is not only your life force, it is the most important tool you have at any given moment to help you navigate your emotions.

I remember as a young girl when I'd have a crying spell. My dad would come in and say, "calm down." Yet I didn't know how to. If only he had come in and said, "take a deep breath." The second you stop and take a deep breath, you let your nervous system know that everything will be okay. You give yourself a moment to pause and slow down. In this slowing down, you can come back to the present and feel more at ease.

Your inhalation is responsible for bringing in fresh air to your body. Every cell is reliant on your breath. Your exhalation empties out waste in the form of carbon dioxide. If you think about it, the deeper your inhalations, the more vital life force you have; the fuller your exhalations, the fewer toxins you carry around.

Somatic breathwork can truly be life altering. Our breath is our life. You can live more fully when you breathe more fully. You can also reduce stress, let go of old habits holding you back, release stored trauma, become more conscious, live in the moment, and connect better with others.

Understanding How Somatic Breathing Works

On a day-to-day basis, how often do you actually pay attention to how you are breathing? Because your breath is autonomic (runs without you thinking about it), you don't need to tell yourself to breathe. Somatic breathing, on the other hand, happens only when you think about it. It's the practice of using your breath to become more connected to yourself. You can use ancient and more modern-day somatic breathing techniques to become more conscious of how you are breathing and control your breath so that you can tap into your emotions and foster a stronger mind-body connection. Later in this chapter, I take you through many different techniques you can try.

REMEMBER

Unlike automatic breathing, somatic breathing requires your full attention. It helps you notice the subtle nuances of each breath. This heightened awareness can help you identify and release physical tension and emotional stress.

Somatic breathing in a nutshell

Incorporating somatic breathing into your daily routine can lead to profound changes in how you experience life. When you apply somatic breathing, you're helping yourself consciously pay attention to your breath and noticing how it affects your mind and body.

Stop what you are doing right now (which is reading this amazing book) and take a deep full breath in through your nose. Next, exhale all the air out through your nose until you are completely empty. Pause and notice how you feel. Feeling what a simple breath can do for you is pretty incredible, and it's available 24/7! You have this magical tool at your disposal whenever you need it!

By practicing somatic breathing, you can influence your nervous system, promoting a state of relaxation and balance. This method is not just about breathing deeply; it's about understanding how your breath can serve as a bridge between your body and emotions. Somatic breathing is a wonderful practice to integrate into your daily life, paving the way to help you

>> Reduce stress and calm yourself

>> Improve mental clarity

>> Strengthen the connection between your physical and emotional health

REMEMBER

When you incorporate simple somatic breathing exercises into your daily life, you positively influence the balance of your sympathetic and parasympathetic nervous systems, which helps you handle stress more effectively and exist in a healthier state of being.

Impact on the sympathetic nervous system

The *sympathetic nervous system*, or SNS, is your fight-or-flight system. It keeps you on high alert. When you breathe shallowly, you trigger the SNS, which raises your blood pressure, increases your heartbeat, and releases *epinephrine* and *norepinephrine*.

>> **Epinephrine is adrenaline:** If you've ever had to race for a bus you're about to miss or you are afraid someone is following you in a dark alley, chances are you're releasing adrenaline. Adrenaline is good in certain situations. It can help you run faster or scream louder, but you don't want to be pumping adrenaline into your system all day long. Studies have shown that chronic elevated levels of adrenaline can lead to an increased potential for heart damage, especially if you have preexisting cardiovascular disease, as well as an inability to sleep and general feelings of nervousness.

>> **Norepinephrine is a hormone that helps you stay focused and alert:** You may want this if you are driving late at night or a surgeon in an operating room, but too much norepinephrine can lead to feelings of anxiety and panic, as well as high blood pressure.

When you aren't cognizant of your breathing, this can lead to taking shallow breaths, which is a common problem in today's world. Did you know that opening up many tabs on your computer or staring at social media can lead to holding your breath? This is due to a psychological response related to feeling overwhelmed or stressed by the sheer volume of information and tasks seemingly present and can manifest physically as a sense of tension, including holding your breath. Many people's current lifestyles and shallow breathing can lead to chronic stress and illness.

WARNING

Poor breathing habits can also have a direct impact on the SNS, including increasing your heart rate, elevating your blood pressure, and releasing epinephrine and norepinephrine. When you breathe under stress for extended periods, your brain cells struggle to get enough oxygen to function efficiently.

For one reason or another as people age, they often move farther from the original deep breaths that they took as a child. Watch a child breathe; it's so natural and amazing. You see their bellies and chests naturally inflate on their deep inhalations and everything relax as they exhale. Whether it's societal pressures or stress in general, few adults are able to breathe this deeply. Coming back to your breath is important for keeping your sympathetic nervous system in check. The sooner you start to cherish your breath and use it to stay balanced, the better off you'll be. You don't want to breathe shallowly or rapidly and constantly incite the sympathetic nervous system.

Impact on the parasympathetic nervous system

When you take long, slow deep breaths, you tap into your *parasympathetic nervous system* (PSNS), known as the "rest and digest" state. The parasympathetic nervous system helps your body relax. The PSNS undoes the work the SNS creates after a stressful situation. The PSNS decreases your respiration and heart rate and aids in digestion.

TIP

Somatic breathwork is one of the best ways to trigger the parasympathetic nervous system. It lets your brain and body know that it is safe and doesn't need to go into fight-or-flight mode.

In this relaxed state, you may experience numerous physical and emotional benefits, including

>> Reduced fear

>> Decreased stress

>> Reduced anxiety

>> Lower blood pressure

>> Improved mental well-being

>> An overall state of calm and relaxation

Somatic memories

Somatic memories are physical sensations of pain that can linger in the body after something traumatic happens. Remember, soma means "of the body." You store all of your experiences in your body and mind (which are connected). You could be unaware of what gets stored or how it's stored. A somatic memory can be triggered by a sound, a smell, a sight, or a feeling:

>> Do you ever get a knot in your stomach when you're in an area that makes you feel unsafe?

>> Maybe you were in a car accident and hurt your neck. Now, every time you get in a car you feel your neck tense up.

>> Did you spend some time in the hospital once, and now every time you smell the lemony scent they used to clean the floors, you feel sick?

>> Maybe you were bullied by someone at school when you were younger and whenever you hear a school bell ring, your shoulders tense up and you find yourself starting to sweat.

These are all examples of somatic memories. These memories can be a sign that your body is still holding physical or psychological trauma (or both). Unresolved events from people's past can come back to haunt them in the present. Your breath can be a very powerful tool for recognizing anything you're holding onto and for helping you move through it and eventually let go of it.

Staying Safe

When you practice somatic breathing or movement, you have the opportunity to bring awareness to your direct felt sense. As you practice somatic breathwork and movement, you tune into your senses and feelings in your body. This heightened awareness allows you to notice areas of tension, discomfort, and emotional stress that you may be unconsciously holding on to. You can invite your body and mind to feel safe enough to open up and then explore what you're holding on to. The deep diaphragmatic breath (discussed in the "Diaphragmatic breathing" section later in this chapter) is key here, because it keeps your nervous system in a relaxed state while you deal with traumatic memories and difficult emotions.

WARNING

If you don't take time to communicate with your body and remind it that you are safe, you risk staying in a state of hyper-alertness or survival mode, which can lead to emotional and physical unease and potentially even disease. Many illnesses today are due to stress. Getting connected to your breath can help you live a long, healthy, and happy life!

Trying Some Somatic Breathing Techniques

You have various somatic breathing techniques at your disposal. Some may resonate with you more than others. Remember to give it time and to set up a regular daily practice to get more acquainted with your breath and how you can manipulate it to your advantage.

Breath awareness

The first thing to practice is becoming aware of your breath. Sit in a comfortable position or lie down on your back. You can close your eyes or keep them open. Start to notice what is happening with your breath. Where do you tend to breathe into? Is it your stomach, is it your chest? Do your shoulders lift up when you breathe? Do you feel more comfortable breathing through your nose or through your mouth? What is the temperature of your breath? Do you breathe more through one side of your nose than the other? As you sit or lie here, just take note of your breath. Don't judge it; just observe it.

REMEMBER

This is a practice of complete awareness and nothing else. You may notice as you pay all attention to your breath that you start to feel more relaxed. Don't focus on achieving any goal; just notice how you breathe. Every one of us in unique so this is your opportunity to get to know yourself better through your breath.

Diaphragmatic breathing

Once you've spent some time getting acquainted with how you breathe (see the previous section, "Breath awareness," for guidance on consciously tuning in to this involuntary process), you can start to work on *diaphragmatic breathing*. This is the kind of breath you used as a baby before you knew how to breathe any differently. I love coming back to this breath because it's like returning home, revisiting that childlike state that was so carefree and easygoing.

Ideally, you can start to reclaim that state more often in your adult life as you breathe in a way that is better for your nervous system and entire being. For example, in yoga, you use diaphragmatic breathing to stay calm throughout the practice, but you don't have to limit it to class. You can use diaphragmatic breathing any time to stay calm. I personally love to do diaphragmatic breathing at night to relax and unwind as I'm falling asleep.

REMEMBER

Diaphragmatic breathing is the most efficient way to breathe. It helps your body exchange oxygen for carbon dioxide and strengthens your abdominal muscles.

To practice diaphragmatic breathing, follow these steps:

1. **Sit or lie down in a comfortable position.**

2. **Take slow, deep breaths using your diaphragm and abdominal muscles.**

3. **Make sure to fill up your abdomen on your inhalation.**

   When you inhale, the diaphragm (a large, thin muscle located just below the rib cage) descends and the stomach expands.

4. **On the exhalation, the diaphragm lifts up and the stomach deflates. Let your stomach relax and release on your exhalation.**

You can place a pillow on your stomach if you're lying down and watch it rise and fall. For younger kids, I often tell them to place a stuffed animal on their stomach.

TIP

Try not to force air into the belly region, just allow it to naturally expand and fill with air. These slow, long breaths help relax the nervous system.

Alternate nostril breathing

Alternate nostril breathing is something I remember learning years ago in my yoga classes. I always love how immediately relaxing it is. Alternate nostril breathing is also known as *Nadi Shodhana* in Sanskrit, and it involves breathing in through one side of the nose while blocking the other side. You then exhale out the opposite side and repeat the process back and forth from side to side. Alternate nostril breathing can

>> Calm your nervous system

>> Give you focus and energy

>> Reduce stress

>> Restore balance to your brain's hemispheres

>> Rejuvenate the nervous system

>> Support your respiratory system

>> Remove toxins

To practice alternate nostril breathing, you can make a *mudra* (a hand gesture in yoga used to seal your nostril) called *Vishnu Mudra*, as shown in Figure 4-1.

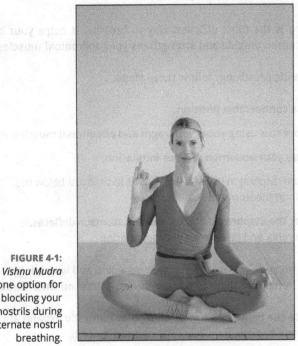

FIGURE 4-1:
The *Vishnu Mudra* is one option for blocking your nostrils during alternate nostril breathing.

Photograph by Guen Egan

Follow these steps to try the *Vishnu Mudra* gesture:

1. **With your right hand, fold your index and middle fingers down. These fingers stay curled in, touching your palm.**

2. **Keep your thumb, ring finger, and little finger extended.**

3. **Place your thumb on your right nostril and close it gently.**

4. **Use your ring finger to close your left nostril when it's time.**

5. **Keeping gentle contact between your fingers and nose the entire time, apply light pressure when closing the nostril.**

TIP

You can also just use your thumb and pointer finger if that's easier.

Try the alternate nostril breathing practice now:

1. **Sit up tall with your shoulders down and back and your neck in line with your torso.**

2. **Make Vishnu Mudra or take your thumb and index finger to your nose.**

3. **Close your eyes or soften your eyelids and gaze.**

4. Gently close your right nostril and inhale through your left nostril.

5. Close both nostrils briefly, and then open only the right nostril.

6. Exhale out of the right nostril.

7. While keeping the left nostril closed, inhale through the right nostril.

8. Close the right nostril, open the left nostril, and exhale out the left.

9. Repeat this process back and forth.

10. After 8-10 rounds of alternate breathing, let your hand relax and breathe evenly through both sides of your nose.

TIP

To establish a rhythmic flow, count your breath in seconds and keep it constant. For instance, inhale for four counts (or seconds), then pause for one count, then exhale for four counts, and pause for one count. You can also use *breath retention*. Inhale for four counts, hold for four counts, exhale for four counts, and stay empty for four counts.

People tend to naturally alternate which side of their nose they breathe out of more during the day. Approximately every 90 minutes, we switch over. Yogis believed that by monitoring this habit, they could get the most out of each day. When the right side is more open, you are more awake and energized. When the left side is more open, you are calmer. When you bring the two together with alternate nostril breathing, you benefit from both!

MOUTH VS. NOSTRIL BREATHING

Breathing through your mouth can lead to more intense sensations and a quicker entry into activation. This method often generates a faster, more powerful release of emotions and physical energy, making it a popular choice in more intensive breathwork sessions where deep emotional work is the goal. However, because it can be so powerful, mouth breathing might feel overwhelming for beginners or those unaccustomed to deep breathwork. It can also cause mouth and throat dryness, so staying hydrated is important if you choose this method.

On the other hand, breathing through your nose provides a more controlled and gentle experience. The nose filters and warms the air before it enters your lungs, which can make the breathing process feel smoother and more calming. This method is ideal for beginners or anyone seeking a more grounded, centering practice. Nostril breathing is also recommended for those who are practicing breathwork for relaxation, stress relief,

(continued)

(continued)

or when you want to maintain a steady, balanced state without triggering intense emotional or physical responses.

In some practices, alternating between mouth and nostril breathing can offer a balanced approach. For example, starting with nostril breathing to center yourself, and then shifting to mouth breathing for deeper emotional work, can help you ease into the process before diving deeper into activation.

When choosing between mouth and nostril breathing, consider what you want to achieve with your breathwork session. If you're looking to explore and release deep-seated emotions, mouth breathing might be more effective. If your goal is to relax, de-stress, or maintain a meditative state, nostril breathing is likely the better choice.

Sound stimulation breathing

Sound simulation breathing is a playful yet powerful way to connect with your body through sound, allowing you to notice how making different sounds feels. I often see my boys growling or humming or just making noises in general. When is the last time you let yourself growl or let out a lion's roar? Although making sounds like this might sound unusual, vocalizing is a great way to free yourself of tension and get familiar with how you make these different sounds and how they resonate in your body. You may feel a little weird at first, but remember: Somatic breathing exercises are all about observation. Pay attention to how you feel before, during, and after you do all your practices.

To practice sound stimulation breathing, follow these steps:

1. **Start in a comfortable position. You can sit, stand, or lie down.**

2. **Inhale through your nose and exhale an audible "shhhhh," as if you're trying to quiet someone down.**

   As you make the sound, place your hands on different parts of your torso to feel the vibrations. Notice how the sound affects each area.

3. **Inhale again, but on this exhale, try a "pssst" sound. Again, use your hands to feel how the vibrations impact different areas of your body.**

4. **Experiment with a growl. Let the growl be deep and low.**

   Does your chest vibrate? How does it feel?

5. **Practice the humming bee breath (also known as *Brahmari*). Close your mouth and let out a hum on your exhalation.**

Notice how the vibration of the hum travels throughout your entire body and your face.

REMEMBER

Your goal with sound stimulation breathing is to explore how these sounds affect your body and mind. Notice any shifts in energy, mood, or physical sensations as you engage in this playful yet insightful exercise.

4-7-8 breathing

4-7-8 breathing is where you breathe in through your nose for four counts, hold your breath for seven, then release the breath through your mouth for eight counts. The goal of this practice is to release stagnant air from your lungs and release built-up tension in your body. People have used the 4-7-8 breathing technique for years to help:

>> Fall asleep at night

>> Regulate cortisol levels

>> Promote calm and relaxation

>> Reduce anxiety

4-7-8 breathing can also help trigger the *vagus* nerve, which is one of the longest and most important nerves in the body, running from the brainstem through the neck and into the chest and abdomen. The vagus nerve activates the rest and digest state.

To practice 4-7-8 breathing, try this:

1. **Sit up straight and tall or lie down.**

2. **Close your eyes or soften your eyelids and gaze.**

3. **Inhale through your nose for a count of four.**

4. **Pause and hold your breath for seven counts.**

5. **Exhale all the air through your mouth for a count of eight.**

You can make a "whoosh" sound when you exhale the air out if you like.

6. **Repeat this process for five minutes or more.**

7. **After completing the cycle, notice how you feel.**

The specific breathing count isn't as important as simply maintaining the pattern of the longer exhalation (it's twice as long as the inhalation). Sometimes if you focus too much on the counting, you can feel even more anxiety. Also, if you feel uncomfortable or anxious holding your breath as long as suggested, adjust the count as needed.

Reset breathing

Reset breathing is like taking an eraser to a chalkboard and leaving behind a nice clean slate. It's an incredible way to rejuvenate yourself whenever you need to. The reset breath can help you:

>> Balance your autonomic nervous system function

>> Eliminate emotional stress

>> Improve focus

>> Restore the oxygen/carbon dioxide ratio in your bloodstream

To practice the reset breath, follow these steps:

1. **Sit or lie down in a comfortable position.**

2. **Close your eyes or relax your eyelids and gaze.**

3. **Place one hand on your stomach and one hand on your chest.**

4. **Take a deep breath in through your nose.**

   Feel the breath rise up from your stomach into your chest like a wave rising up.

5. **Exhale out of your mouth and feel the wave receding.**

6. **Repeat this ten times.**

7. **On the tenth breath, hold your breath in for as long as you can, and then exhale all the air out.**

You'll notice an immediate difference in your nervous system.

Coherent breathing

Coherent breathing is a breathing technique where there is no pause between inhalation and exhalation. It's a steady state flow of breathing in on a count of six and breathing out for a count of six, resulting in breathing at a rate of approximately five breaths per minute. I often think of this breath like a figure eight or infinity sign where one thing flows into the next.

Coherent breathing can bring you relaxation in a very short amount of time. You can sit or lie down when doing this exercise. Regular practice can:

>> Create a sense of calm

>> Facilitate circulation

>> Help with focus

>> Induce relaxation

>> Restore autonomic nervous system balance

Try coherent breathing by following these steps:

1. Find a comfortable position.

You can sit or lie down, ensuring that your spine is straight and your body is relaxed.

2. Close your eyes or soften your gaze.

This helps you focus inward and become more attuned to your breath.

3. Inhale slowly through your nose for a count of six.

Imagine your breath filling up your lungs completely and evenly.

4. Exhale gently through your nose for a count of six.

Allow the breath to flow out smoothly without any pause.

5. Continue this breathing pattern.

Aim to maintain this rhythm for several minutes, allowing your breath to flow effortlessly from one cycle to the next.

6. Focus on the sensation of your breath.

As you breathe, imagine the air moving in a continuous loop, like a figure eight, creating a sense of harmony and balance in your body.

Connected breathing

Connected breathing is a powerful technique usually best facilitated under an experienced guide; however, if you feel comfortable, you can try this on your own. This conscious, connected, circular breathing pattern eliminates the natural pauses at the bottom of your exhalation and the top of inhalation. The idea is to create a continuous flow of breath that can help you access deeper emotional and physical states.

WARNING

This technique can be intense and may lead to strong emotional or physical reactions. If you are new to connected breathing or have a history of trauma, it's best to practice under the supervision of a trained facilitator at first.

To practice connected breathing, follow these steps:

1. Start by sitting or lying down in a comfortable position.

2. Inhale through your nose then exhale out your nose.

3. Immediately inhale again without taking a pause at the bottom of the exhalation.

4. Continue this pattern for 10-20 rounds.

WARNING

If you start to feel lightheaded or dizzy, you may be dropping into *activation* and the healing process. That's a good thing, but it's only safe to continue with it if you're experienced or with a trained facilitator. If you are new to this and are alone, resume normal breathing and just observe how you feel.

Activation refers to the heightened state that can occur during connected breathing or other intensive breathwork practices. This state can produce:

>> A heightened state of energy

>> Altered levels of consciousness (like a trance)

>> Changes in blood chemistry

>> Changes in brainwaves

>> Emotional release (bringing up suppressed emotions or memories)

>> Euphoric state or feeling of being at one with the universe

>> Periods of yogic sleep

>> Surfacing of past emotions

>> Tingling, numbness, or feelings of hot or cold

Activation can be very therapeutic because it helps you access and release deep-seated emotions, traumas, or physical tensions. When guided by a trained facilitator, this process can lead to significant emotional and psychological breakthroughs.

If you're with a trained facilitator, they may have you continue activation to go even deeper into your emotions, carefully monitoring your responses and providing support to help you navigate the experience. Here's what might happen:

>> **Guided exploration:** The facilitator may encourage you to stay with the feelings or sensations that arise, helping you explore them more deeply. They might ask questions to help you verbalize what you're experiencing, which can lead to important emotional insights.

>> **Emotional release:** As you continue breathing, you may experience the release of emotions such as crying, laughter, or even anger. The facilitator will hold a safe space for you to express these emotions, allowing for catharsis and healing.

>> **Physical release:** The facilitator might use gentle touch or movement to help release physical tension that surfaces during activation. This could involve guiding you to stretch, move, or change your breathing pattern to release blocked energy.

>> **Integration:** After the activation phase, the facilitator will guide you back to a more regular breathing pattern and help you integrate the experience. This may involve grounding exercises, such as focusing on your body's contact with the floor or deep, slow breaths.

>> **Reflection:** The session often concludes with a period of reflection where you can discuss what came up during the breathwork. The facilitator may offer insights or suggestions for continuing the healing process outside of the session.

Coordinating Your Breath and Movement

Vinyasa yoga is a popular style of yoga and moving meditation that focuses on synchronizing breath with movement, which I love. Moving to your breath can feel very therapeutic. You start to find a rhythm and flow that helps you get into a very focused, very relaxed state.

The word *vinyasa* means "to place in a special way." In practice, this means you connect your breath with your movement as you move from one pose to the next, or hold a pose for a certain number of breaths. For example, you might inhale as you raise your arms overhead and exhale as you fold forward. This breath-to-movement connection is what makes *vinyasa* a dynamic and flowing practice (see Figure 4-2).

However, you don't have to be flowing through yoga poses to coordinate your breath and movement. Take swimming. As you turn your head to the side, you inhale through your mouth and as you put your face back in the water, you exhale out your nose. Boom — coordinated movement and breath. If you watch an accomplished swimmer, they make it look effortless. Same goes for an experienced yoga practitioner.

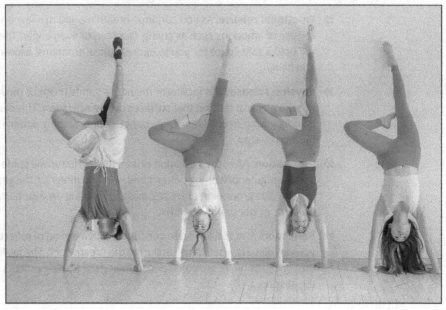

FIGURE 4-2:
A *vinyasa*-style
yoga class is a
good way to
coordinate breath
with movement.

Photograph by Guen Egan

You can also try coordinating your breath with your movement as you walk. For instance, take in inhalation as you step on one foot and an exhalation as you step on the other foot. This mindful breathing helps create a rhythm that can make walking feel more meditative and relaxing. Play around with coordinating your breath and movement as you move throughout your day.

Dance is yet another example where breath and movement come together. In dance, breathing often follows the rhythm of the music, helping you stay connected to both your body and the beat.

TIP

If you've never taken a *vinyasa*-style yoga class, I encourage you to try it! You'll experience the ultimate in breath-movement connection!

Practicing Somatic Breath Therapy with a Therapist

Somatic breath therapy with a therapist can be transformative. You usually do it in a series of sessions with a skilled therapist who helps you utilize your breath to release pent-up emotions and stored trauma. Unlike general breathwork practices, somatic breath therapy is a structured, therapeutic approach designed to support deep emotional healing and personal growth.

Somatic breath therapy includes activation (see the earlier section in this chapter called "Connected breathing" for more insight into activation) and other elements. Somatic breath therapy enables you to bring your awareness to your breath and engage in different breathing exercises, which can reduce stress, help you heal emotionally, and enable you to develop a better awareness of yourself.

TIP

To find a somatic breath therapist, you can use a directory like the one in *Psychology Today* to search for therapists specializing in somatic therapy. You can specifically ask about their experience with breathwork techniques. Check with organizations like Somatic Experiencing International for certified practitioners or inquire with local mental health clinics to see if they have therapists trained in somatic practices.

You always want to verify their credentials and training in somatic breath therapy before booking an appointment. Many yoga teachers are trained in pranayama practices and breathwork but they may not have the additional therapist license.

The philosophy behind somatic breath therapy builds on several principles:

>> Breath awareness happens in the here and now. It roots you in the present moment.

>> Breathing helps you relax on a deeper level and opens you up to a stress-free way of living.

>> Conscious breathing elicits conscious awareness.

>> Consciously breathing together with others can establish a better community.

>> Everything breathes.

>> Your breath is your communication with yourself and the outside world.

>> Somatic breathing can help your body heal itself by removing blocked patterns and poor breathing mechanics.

Chapter 5

Step by Step: Somatic Movements

Have you ever thought about movement for the sake of movement? So often people are fixated on movement as a goal. We think we have to walk a certain number of steps or we are training for a race or we are playing on a team and want to beat our opponents. Somatic movement is the exact opposite. When you practice somatic movement, you aren't interested in any end result. You move for the sake of movement. You explore how your body and mind feel. You are getting to know yourself better and are using movement to connect to your emotions.

Movement is an integral part of being human. It feels good to move, yet we sometimes place expectations on why or how we should be moving. What if you took time every day to explore how movement makes you feel? Somatic movement gives you the opportunity to stay present and release things that you may be storing in your mind and body. The goal is not to let go of trauma stored in your musculature, although that may happen. Remember — there is no goal.

Releasing and Relaxing: Somatic Movement Fundamentals

Like taking a big stretch when you wake up first thing in the morning or massaging your feet after taking your shoes off at the end of the day, somatic movement is often organic, intuitive movement that your body naturally craves. But somatic movement doesn't stop at the physical; it goes beyond your body and into your mind.

Discovering what somatic movement is

Somatic movement is any movement that helps you create full-body awareness. Performing somatic movement helps you get in tune with your body, release built-up emotions, let go of trauma, and manage your mental health. You perform somatic movement deliberately rather than unconsciously, and — instead of focusing on the physical outcome of the movement — you home in on your internal feelings.

Some examples of somatic exercises include:

>> Focusing on each inhalation and exhalation when you breathe

>> Choosing to move your body in any way that feels good to you

>> Noticing how it feels to tense and then release parts of the body

>> Grounding by feeling the connection of your body to the ground or other surface

Applying these fundamentals of somatic movement helps you grow a strong connection between your mind and body:

>> Practice movement slowly and intentionally

>> Be exploratory with your movement

>> Focus on the internal experience and process of your movement

>> Be present and aware of what is happening in the moment and during the movement

Somatic movement reconnects you to yourself and to movement that can make you happy and whole. Somatic movement is fun and playful and often the types of things you may see a baby doing. Animals and young children often react instinctively to their body's signals, like feeling hungry and seeking food, feeling tired and wanting to sleep, or sensing danger and fleeing. As adults, we tend to lose touch with our inner compass and inner guide. We force ourselves to do certain movements that we hate because we think we have to. We become result oriented and lose sight of the joy of being.

TIP

To reconnect with yourself somatically, sit and observe the way a young child or animal moves and how they explore things with their entire being. Simply observing them can help you consciously remember to do the same.

We take in most information through our vision, which is helpful and essential, but in doing so, we sometimes forget the powerful internal net of communication happening inside of us. Your body intuitively knows what it needs, if you slow down enough to listen to it. The problem is today that people are always on the go and often in their heads.

Understanding how somatic exercise differs from other exercise

Somatic movement is different from traditional strength workouts or result oriented workouts. It is less about the quantity of a move or the intensity of a run and more about the quality. Even running can be a somatic exercise if the intention is to feel your body from the inside out. Not needing to make a goal time or run a race, but rather checking in with yourself when you're propelling your body forward in space.

I recently trained for my first marathon. Since I love somatic type movement, I never listened to music or wore headphones. Everyone thought I was insane. "How can you just run? You really don't listen to music? Oh, you have to start listening to music" were some common comments I'd get. I don't want to listen to music while I run. I want to run free. I like to observe my body and mind when I go out for a jog. I notice how my feet hit the pavement, where my breath enters my body, how my shoulders tense up, and how I can find a way to release them.

REMEMBER

Any movement, even a pushup or squat, could be somatic in nature if it's about the exploration of the exercise and conscious attention to your body, mind, and breath as you perform the workout.

Another defining example of somatic movement is that it is usually performed slowly. However, as you will learn, there are some movements that are faster. For example, running isn't extremely slow, but the goal of someone running for the sake of internal exploration as opposed to a goal or finish line is completely different.

Considering the benefits of somatic movement

Somatic movement can benefit your mind and the body in many ways. Somatic movement allows you to connect your emotions to your physical self. You'll build *interoception* (the ability to *self-sense* or be aware of how you're feeling), which not only helps you feel good, but can also help you get to know yourself better. You'll learn to connect feeling a certain way with how it makes your body react. You'll also notice that a lot of your "issues are stored in your tissues." We hold on to memories in our musculature; somatic movement can help us process and release trauma. Somatic movement can also help us cherish our bodies for what they do for us as opposed to how they look. It's an inside-out job.

For lots more about the benefits of somatic exercises, see Chapter 2.

REMEMBER

There is no need to observe yourself in a mirror when practicing somatic movement. This is the time to drop into your heart and listen to what your body is telling you.

Starting with Gentle Stretches

Many people for some reason hate to stretch. It's like core work and stretching are always saved for the end of the workout and always skipped or done rapidly. Somatic stretching can help you fall in love with stretching. When you find more freedom of movement in your physical being, you'll also find more freedom in your mental being.

Somatic stretching helps you slow down your brain so you can feel the sensations in your body. It's not natural to experience discomfort and stay with it. Our immediate reaction is to stop — the fight-or-flight response. We immediately stop the movement, fight it by tensing up, or completely avoid it all together (mentally and/or physically).

When you begin to practice gentle, controlled movements like stretches and breathe into the areas that feel intense at first, you can reconfigure muscle length. You'll gain more flexibility and with regular somatic movement practice, you can also improve your posture, balance, and mobility.

REMEMBER

When you do somatic stretches, don't look for an immediate result or set a fitness goal. Practice these stretches simply to feel better in your body. Over time, you'll possibly notice the benefit, but while you're doing these, just be in your body and be with your breath. Observe how you're feeling and relax into the movements.

Try these gentle somatic stretches to start your somatic journey, but before each exercise, start with an awareness exercise, such as connecting with your breath, doing a body scan, or trying a grounding exercise.

TIP

Either while standing, seated or lying down, close your eyes and check in with your breath. Feel your body in space. Relax and connect internally.

The Hang Your Head exercise

Did you know that the human head weighs eight pounds? If you've seen the movie *Jerry Maguire*, you most likely do! We carry a lot above our shoulders, not just mentally, but also physically. It doesn't help that many people are constantly on their phones and computers. "Forward head syndrome" is a common postural issue when someone's head is forward of their midline and "tech neck" is pain from prolonged use of electronics. These are too common and can lead to discomfort and misalignment.

This exercise (Hang Your Head) can help relieve tension and tightness in your head, neck, and shoulders and alleviate imbalances created from forward head syndrome and other ailments.

Follow these steps to try the Hang Your Head exercise:

1. **Stand up straight with your feet grounded on the floor hip-width apart.**

2. **Slowly let your head hang down comfortably, feeling a slight stretch.**

3. **Observe how your neck muscles feel, and how the movement affects the muscles in your upper back and shoulders. Also note what comes up emotionally.**

4. **As you identify tight areas, move your head gently to stretch those muscles.**

5. **Breathe and feel the tension release.**

6. **Come back up to neutral and repeat three to five times.**

The Seated Spinal Twist exercise

One of my favorite quotes from Joseph Pilates is that you're only as young as your spine is flexible. Seated Spinal Twists create flexibility in the spine and are wonderful to incorporate into your day. Seated Twists in particular are great. You get a 360-degree view of things after you twist to both sides.

Twists can have a cleansing and therapeutic effect on the mind and body because they release tension and calm the mind. You may find that twists also:

>> Help relieve back and neck pain

>> Massage the internal organs

>> Allow you to find more range of motion in your torso

If you're ever stuck in one position for a while, gently twist it out and see how much better you feel afterward. Here's how:

1. **Sit on the floor with both legs straight in front of you, as shown in Figure 5-1.**

2. **Bend your right knee and place your right foot on the floor, as shown in Figure 5-2.**

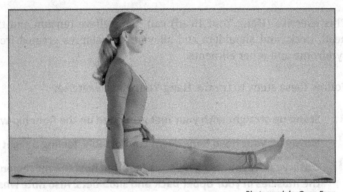

FIGURE 5-1:
Start the Seated
Spinal Twist with
legs extended.

Photograph by Guen Egan

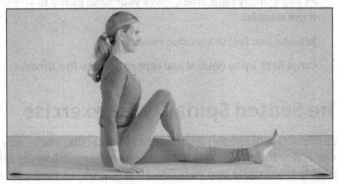

FIGURE 5-2:
Bend your right
knee with your
foot flat on the
ground for the
Seated Spinal
Twist.

Photograph by Guen Egan

3. **Place your right hand behind you on the floor near the small of your back to help lift up out of this area (or prevent slouching), as you can see in Figure 5-3.**

   If you need to sit up on a blanket or folded towel you can.

4. **As you exhale, twist to the right, placing your left elbow outside of your right knee, as shown in Figure 5-4.**

5. **Every inhalation, feel yourself lengthening your spine, every exhalation, twist a little deeper. Hold the position and breathe for four or five breaths.**

6. **Release the twist and come back to center. Observe any changes in your body and mind.**

7. **Repeat on the other side.**

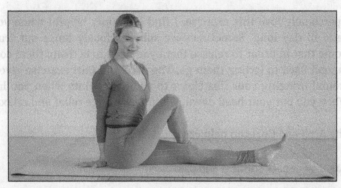

FIGURE 5-3:
Place your right hand near the small of your back.

Photograph by Guen Egan

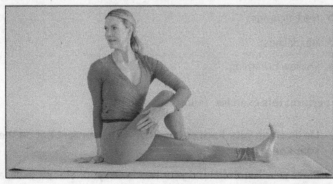

FIGURE 5-4:
Keep your left elbow outside of your knee while twisting to the right.

Photograph by Guen Egan

You can adjust the movement slightly to meet your specific needs:

>> If you are more flexible, fold the opposite leg underneath you to feel your hip open more deeply.

>> If you are less flexible, try this exercise by sitting on a folded towel or blanket.

>> If you are stuck at work or have limited range of motion, you can perform the twist in a chair. See Chapter 7 for step-by-step instructions on doing this movement in a chair.

REMEMBER

Before you rotate, you need to find the length first, so be sure to complete the steps in this order!

The Arch and Curl exercise

I personally love this exercise. I find it's super helpful when you're sitting at a desk all day long. Sometimes we subconsciously tense our front muscles. It's ironic that in order to release them you need to activate them consciously so you can get used to letting them go. The Arch and Curl exercise gives you awareness around bringing your ribs closer to your hip points when you lift your head up. When you put your head down, you'll feel a huge relief and relaxation.

The Arch and Curl can help ease:

>> Lower back stiffness and pain

>> *Hyperkyphosis* (rounded shoulders)

>> Forward head syndrome

>> Neck tightness

>> Headaches

>> Shallow breathing

To perform this exercise, follow these steps:

1. **Lie down on your back on the floor with your feet flat on the mat and your knees bent.**

2. **Place your hands behind your head with your elbows wide, as shown in Figure 5-5.**

3. **Arch your lower back by letting the tailbone rest forward into the mat. You should feel some space under the small of your back.**

4. Lift your head up and narrow your elbows, as shown in Figure 5-6.

5. Hold for a second to feel the contraction (different from doing a crunch).

6. Lower your head and neck back down and release back into an arched position in the lower spine, as shown in Figure 5-7.

FIGURE 5-5:
Start the Arch and Curl by lying on your back. Keep your elbows wide.

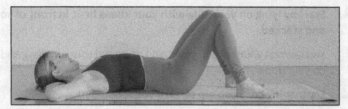

Photograph by Guen Egan

FIGURE 5-6:
Bring your elbows together while lifting your head.

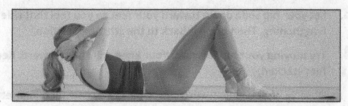

Photograph by Guen Egan

FIGURE 5-7:
The final resting position of the Arch and Curl.

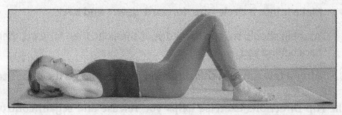

Photograph by Guen Egan

REMEMBER

When you are performing these exercises, make sure you're not only observing your body but also your mind and emotions.

The Hip Directions exercise

I often say our hips are like the basement of the house. We store a lot of "junk in our trunk," so to speak. Somatic exercises for the hips can help you clean out the dusty cobwebs downstairs. The hips are important for walking and movement. When your hips are tight, your whole body gets thrown off.

The Hip Directions exercise is a great way to realign your hips, clean house, and create freedom and space down below. Think of how freeing it can be to clean out the basement and let go of things that are taking up room. When you have a nice clean solid base, everything feels much better.

To perform the Hip Directions exercise, follow these steps:

1. **Start by lying on your side with your knees bent in front of your hips and stacked.**

   You can rest your head in your hand or extend your arm long and rest your ear on your upper arm.

2. **Try moving your top hip toward your shoulder.**

   You'll feel that side engage or the oblique muscles turn on as it pulls the hip upward. Let your hip slide back to neutral and chest in.

3. **Let your hip slide down toward your feet so you feel that side lengthening. Then bring it back to the starting position.**

4. **Try moving your hip forward. Your knee will shift forward. Keep your feet stacked.**

   Observe what happens when you come to the center and then let the hip slide back before coming back to starting position. Each time you come back to the first position, notice how your hips and back feel.

5. **Make it into a circle—up, forward, down, and back.**

   Your hip should shift up toward your shoulder, then forward, then down, then back behind you.

6. **After a few times in this direction, switch and go the opposite way.**

The Hip Directions exercise helps you release and regain control of the muscles that laterally tilt the pelvis, laterally flex the spine, and rotate the spine:

>> *Quadratus lumborum*: The deepest back muscle that runs from the *iliac crest* (a curved, bony ridge located at the upper edge of the ilium, the largest bone in the pelvis) and inserts on L1-5 and the lower part of the twelfth rib.

>> **The internal and external obliques:** The external obliques twist the trunk from side to side and the internal obliques lie on top of the external obliques. Both are on the sides of the rectus abdominis.

>> **The erector spinae muscles:** A group of muscles that run alongside both sides of the spine. These muscles help with strengthening and rotating the back.

>> *Intertransversarii*: These are a set of deep muscles in the back.

>> *Psoas* **major:** I think of the psoas as the "filet mignon" of the body. It is a long, ribbon-shaped muscle and it runs from the lower back to the top of the hip on each side of the spine.

>> **The *iliopsoas* muscle:** This is a group of muscles made up of the *psoas* major, *psoas* minor, and *iliacus* muscles and it is one of the most important abdominal muscles. It attaches at the lumbar spine to the upper inner thigh bone. It is responsible for many functions, including:

- Flexing the hip or bringing the knee in toward the stomach. If you spend a lot of time in your seat, your iliopsoas is most likely tight.

- Rotating the hip laterally so that you can turn your feet out (like a penguin or first position in ballet).

- Helping in the lateral tilting of the pelvis (hiking the hips up one at a time) and lateral flexion of the spine (bending the spine to one side).

WARNING

A tight *iliopsoas* can result in back pain, constipation, menstruation issues, and even indigestion. When the *iliopsoas* is in a shortened state, it can throw the back into *lordosis* (or an overly arched position) and shorten the rest of the back muscles.

You can relax these muscles when you are standing by performing the *Iliopsoas* Release. You will feel relief in your back and even have a better control over your breath. To perform this exercise, follow these steps:

1. **Lie down on your back with your feet flat on the mat and your knees bent, as shown in Figure 5-8.**

2. **Place your hands behind you your head with your elbows open to each side.**

3. **Close your eyes or keep a soft, steady gaze and focus on what is happening in your mind.**

4. **Flatten your back and, upon an exhalation, lift your head up as you also lift your right leg up. See Figure 5-10.**

5. **Release everything and notice how you feel.**

6. **After three to five times on the right side, repeat on the left.**

TIP

Start with the easier side first. Your body *neuromuscularly* remembers the last thing you did. (This is the unconscious trained response of the muscle when it signals the last thing you did.) If you finish with the tighter side, chances are you'll feel the effects more.

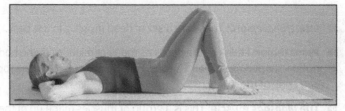

FIGURE 5-8: Start on your back with knees bent to perform the iliopsoas release.

Photograph by Guen Egan

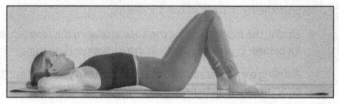

FIGURE 5-9: Place hands behind you your head with your elbows open to each side.

Photograph by Guen Egan

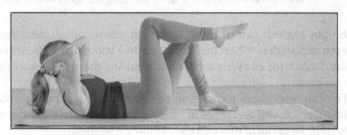

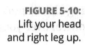

FIGURE 5-10: Lift your head and right leg up.

Photograph by Guen Egan

The beauty of somatic movement is that it puts you in touch with your body so you can recognize what it causing misalignment, tension, and pain.

Child's Pose

Child's Pose feels like a warm hug from within. It can help you down-regulate when things feel overwhelming. This is one of my favorite somatic poses. I feel like once I am in Child's Pose I am in a little cocoon. I can hear and feel my breath, and the outer world disappears.

Child's Pose is a restorative pose in yoga that stretches your back and hips. It's calming and relaxing and it can help manage stress levels by activating the *parasympathetic nervous system* (known as the "rest and digest" state, it helps your body relax) and regulating your blood pressure.

To do Child's Pose, follow these steps:

1. **Start in a kneeling position, as shown in Figure 5-11.**

2. **Either walk your hands forward while keeping your hips on your heels or keep your hands back by your hips.**

Choose the position that feels most comfortable for you.

3. **Rest your forehead on the floor or on a blanket, as shown in Figure 5-12.**

4. **Feel your spine lengthen and your shoulders open. See Figure 5-13.**

5. **Allow your chest and stomach to release toward the floor between your legs.**

6. **Hold for two to five minutes.**

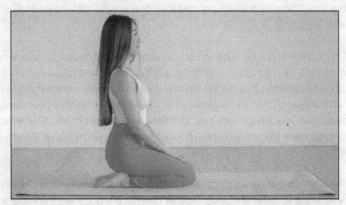

FIGURE 5-11: For Child's Pose, start in a kneeling position.

Photograph by Guen Egan

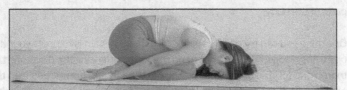

FIGURE 5-12: Rest your head on the floor to fully feel the stretch of Child's Pose.

Photograph by Guen Egan

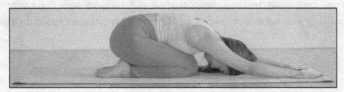

FIGURE 5-13: For a more challenging stretch, try walking your arms out in front of you.

Photograph by Guen Egan

TIP

You can always fold up a blanket and place it between your calves and thighs for extra support. Experiment with placing a bolster between your legs or using a large, firm couch cushion or pillow.

REMEMBER

When you come up out of the pose, take note of how you feel. With all of these somatic exercises, observation is really important. Notice how you move, where you are moving from, and how the movement affects you.

TIP

CARPAL TUNNEL RELIEF

Carpal tunnel syndrome is a numbness and tingling in your hand that comes on when your median nerve is compressed as it passes through the carpal tunnel of your wrist. This compression can occur anywhere from the spinal cord, to the upper arm, to the forearm. Doing repetitive tasks over long periods of time with your hands or arms often triggers it.

A very common cause of nerve compression are tight muscles. I had nerve compression in my toes. I went through months of physical therapy to figure out what was going on. I finally discovered that my left hip and lower back were extremely tight. If you have a nerve sensation that you experience in your wrist and hand, it could be a result of tight muscles in your neck — or chest, shoulder, arm, wrist, or hand. Our wrists are not meant to take the brunt of the work, but when everything else is clenched, they may end up doing more than need be.

The interesting thing about carpal tunnel syndrome is that you can often alleviate it by relieving stress and tension in other parts of the body, like the shoulders, head, and neck. By practicing the Hang Your Head, Spinal Twist, Arch and Curl, and the Hip Directions exercises described in this chapter, you can begin to let go of tightness in all parts of the body.

One thing you can try specifically for carpal tunnel pain is to press your thumb and pinky finger together with your hand that is experiencing the discomfort. Now press the thumb and forefinger together on the other hand and bring it between the thumb and pinky finger of the opposite hand. Slowly try and release the pinky and thumb until the hand is eventually spread open. Repeat.

If you can't avoid the movements that caused the syndrome, you can relieve symptoms by fixing your habitual movement patterns that may have caused the pain to begin with.

Enhancing Balance and Coordination

Improving balance and coordination largely comes down to regularly practicing. I can't even tell you the number of times I've had to fall out of balance to find it again. Each time, I become a bit more coordinated by practicing exercises that test my balance and refine my coordination.

Several other techniques can support these skills:

>> **Body scanning:** A body scan increases awareness of how each part of your body feels, helping you stay grounded and connected.

>> **Diaphragmatic breathing:** This deep breathing technique engages the core muscles, which are essential for stability and coordination. For more on breathing techniques, see Chapter 4.

>> **Grounding techniques:** Grounding roots you in the present moment, helping to deregulate the central nervous system. It's challenging to stay balanced when your mind is distracted, so grounding can improve both focus and stability.

>> **Pilates and dance:** Pilates and dance are both excellent for balance and coordination due to their core-focused movements and complex sequences. For somatic Pilates practices, see "Trying Pilates Somatically" later in this chapter.

>> **Progressive muscle relaxation:** This method helps you release tension in tight areas that may be holding you back from achieving better balance and coordination.

>> **Somatic yoga:** Somatic yoga improves motor control and coordination by helping you develop a deeper mind-body connection. For additional somatic yoga practices, see the section "Practicing Yoga" later in this chapter.

Simple routines to improve stability

To improve your stability, incorporate single-leg stands, heel-to-toe walking, calf raises, lunges, planks, bridges, side leg lifts, and sit-to-stand movements. You can even try sitting down on a stability ball and standing back up. While you do all of these, engage your core and gradually increase the duration of your holds. Set a timer and see how long you can stand on one leg while holding the other leg into your chest. Over time, you'll see remarkable improvement as you learn to work all the little stabilizing muscles in your body and your core and your focus and your breath.

Focus on your core engagement by working through this routine, which starts with easy exercises and progresses in difficulty:

1. **Single-leg stands:** Stand on one leg while pulling the opposite leg up to your chest. Hold for as long as you can then switch sides.

2. **Heel-to-toe walks:** Walk in a straight line placing the heel of one foot directly in front of the toes of the other as if you're walking on a plank.

3. **Calf raises:** These help with ankle and foot mobility and strength; they are also great for balance. Stand on the balls of your feet, lift your heels off the ground, then slowly lower back down. Build up to one leg at a time.

4. **Lunges:** Lunges improve everything in my opinion. Step forward with one leg, lowering your body until your front knee is bent at a 90-degree angle then stand up and step back to start (see Figure 5-14). Repeat on the other leg. You can also do walking lunges. Make sure your knee doesn't go past your toes, and that you're using your core. If this is too advanced, hold on to a chair in a lunge position and lower and lift a little.

5. **Planks:** Planks strengthen your core which will help with everything. Hold the top of a pushup position with your hands on the ground and your arms straight. Or you can place your forearms on the ground. Keep your body in a straight line and breathe deeply. See Figure 5-15.

6. **Bridges:** Lie on your back with knees bent. Lift your hips off the ground, hold for 30 seconds, lower down, and repeat.

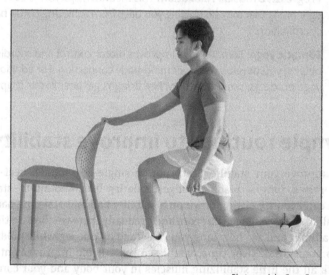

FIGURE 5-14: Lunges strengthen your legs and core.

Photograph by Guen Egan

7. **Side leg lifts:** Standing on one leg, lift your leg out to the side keeping your hips stable and your toes turned forward. Repeat ten times on each side. You can hold on to a chair or the wall or place your hands on your hips.

8. **Sit-to-stands:** From a chair or physio ball, stand up without using your hands. Focus on your legs and core to lift you up.

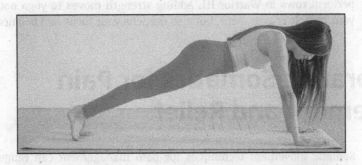
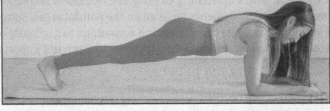

FIGURE 5-15: Planks strengthen your core and shoulders.

Photograph by Guen Egan

TIP

As you work through these exercises, focus on engaging your core and progressing in difficulty by starting with simpler movements before moving on to more challenging variations. Regular practice will lead to noticeable improvements in stability.

Combining balance with strength training

Many exercises in strength training already incorporate single-legged or single-armed movements, which naturally engage your core and challenge your balance. For example, performing a lunge or a single-arm alternating chest press requires you to stabilize your body, activating the core to maintain alignment.

TIP

To take your balance challenge further, try standing on a squishy pad or balance pad when doing exercises like deadlifts. Using an unstable surface increases the demand on your stabilizing muscles, enhancing both balance and strength.

You can also incorporate a stability ball (also known as a physio ball) into many exercises as you progress. For instance, lying on a stability ball while performing chest presses engages your core and helps improve balance.

Another way to blend strength and balance is by incorporating weights into yoga poses. In a yoga sculpt workout, you can do bicep curls while holding Tree Pose or perform rows in Warrior III. Adding strength moves to yoga not only enhances your muscle engagement, but also deepens your focus and balance.

Incorporating Somatics for Pain Management and Relief

Somatic movement techniques for pain management can range from mindful breathing to gentle stretching to progressive muscle relaxation, body scans, and slow, deliberate movements targeted on the painful areas. Somatic exercises focus on deep body awareness and noticing sensations to gradually release tension and retrain the nervous system. When it comes to pain, it's important to move slowly and mindfully:

>> **Breathwork:** Using focused breathing techniques can help to calm your nervous system and reduce muscle tension, which can be especially beneficial for pain relief. See Chapter 4 for more on breathwork.

>> **Mindfulness practices:** Developing awareness of how your body feels is key to managing pain mindfully. Consider practicing body scans and mindful movement. These practices can help you stay attuned to areas of discomfort and respond with gentle adjustments. See Chapter 10.

>> **Self-massage:** Gentle self-massage techniques can increase blood flow and alleviate tightness. See Chapter 7.

>> **Somatic movements for tension release:** Small, gentle movements can mobilize your joins without straining them, helping to release chronic tension. See Chapter 7.

>> **Visualization techniques:** Visualization can be a powerful tool for managing pain by helping you focus on relaxation and calm. If you're interested in using imagery to reduce discomfort, Chapter 10 provides visualization techniques and mindfulness practices that can be adapted to address pain in specific areas. Use somatic breathing and visualization together to deepen your relaxation. Breathing mindfully into areas of pain, combined with visualizing the release of tension, can also significantly reduce discomfort over time.

TIP

Regularly practicing these techniques can enhance your body's natural ability to manage pain. Use them proactively to prevent pain from building up and to promote overall hip health. Chapter 13 addresses specific pain areas with exercises you can incorporate to alleviate pain.

Dancing as Somatic Movement

I grew up dancing. As a young girl, I loved the way I felt after dance class. I practiced tap, ballet, and jazz. I ultimately performed my choreographed pieces. I loved to show off my moves, but I also felt more pressure when I was in class.

Somatic dance is the opposite of the kind of performative dance I did in my early years. When I started as an acting major, I took some experimental theater classes. In one of them, I remember being asked to feel our bodies and explore what they could do. My fellow students were rolling on the floor, gyrating their hips and flailing their bodies in some unique ways. I closed my eyes and tried to get out of my head and start moving from some place inside of myself. It was foreign to me at first, but overtime I felt more comfortable. The goal was to get out of my own way and let go of rigidity.

Somatic dance has similar effects. It helps you free yourself from programmed ways of moving. You essentially sense your internal experience and respond to what your body is signally you to do. It isn't about choreography but more about your own intuitive movement.

It's a wonderful way to connect with your body and emotions through mindful movement. It's all about tuning into your inner sensations and letting your body express itself naturally, without worrying about specific dance steps. If you let go, you'll find yourself exploring your body's natural rhythms and discovering new ways to move that feel right for you. This practice not only helps you become more flexible and strong, but also promotes emotional healing and mental clarity. Whether you're a seasoned dancer or just starting out, somatic dance offers a warm and welcoming space for personal growth and self-discovery.

REMEMBER

Somatic dance is for everyone. The beauty of somatic dance for adults is that they become more aware of their emotions, and they can use this type of movement to process all sorts of things from grief to joy to anxiety to fear to intense love. For more detailed information and specific steps for trying somatic dancing, see Chapter 7.

Practicing Somatic Martial Arts

Two forms of martial arts are very somatic in their nature. One is Akido and the other is Tai Chi.

Akido is a nonviolent form of martial arts with an emphasis on flow, coordination, meditation, and breathing. Akido focuses on the mind/body connection as well as relaxation and compassion. I think all somatic movements have a very compassionate component in the fact that they help people become more caring and kinder toward themselves and others by releasing stress through movement.

To practice Aikido, start by learning the basic stances and movements from a qualified instructor. These include techniques for blending with an attacker's motion and redirecting their energy. Regular practice involves *kata* (forms) and partner exercises that emphasize timing and fluidity.

REMEMBER

Focus on your breathing and stay relaxed to fully integrate the mind-body connection.

Over time, Aikido can help you develop greater physical coordination, mental clarity, and emotional calmness.

Tai Chi is also somatic in nature, with its emphasis on posture and movement, breathing techniques, self-massage, and meditation. There are 108 moves that are all in motion, making Tai Chi a moving meditation practice. There are also shorter forms of Tai Chi that can be practiced. Have you ever witnessed someone practicing Tai Chi? It is beautiful! I often see people up early in the park doing Tai Chi. It is quite an art form, and everyone always seems very calm. Tai Chi is one of those somatic type movements that helps you stay in the here and now. The wave-like flow and concentration that comes from doing Tai Chi is beneficial for your nervous system. You can enter into a state of "oneness" with yourself and the world around you.

To get started with Tai Chi, find a quiet space and begin with simple warm-up exercises to loosen your joints and muscles. Learn the basic Tai Chi postures and movements, focusing on slow, deliberate motions and deep, even breathing. Practice regularly, ideally under the guidance of an experienced instructor, to refine your technique and deepen your understanding. Tai Chi can be practiced alone or in groups, and with consistent practice, you'll notice improvements in your balance, flexibility, and overall sense of well-being.

If this has piqued your interest, check out *T'ai Chi For Dummies* by Therese Iknoian.

Trying Pilates Somatically

Pilates is one of my favorite forms of exercise. It was created by Joseph Pilates, who was ahead of his time and believed that every movement should initiate from the core or what he called the "powerhouse." Our core is our center. When we move from the center, it has lasting effects on our minds and bodies. Over time, we may start using our limbs to stabilize our bodies as opposed to our core. Instead, your core should help you stay strong and stable while your limbs become flexible and mobile.

Originally called "Contrology," Pilates is about learning how to control your body in a way that is efficient and beneficial. When you practice strengthening your core, you support your spine. Joseph Pilates would say, "you're only as young as your spine is flexible." Having a flexible spine can do wonders for mood, posture, and quality of life. When you practice Pilates as a somatic movement, it is all about having a mind–body connection and tapping into your deep core.

REMEMBER

Pilates is not about strengthening the superficial abs (or six pack ab the rectus abdominals); it's about using your *transverse abdominals*. The transverse abs act like an inner corset and support you in all you do. They also work together with your diaphragm, which helps you take deeper fuller breaths.

If you're starting out, try these three Pilates moves:

>> **Roll-Up:** Start by lying on your back with your arms stretched overhead. Inhale and start to roll up one vertebra at a time. As you sit up, reach forward toward your toes as you pull your abdominals in and up and C curve your spine. Slowly lower back down with control. Repeat six to eight times.

>> **Leg Circles:** Lying on your back, lift one leg in the air. Imagine you are holding a marker with your big toe and draw a big circle with it — clockwise and then counterclockwise. After eight circles in each direction, repeat with the other leg. Keep the circle small enough so that your hips don't wobble.

>> **Rolling Like a Ball:** Curl into a small ball with your feet suspended off the floor and hold onto the front of your shins. From your core, rock back to your shoulders, then rock back up to a sitting position without touching your feet to the floor. Repeat six to eight times. Try not to use momentum and instead control the movement from your abdominals.

As you practice Pilates, you'll get more and more in touch with your deep core. On a somatic level, your core is your center. When you move from your center and feel connected to your center, you feel more at ease, more confident, and more stable.

Practicing Yoga

Yoga is an age-old practice that has been around for over 5,000 years. The word *yoga* means to unite or join. In yoga practice, you connect your mind and your body through your breath. Yoga is all about turning inward and finding more peace and clarity. Practicing yoga is not only a personal practice but also a universal practice. You'll feel more united with others when you feel more integrated within.

The physical practice of yoga is called *Hatha*. In Hatha, *yoga asanas* (or postures) are made with the body and help with flexibility, strength, balance, and focus. I have been practicing yoga for 30 years. I discovered yoga in acting school. I was an acting major, and we did yoga to warm up before we went on stage. Yoga and theater acting are intimate and immediate experiences. You have to be present for both. If you start thinking about something else, you may fall out of a pose or disconnect from the sensations in your body. Yoga keeps you focused and in the present moment.

Somatic exercise is all about staying present and sensing what is going on while it is happening. All yoga postures are somatic in nature because what makes yoga different from just stretching is its deep emphasis on the breath. Each breath is an opportunity to connect with your body and to feel what is happening on the inside.

The beauty is you don't need to wrap yourself into a pretzel to feel things. You can simply practice the Mountain Pose, also known as *tadasana*, where you stand still in an upright posture with your spine aligned, as shown in Figure 5-16. It's harder than it seems! It gives you the opportunity to scan your body and find your midline. You'll notice what foot you put more weight on and if your head is jutting forward or your shoulders are rounding forward. For detailed instructions on trying the Mountain Pose, see Chapter 7.

You can start with the Mountain Pose and transition to more advanced postures. Regardless of the posture, you apply the same attention to the information your body is giving you.

Types of yoga suitable for somatic practice

Exploring different types of yoga can greatly enhance your somatic practice by helping you connect more deeply with your body and mind. Each style of yoga offers unique benefits that support mindful movement, emotional release, and physical well-being. For more detailed instructions on incorporating yoga for stress relief, see Chapter 7.

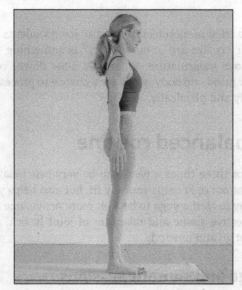

FIGURE 5-16:
The Mountain
Pose (*tadasana*) is
a wonderful way
to become aware
of your mind-
body connection.

Photograph by Guen Egan

Let's take a closer look at three yoga styles particularly suited for somatic practice: Hatha, Yin, and Restorative yoga.

» **Hatha yoga** is a slower version of yoga where you practice different asanas. "Ha" means sun, which represents the physical body, while "tha" means moon and represents the mind. It's a practice of balancing the two. We are often only in our heads. Yoga lets you drop into your body and notice what is going on as you form various shapes that challenge your balance, flexibility, and stamina. Every yoga posture can be considered a somatic exercise.

» **Yin yoga** is a type of yoga where you hold a posture for up to three minutes or more and work on opening connective tissue as opposed to muscle. Yin gives you the chance to unlock areas that are very blocked. We forget how important it is to open up space between our joints. I always feel so refreshed after a Yin class. In Yin, each posture can have a different emphasis, whether it's on the heart opening, or releasing trauma from the hips, or taking pressure off of your shoulders.

» **Restorative yoga** helps you relax and tap into your parasympathetic nervous system, the "rest and digest" system. You use props to help assist your body as it rests in a shape. Your breath slows down, your body releases tightness, and your mind relaxes. Only when you can find some stillness, are you able to truly listen. I find Restorative yoga a wonderful way to let go and release any negative energy I am holding on to.

In my practice, I have cried numerous times. I also have students who've had the same experience. Our "issues are in our tissues" is something I often say. We store everything in our musculature. When you slow down, connect to your breath and unite your mind and body, you have a chance to process emotions and release them mentally and physically.

Creating a balanced routine

Practicing yoga two or three times a week can be very beneficial. It's a somatic type of movement that not only helps you stay fit, but also helps you tune in. You could dedicate one day to Hatha yoga to be a bit more active, one day to Yin yoga to open up the connective tissue and take care of joint health, and one day to Restorative yoga to let go and unwind.

Scheduling yoga and somatic sessions

Make sure to schedule your classes in advance, maybe in a notebook or on your calendar in your phone. Find a studio you like, take class on an app, or follow some of the postures in this book. The more you plan ahead and schedule, the more likely you will keep to a schedule and make these practices a priority.

Balancing intensity and relaxation

By balancing intensity in the Hatha classes and relaxation in the Restorative classes, you give your body and mind the opportunity to process all types of emotions. In more intense yoga classes, you may feel frustration, anger, determination, courage, confidence, and heat. In the Restorative classes, you'll find more peaceful, mellow, sad, or joyful moments. In Yin classes, you may have "aha" moments where you truly let go in a way you never thought possible.

There is no goal, just observation. Each time you engage in somatic exercise, remember that you are getting to know yourself better so you can treat yourself better.

REMEMBER

The more stressed you are, the more likely you are to lash out. I know this firsthand as a single mom of three boys. I love them more than anything, but if I haven't found a way to release the physical tension in my body or stored emotions, I'm more likely to become agitated and reactive. When I take time to do somatic movements, whether it's dance or yoga or breathing exercises, I am more responsive, loving, and caring toward myself and my boys.

IN THIS CHAPTER

» Improving posture and balance with Standing Awareness exercises

» Using body scanning to enhance relaxation and self-awareness

» Mapping your body to uncover emotional connections and improve movement patterns

» Relieving pain and fixing alignment with Rolfing

» Managing stress and emotional balance with Emotional Freedom Techniques (EFT)

» Applying Proprioceptive Neuromuscular Facilitation (PNF) techniques to boost flexibility, strength, and rehabilitation

Chapter **6**

Other Somatic Practices

Embarking on a somatic journey often begins with familiar practices like Pilates, yoga, meditation, Tai Chi, or breathwork. But there's a whole world of other somatic practices just waiting for you to discover them. These lesser-known practices have just as many benefits and offer a wide range of options for all fitness levels and body types.

What's amazing about somatic exercises is the variety — different methods help you connect deeply with your body, improve your posture, and boost your overall sense of well-being in different ways. This chapter introduces you to these incredible techniques and guides you on how to incorporate them into your daily life.

Throughout this chapter, I share practices like Standing Awareness, body scanning, Rolfing, and even Emotional Freedom Techniques (EFT). Each of these methods offers its own way to enhance your sensory-motor awareness, align your body, and reduce stress. Whether you're looking for physical relief or a deeper emotional connection, there's something here for you. Get ready to explore new ways to move, relax, and feel more in tune with your body.

Practicing Standing Awareness

Standing Awareness is a simple yet powerful exercise you typically do at the beginning and the end of a somatic practice. The goal is to notice how your body feels internally while you're standing still. Think of it as your way to touch base with yourself before you start and after you end your exercises. Ask yourself questions like, "How am I doing? Where is my body today? What is my body telling me? How do I feel now? Can I sense things are different?"

If you've never taken the time to connect with your body in this way, it might feel unfamiliar at first, but think about how you approach other activities. Before exercising, do you ever ask yourself how you're feeling? Do you notice how you feel when you return? Maybe you think to yourself, "I really don't feel like working out." Afterward, you might feel energized, exhausted, or somewhere in between. Now imagine taking a few moments before and after your activity to scan your body from head to toe — you'd have a lot more information.

Try the Standing Awareness exercise to connect your mind and body by following these steps:

1. **Stand comfortably, letting your arms hang slack by your sides. Relax all of your muscles as much as you can.**

2. **Close your eyes or keep a soft gaze.**

3. **Starting at your feet, focus on your internal sensations.**

   Notice your feet and feel them inside your socks or shoes; or if you're barefoot, feel how your feet meet the floor. Sense the bottoms of your feet, your toes, the tops of your feet, and your heels.

4. **After a few seconds, move your attention up through your body.**

   Notice internally how each part of your body feels. Is your weight more in one foot than the other? Does your pelvis feel even from side to side and from front to back? If your pelvis were a bowl, would the water rest evenly in it? Is one shoulder more tense than the other? Is your head jutting forward in space? Ask yourself questions as you make your way up from your feet to the crown of your head.

5. **If you want to compare your body sensations before and after a workout or somatic movement, do this process pre-and post-movement. Stand with your eyes closed and your muscles relaxed and try to remember what you felt like before.**

Do you notice any changes or new sensations? How are you holding your head now? This post-movement check-in helps you become more aware of how the exercises have shifted your alignment and sensations.

6. **When you feel ready, open your eyes or release your gaze.**

TIP

You can perform the Standing Awareness exercise any time you want to check in with your body, not just before and after physical activity.

Benefits of the Standing Awareness exercise

Standing Awareness offers several benefits that can positively impact your body and daily life:

>> **Builds internal sensory-motor awareness of your body:** By learning to sense your muscle tension, posture, and movement, you can realign or adjust where you need to. This practice helps you become more aware of how your body feels from the inside, allowing you to correct imbalances before they lead to discomfort.

>> **Improves posture and movement:** Once you sense your imbalances, you can work to come back to a state of harmony in your body. Maybe you notice one hip is higher than the other, or that you lock out your knees when you stand. Once you recognize these patterns, you can work to correct them. You'll find a way to stand with your head over your heart and your heart over your hips. This awareness carries into everything you do, helping you maintain better posture when walking, sitting, standing, or moving throughout the day.

>> **Prevents injury:** Repeating the same movements with misalignment or poor form can lead to injury. Standing Awareness helps you catch these imbalances before they become problematic. For example, you might tear your rotator cuff because of repetitive overhead motion without proper form or core support. Or maybe you hurt your back because you've become accustomed to standing with your hips too tucked under or your back too arched. With regular practice over time, you can correct these misalignments and prevent injury.

REMEMBER

It may take time to build awareness and notice how you feel before and after practicing your exercises, but you will get better. You can always improve your sensory-motor awareness with practice and dedication.

Techniques for improving posture and balance

Improving your posture and balance through Standing Awareness begins with simple observation. By closing your eyes and noticing where you shift your weight, you can become aware of all the little micromovements your body makes to keep itself upright. Ideally, you want to relax your muscles and let your bones come back to their natural position, allowing yourself to release tension.

The more you develop the ability to sense your body's position, the better you can adjust your posture, allow your muscles to relax, and allow your bones to come back to their natural positions. If you have a muscular imbalance, like pulling one hip out of alignment or jutting your head out when using electronics, you can make gradual adjustments over time. As you stand and become aware of the misalignment, you can shift your hips back into alignment and rest your head more squarely on your spine. This balanced posture requires less effort from your muscles, allowing you to stand with greater ease.

You can balance better when you have good posture. If you observe a dancer or gymnast, you'll see years of body awareness and balance reflected in their posture. But good posture isn't just about standing tall — it also requires core strength and proper breathing. When you connect to your center, you stabilize from your abdominals instead of using your legs (overgripping the quadriceps) or your shoulders (tensing them up to your ears).

Pilates is a great example of a practice to learn to move from and strengthen your center. For information about getting started with Pilates, see Chapter 5.

A few techniques to help with posture and balance include:

>> **Strengthen your core:** Engage your abdominal muscles throughout the day. You can do this by pulling your belly button toward your spine as you stand or sit, creating a steady support system for your posture.

>> **Relax your shoulders:** Let them fall away from your ears to avoid tension.

>> **Tuck your chin:** Periodically bring your chin back in space to align your head with your spine.

>> **Stretch tight muscles:** Regular stretching different muscles prevents imbalances. Turn to Chapter 5 for step-by-step instructions on how to do various stretches.

>> **Deepen your breath:** Focus on diaphragmatic breathing to support your core. Chapter 4 walks you through how to do it.

>> **Practice standing on one foot:** Alternate throughout the day to improve your stability and balance.

>> **Check your posture throughout the day:** Regularly remind yourself to realign your posture.

>> **Get up from your seat:** Sitting too long compromises your posture, so take frequent breaks to stand or walk.

Incorporating Standing Awareness into daily life

Incorporating Standing Awareness into your daily life is easy if you use "habit stacking," where you pair a new habit with one you already do regularly. For instance, you may want to do Standing Awareness in the morning and evening, before and after you brush your teeth. If you habit stack Standing Awareness into your routine, you'll reap its benefits without needing to carve out extra time.

Another great opportunity to incorporate Standing Awareness exercises is when you're standing in line — at the grocery store, waiting for a bus, or even on the sidelines of a game.

TIP

Instead of scrolling through your phone or feeling impatient, you can use this time to check in with your body. Ground yourself by noticing how you're standing and where your weight is shifting. Take a few deep breaths and do a quick internal scan.

You can also integrate Standing Awareness into your movement practices like yoga, Pilates, or Tai Chi. Any time you have a few extra moments, try adding it. Even during everyday tasks like unloading the dishwasher or folding laundry, you can take a moment to pause, check your posture, and reconnect with how you're holding your body. This simple awareness can make you more present and engaged in whatever you're doing.

Body Scanning

Body scanning is a meditative practice that helps you become more aware of your sensations and feelings within your body. Your body processes all of your experiences, and body scanning allows you to explore these sensations without judgment. By mentally scanning each part of your body, you can increase somatic awareness and tune into what's happening inside.

When I teach, I often lead people through a body scan at the end of a yoga practice while they are in *savasana* (final relaxation), but you don't need yoga to benefit from a scan. You can do a quick body scan whenever you need to go deeper into yourself — before giving a speech, taking a test, or even going on a first date. When you bring your awareness to your body, you can relax more easily by noticing where you're holding tension and gently reminding each part of your body to let go.

TIP

Sometimes, repeating a mantra like "let go" can enhance your experience as you move through the parts of your body.

Even if you only have five minutes, you can still reap the benefits of a mindfulness body scan. When you have time for a longer body scan, you can spend up to 30 minutes engaged in mindful exploration of your physical state, going deeper into your body's sensations. Each time you practice, you connect with the present moment, observing where your body is today and how it feels in that moment.

As you incorporate body scans into your regular routine, you may start to feel more anchored, connected to your body, and resilient and relaxed. Body scanning helps reduce physical and psychological stress and even helps you manage your emotions better.

Principles of body scanning

Body scanning is a flexible practice, and there is no right or wrong way to do it. The main goal is to connect with your body by feeling each part without judgment. Just be a witness. Allow thoughts, emotions, and sensations to rise while simply observing them without reacting.

TIP

You can always journal afterwards if you need to, but ultimately, keep the body scan in and of itself relaxing so it puts you in a restful state.

By focusing on your body, you quiet your mind. Body scanning is an act of self-compassion, where you observe your body from the inside rather than judging it based on external appearances. This practice helps you build a kinder, more intuitive relationship with your body.

Steps for effective body-scanning practice

To get the most out of your body scan, follow these simple steps:

1. **Find a quiet, comfortable space where you won't be disrupted.**

You can sit, stand, or lie down, but I recommend either sitting or lying down.

2. **Close your eyes and connect with your breath.**

Take slow deep breaths in and out through your nose.

3. **Start at your feet.**

Focus your attention on each part of your foot, starting with your toes and working your way up to the sole, the top of the foot, and so on. If you like, you can scan one foot at a time, paying attention to each individual toe.

4. **Notice any tension or other sensations.**

If you notice any tension as you move through each part of your body, stay with it a little longer, breathing into the tightness. You can also gently move that part if you need to.

5. **Don't censor or judge yourself.**

As thoughts or sensations arise, allow them to come and go without judgment. If you feel the need to shift or adjust, follow your impulses, but see if you can eventually relax and let go completely.

6. **Finish at the crown of your head.**

Continue your scan all the way to the crown of your head, including your face, lips, mouth, throat, jaw, and forehead. Don't forget these small areas, as they often hold tension.

7. **Stay in the moment.**

Before finishing your scan, linger for a bit in stillness. When you're ready, deepen your breath again and ease back into your surroundings.

You can also reverse the process, going from the top down, if you want to. Another variation is to scan one side of your body, then the other, and finish with your back and front.

TIP

You can use a guided body scan if you'd like more help. To find good body-scan guides, explore meditation apps like Insight Timer, Headspace, or Calm. These offer a variety of guided body-scan meditations from different teachers. You can also find detailed body-scan scripts and instructions on websites like Greater Good Science Center at UC Berkeley, Mindful.org, and HelpGuide.org. I like books such as *The Mindfulness Guide for the Modern World* by Jonathan Harris *and The Four Foundations of Mindfulness* by Bhante Gunaratana as well. I also have some body-scan meditations on my website, www.kristinmcgee.com. You might have to try a few until you find one that resonates with you. When you're comfortable, you can do a self-guided body scan.

Using body scanning to enhance relaxation and awareness

Body scans are a great way to enhance relaxation and awareness. By turning your attention inward, you focus on your physical self and begin to release the tension that you hold subconsciously. You can use your breath and imagination to feel your body letting go. Imagination is a wonderful tool that you probably used a lot when you were younger to daydream and allow yourself to be curious. Many people lose touch with their imagination as they get older, but when you engage your imagination during a body scan, you tap into that curiosity and freedom once again.

Your mind is your greatest asset, but it can also become a barrier if you allow it to block your ability to relax. As you scan your body with a sense of acceptance and non-judgment, begin to eliminate harsh thoughts or self-criticism. Instead, simply observe. You allow yourself to become more aware of who you are, and in doing so, you relax into your own unique beauty.

Your mind and body are connected. As you let go of physical stress, you can enhance your mental relaxation as well.

REMEMBER

Your only task is to observe and soften, then observe some more and soften even further. How wonderful it is to give yourself this gift of peace and rest.

Body Mapping

Body mapping is a fascinating and deeply personal technique used in somatic movement and therapy. It involves exploring your physical sensations in a creative and contemplative way, often by drawing, painting, or sketching a life-sized representation of your body. Through this process, you explore your body's stories, paying close attention to the sensations and feedback it gives you and how certain emotions may contribute to physical tension and discomfort. It also helps you reconnect with your sense of self, reflect on past experiences, and gain a deeper understanding of your relationship with your body. This form of movement can also help you access a deeper intuitive wisdom and feel the impact of significant things that have happened in your life.

My first experience with body mapping goes all the way back to when I was a young girl in elementary school, and we did a project where we laid down on a big sheet of paper and someone traced us. I remember standing up and seeing my outline — it was surreal, almost like meeting myself for the first time. I saw my hands, feet, and head all mapped out, and it made me appreciate my body in a whole new way. It put things into perspective and left me in awe.

When you see yourself in your full expression, you may feel a powerful sense of self-awareness. Your intuition kicks in and you can examine those areas that give you feedback. You may have an aha type moment like I did when I was a young girl in school. It's like seeing a map of the city you live in and getting a bird's eye view instead of walking or driving around inside town.

TIP

Use body mapping to shift your perspective, allowing you to see familiar terrain in a whole new light and revealing details you might otherwise miss. By engaging with your body in this way, you open up a path to greater self-discovery and healing.

Understanding the benefits of body mapping

Body mapping offers numerous benefits that can enrich your self-awareness and emotional well-being. As you map your body, you start processing feelings tied to past events, whether joyful or painful. This process allows you to explore difficult emotions and gradually release what you've been holding onto, making body mapping a powerful therapeutic tool.

I also love body mapping for its ability to help spark creative expression. You can express your feelings and thoughts through stories, images, and art. You can also tell your story and create meaning from the experiences you've had in your life. Body mapping gives you a sense of empowerment as you get to tell your story from your perspective. You can also make it a collaborative experience and engage with others going through a similar process. When we each drew each other's body outlines in school, we didn't just stop at the drawing; we got to look at them and talk about it. We also got to fill in our outline. It was a creative process.

Body mapping:

>> **Enhances self-awareness:** Body mapping helps you recognize how your body stores emotions and experiences, allowing you to process and release them.

>> **Provides therapeutic effects:** It offers a safe space to explore and let go of difficult emotions or past traumas.

>> **Fosters creative expression:** Through art, you can express your inner thoughts, feelings, and personal narratives in a visual, tangible way.

>> **Empowers storytelling:** You get to tell your story from your perspective, creating meaning and understanding from your experiences.

>> **Encourages collaboration:** Body mapping can be shared with others, fostering connection and shared understanding.

>> **Offers a new perspective:** It helps you see your body from an outside view, revealing unexamined areas and allowing you to connect more deeply with yourself.

Body mapping encourages you to see your body from a new vantage point, prompting you to go deeper inside yourself. This painted or drawn representation of your body allows you to explore parts of yourself that have been holding energy for a long time or that have gone unexamined. Whether you're moving, breathing, dancing, or creating, body mapping helps you connect with those hidden places, letting go of what no longer serves you and making room for healing and freedom.

Techniques for creating an accurate body map

Creating a body map is a personal and insightful process, and there are several techniques you can use to make it as accurate and meaningful as possible. In addition to using the outline drawing, you can also use self-observation and self-inquiry. You can use a mirror, books, pictures, and other people to help you learn more about your body's structure and movement. Your body map is essentially your brain's perception of your body. When this map is accurate, your movement is natural and balanced. If it's inaccurate, your movement can be inefficient or even lead to injury. Figure 6-1 shows an example.

TIP

You can correct your body map by gaining accurate information about yourself using a mirror, or looking at an anatomical model, using pictures, teachers, and books. You replace harmful movement with proper biomechanics based on your own structure and size.

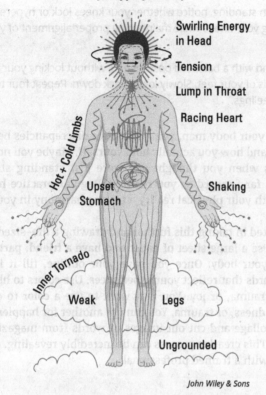

Body Mapping Anxiety

- Swirling Energy in Head
- Tension
- Lump in Throat
- Racing Heart
- Hot + Cold Limbs
- Upset Stomach
- Shaking
- Inner Tornado
- Weak
- Legs
- Ungrounded

FIGURE 6-1: Body mapping can help you reconnect with your sense of self, reflect on experiences, and gain a deeper understanding of your body.

John Wiley & Sons

Body mapping can be organized around six points of balance:

>> **Where the head meets the spine:** Gently place your fingers in your ears and move your head up and down with tiny movements. Notice the sensation and see if you can release tension in the back of your neck. Your chin may drop slightly as you relax.

>> **Shoulders:** Stand in front of a mirror and observe the height of your shoulders relative to your ears. Slowly raise your shoulders up, hold for 20-30 seconds, and then gently release them. Repeat three to four times to notice whether your shoulders relax into a lower position.

>> **Lumbar spine:** Place one finger on your navel and another at the same level on your side. Rock your pelvis back and forth, and then in a circle, feeling the movement. Alternate between a hunched position and upright posture until you find your neutral midline.

>> **Hips:** Check that your pelvis is centered over your feet and your head is aligned with your spine.

>> **Knees:** When standing, notice whether your knees lock or hyperextend. Try softening your knees while maintaining proper alignment of your pelvis and spine.

>> **Ankles:** Stand with a balanced posture and, without locking your knees, rise onto the balls of your feet. Slowly lower back down. Repeat four to five times, noting the feelings.

TIP

As you examine your body map, you may notice discrepancies between how you think you stand and how you actually hold yourself. Maybe you notice you always lock your knees when you thought you were just standing straight. Or your midline isn't as far forward as you realized. Regular practice helps align your internal map with your physical reality, creating harmony in your movements.

If you're interested in taking this further and drawing a life-sized outline of your body, you can. Use a large sheet of paper and have a friend, partner, teacher, or therapist trace your body. Once you have your outline, fill it in with images, symbols, and words that reflect your experiences. Use colors to highlight areas of grief, sadness, trauma, or joy. You may want to use a color to draw in specific areas of grief, sadness, or trauma. You can use another for happier memories. You can also use a collage and cut out images or words from magazines to decorate your body map. This creative process can be incredibly revealing, and it's one you can do alone or with a trained professional.

Rolfing

My first experience with Rolfing came in my 30s, when I was living in the West Village in Manhattan. I met a woman who was an experienced Rolfer, and out of curiosity, I signed up for the ten-session bodywork package. It was an interesting and incredible process. Rolfing is like massage on steroids! You go *deep*. I mean, you get into places you'd never imagine.

Rolfing, also known as structural integration, is a form of bodywork created by Dr. Ida Rolf. This technique aims to reorganize the *fascia* — the connective tissue that weaves throughout your entire body. Dr. Ida Rolf believed that misalignments in the body caused various health problems. Fascia is like a webbing that is woven throughout your body. It lies above the muscles.

Someone once explained it to me like the film that's between the white of a hard-boiled egg and the shell. Have you ever noticed when you try to crack a hard-boiled egg and the pieces get stuck? Other times you can crack it in one easy piece and when you remove the shell from the egg the layer of film comes off easily. You have this layer of film that wraps around your entire body. When it gets sticky or stuck, it can create fractures or imbalances. Everything is connected. Dr. Rolf recognized this and created a form of bodywork that works on the fascia to release, realign, and balance the whole body.

TIP

By addressing these deep-seated fascial restrictions, Rolfing can alleviate pain, reduce compensation patterns, and enhance overall flexibility and ease. When your body regains its natural integrity, your posture improves, and you move with more freedom.

Fundamentals of Rolfing

Rolfing is a form of somatic bodywork that aims to realign the body's architecture and relieve tension. Rolfing works on your body's fascia to release adhesions and improve mobility. The phrase, "your issues are in your tissues," is applicable here. This is particularly true with fascia, which holds onto the memories of your experiences — physically, emotionally, and mentally. Fascia, muscles, and even organs can store tension from past events, sometimes without you even realizing it. Your mind does a good job of ignoring the body until you have something really wrong with you and you need medical treatment, or you've had enough of living with discomfort and you need to solve the problem.

Unlike quick fixes, somatic exercises and therapies like Rolfing aim to change the root of the problem, process stored emotions, and get you back to your natural aligned state. You learn to deal with the trapped tension and trauma and move through it to a better place physically and mentally. Rolfing can also help you improve performance in your professional and daily life.

The goal of Rolfing is to create lasting change by realigning your body's structure through a series of sessions that build on one another. Unlike a regular massage, which provides temporary relief, Rolfing integrates your whole body, working with the fascia that surrounds your muscles, nerves, and organs. When your fascia is healthy, it is hydrated and can stretch easily. If your fascia is dry or rigid, it can restrict movement and pull you into misalignment.

Rolfing sessions typically last around 60 to 90 minutes, and unlike traditional massage where you mostly lie face down or face up, you may be asked to move, stand, sit, or lie in different positions. The standard Rolfing series involves ten sessions, each focusing on a different part of the body and building on the progress of the previous session. Depending on your needs, additional sessions may be recommended.

WARNING

Rolfing can be intense and sometimes uncomfortable, especially as it works deeply into areas of tension. However, the discomfort is short-lived, and the benefits of completing the full series can be significant, leading to improved balance, posture, and overall movement.

Structural alignment and pain reduction

Rolfing addresses imbalances in the fascial network, starting with the most superficial layer and then moving into deeper restrictions. If you can handle the intensity as the practitioner goes deeper, you'll soon feel the release of bound-up tissue and start to move with more ease and feel better.

TIP

Speaking with a professional Rolfer ahead of time ensures that this is right for you, as the benefits on your structural alignment and pain reduction can be significant.

REMEMBER

Since Rolfing's goal is to realign the body's structure, it can help reduce tension and improve flexibility. Your therapist will work on loosening your fascia. When you release the connective tissue, it can help reorganize the body and help you get realigned. When you are in alignment you move better and have less pain. The slow deep strokes of Rolfing can also stimulate sensory neurons in the muscle nerve, which tells the nervous system to relax.

Rolfing also addresses your posture, breath and movement. I remember when my Rolfer worked on my psoas muscles (long muscles in your back) — afterward, I felt I could breathe so much easier. Each session invites you to create new movement patterns and options, and you'll often be asked to stand, sit, or walk around after your session to notice how your body feels.

Incorporating Rolfing techniques into your routine

Even if you don't have the time or money to do a full ten-session Rolfing treatment, you can still apply some of the techniques into your current routine. One of the best ways to work on your fascia at home is using foam rolling. Foam rolling targets the fascial tissue, helping to release tightness and restore movement, much like Rolfing. Keeping a foam roller handy can serve as a reminder to use it regularly, whether before or after workouts — or anytime you feel tension building up.

Here's a quick guide to foam rolling your fascia:

1. **Start with your IT band.**

   Begin by rolling the side of your legs along the *iliotibial* (IT) band, which runs from your outer hip to your shinbone. This band often gets tight due to its role in knee extension and flexion.

2. **Move to your other muscles.**

   After addressing your IT band, continue to your hamstrings, calves, quads, and glutes, spending a few minutes on each muscle group.

3. **Open up your upper back and chest.**

   Lie over the roller with it placed horizontally under your shoulder blades (parallel to the top of your mat). Roll gently to release tension in your upper back and chest.

4. **Target your shoulders and arms.**

   With your head lifted and hands behind your head, roll along the back of your arms and shoulders, focusing on any tight spots.

TIP

Foam rolling is highly customizable — you can adjust pressure and timing to suit your needs. Explore different areas of your body and spend extra time on spots that feel particularly tight.

Rolfing principles can also encourage you to be mindful of how your everyday movement patterns affect your fascia. If you sit for long periods, make a habit of getting up frequently to move around. Incorporate deep breathing, maintain postural alignment, and keep your body hydrated — hydration, movement, and stretching are essential to keeping your fascia healthy and flexible.

Emotional Freedom Techniques (EFT) (Tapping)

I first learned about Emotional Freedom Technique (EFT), commonly known as *tapping*, from a friend who is trained in EFT. Tapping is a method that involves gently tapping on specific places on the body while focusing on uncomfortable thoughts and/or feelings. The idea is to manage emotions and stress. You can try EFT on your own or look into hiring someone who has trained in EFT tapping, but this mind-body somatic method is a wonderful self-help tool that's simple enough for everyone to use.

The tapping points are similar to the acupuncture points located on your hands, face, and body. As you tap with your fingertips, you focus on specific thoughts, feelings, or issues you want to address. When overwhelming emotions like guilt, anger, or hurt arise, tapping provides a way to confront and process these feelings rather than suppressing them. Often, just a few rounds of tapping can bring noticeable relief — you might feel lighter, calmer, or find it easier to breathe.

You can use EFT to address deep-seated problems and eventually make progress in moving through trauma and living more freely. You can make lasting changes in your patterns and address your issues through tapping.

TIP

EFT can be an alternative treatment for physical pain and emotional distress and can be used to create a balance in your energy. According to EFT founder Gary Craig, disruptions in the body's energy system are the root cause of negative emotions and physical pain. Tapping helps to restore balance, making it a powerful tool for moving through trauma, shifting emotional patterns, and fostering greater freedom in your daily life.

EFT tapping basics

EFT, like acupuncture, focuses on meridian points — specific areas where energy flows through your body. This energy-based approach helps restore balance, relieving symptoms caused by negative experiences. Meridians are based on Chinese medicine and are areas of the body where energy flows through. When you tap, you hit each one of these areas. When these pathways are balanced, the idea is that you can maintain your health, and any imbalance may result in disease.

Although there are 12 major meridians that correspond to different organs, EFT focuses on nine key points, making it a simple yet powerful practice for maintaining health and emotional well-being (see Figure 6-2). The nine major meridians that EFT focuses on are as follows:

>> Side of the hand (small intestine meridian)

>> Top of the head (governing vessel)

>> Eyebrow (bladder meridian)

>> Side of the eye (gallbladder meridian)

>> Under the eye (stomach meridian)

>> Under the nose (governing vessel)

>> Chin (central vessel)

» Beginning of the collarbone (kidney meridian)

» Under the arm (spleen meridian)

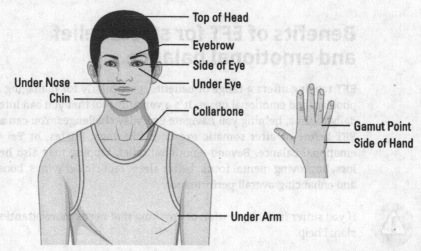

Top of Head

Eyebrow

Side of Eye

Under Nose

Under Eye

Chin

Collarbone

Gamut Point

Side of Hand

Under Arm

FIGURE 6-2:
The nine main
tapping points/
meridians
associated
with EFT.

John Wiley & Sons

EFT tapping is easy to try on your own by following some simple steps:

1. **Start by thinking about an issue or problem that is bothering you. Rate how intense you feel on a scale from 1-10.**

2. **Create a statement that describes the issue and then follow it up with a statement or affirmation of self-acceptance.**

    An example could be, "Even though I'm upset that my job is uncertain, I completely accept and love myself."

3. **Start tapping, beginning with the side of your hand.**

    Tap on the edge of your palm, below your pinky finger, as you repeat your statement three times.

4. **Continue through the nine tapping points shown in Figure 6-2.**

    Move through the sequence of nine tapping points described in this section, tapping each spot about seven times.

5. **Focus on your reminder phrase.**

    As you tap each point, repeat your reminder phrase, such as, "I'm upset my job is uncertain."

6. **End at the top of your head.**

   After finishing the sequence, pause and check in with yourself. Rate the intensity of your feeling again and repeat the sequence as needed until you feel more relaxed.

Benefits of EFT for stress relief and emotional balance

EFT tapping offers a range of benefits, particularly for managing stress, anxiety, phobias, and emotional upset. It's a versatile tool that you can integrate into your daily routine, helping you navigate everyday challenges. You can also incorporate EFT before or after somatic exercises like yoga, Pilates, or Tai Chi to enhance emotional balance. Beyond emotional relief, tapping may also help with weight loss, improving mental focus, better sleep, reducing cravings, boosting creativity, and enhancing overall performance.

WARNING

If you suffer from depression or anything that needs more attention, seek professional help.

Practicing Proprioceptive Neuromuscular Facilitation (PNF)

Proprioceptive Neuromuscular Facilitation (PNF) is a hands-on therapy technique that combines stretching and contracting muscles to enhance flexibility, coordination, and range of motion. Originally developed by physiotherapists for rehabilitating stroke victims, PNF has evolved into a widely used method for performance enhancement and injury rehabilitation.

PNF and somatics are not exactly the same things. Somatics typically places a greater emphasis on subtle, mindful movements and addressing underlying tension patterns through techniques like pandiculation. PNF often involves more active muscle contractions during stretching. However, they can both be considered somatic in nature. These practices focus on enhancing body awareness and movement control by utilizing neuromuscular mechanisms to improve flexibility and range of motion.

PNF improves flexibility by stimulating your neuromuscular system. When you stretch and contract your muscles, you activate sensory receptors in the muscles and tendons, which help improve mobility and inhibit the stretch reflex. This also triggers the inverse *myotatic reflex* — a protective response that encourages your muscles to relax further, allowing you to deepen your stretch and expand your range of motion. PNF is particularly beneficial for athletes, dancers, and anyone recovering from surgeries or injuries involving soft tissue damage.

WARNING

PNF is an advanced technique that often involves manual resistance, repeated stretches, and compressions, making it essential to practice with a trained professional or approach slowly if you're new to stretching.

PNF improves muscle elasticity by integrating passive and active stretching techniques. The process typically involves passively stretching the muscle, then contracting it isometrically against resistance while still in the stretched position, and finally relaxing it to deepen the stretch further. This combination not only increases flexibility but also strengthens the muscles involved.

PNF techniques can involve a variety of actions, including:

>> **Manual resistance:** A partner or therapist provides resistance while you contract the muscle.

>> **Repeated stretches:** You stretch, contract, and stretch again, each time gaining a bit more flexibility.

>> **Distraction and compression:** Using techniques like pulling or pushing on a joint to increase the stretch's effectiveness.

Four key mechanisms contribute to increasing your range of motion:

>> **Autogenic inhibition:** This reflex helps your muscle automatically relax under tension to protect it from tearing.

>> **Reciprocal inhibition:** This occurs when muscles on one side of a joint relax to allow the muscles on the opposite side to contract. For example, when your hamstring relaxes, your quadricep engages and vice versa.

>> **Stress relaxation:** This happens when the musculotendinous unit (MTU) — the muscle and tendon complex — is under continuous stress for an extended period, gradually allowing the muscle to lengthen. Your muscles are gently stretched to a comfortable length and held for a period of time, allowing the tension in the muscle to gradually decrease, effectively releasing built-up stress and promoting relaxation in the body. The muscle fibers relax while being held at a fixed length, reducing the force needed to maintain that stretch.

>> **Gate control theory:** A neurological concept that explains how pain signals are controlled in the spinal cord, essentially acting like a "gate" that can either allow pain signals to pass through to the brain or block them. Non-painful stimuli like rubbing can sometimes reduce perceived pain by "closing the gate" on pain signals.

REMEMBER

While PNF can be highly effective, it's important to approach it with care. Stretching too forcefully can lead to injury, so listen to your body and never push beyond your comfort zone. Always consult with a professional if you're new to PNF or recovering from an injury.

PNF techniques for improving flexibility and strength

PNF offers two main techniques that can help you enhance flexibility and build strength: The contract-relax method and the contract-relax-antagonist-contract method. The following sections break down these techniques and explain how they work.

Contract-relax method

This method focuses on contracting the target muscle while it's in a stretched position. Here's how to do it:

1. **Choose your target muscle.**

   Begin by stretching the muscle you want to work on.

2. **Contract the muscle.**

   In the stretched position, contract the muscle at about 50 percent of your maximum effort and hold isometrically for four to six seconds.

3. **Release and relax.**

   Relax the muscle for a few seconds, then gently stretch further into the new range of motion.

4. **Hold the final contraction.**

   Hold the final contraction for about ten seconds, then release and stretch into your full range of motion for at least 20 seconds.

You can perform this method with or without assistance. If you're working on your hamstring, you might press your heel into a bench or use your hands behind your thigh for resistance.

Contract-relax-antagonist-contract method

This variation engages the target muscle (agonist) and its opposing muscle (antagonist).

1. Stretch and contract the target muscle.

Begin by holding the target muscle in a stretched position and contracting it isometrically for five seconds.

2. Switch to the opposing muscle.

Immediately contract the opposing muscle group (for example, contracting your quadriceps after stretching your hamstrings) for another five seconds.

3. Relax and repeat.

Relax for 20 seconds and repeat the sequence as needed.

Using PNF for rehabilitation and performance enhancement

PNF began as a rehabilitative technique and quickly found its way into the athletic world due to its remarkable effectiveness. By alternating between static stretches, holds, and isometric contractions, PNF improves both active and passive range of motion. When used alongside traditional static stretching, it helps increase flexibility and strength, making it a powerful tool for both rehabilitation and performance enhancement.

Originally developed for stroke victims, PNF can aid in improving lower-body strength, walking speed, and overall balance. The technique retrains muscles to engage and relax effectively, making it ideal for anyone easing back into movement after a setback.

Athletes often incorporate PNF into their routines to enhance performance. The targeted stretching helps to realign muscle fibers and connective tissue, reducing knots and aiding recovery after intense workouts. Studies have shown that athletes who perform PNF twice a week see more than double improvement in activities like jumping and throwing within eight weeks.

TIP

The greater your range of motion, the more strength you can build. For example, deeper squats can lead to increased glute strength, and better shoulder mobility allows for faster, more powerful throws.

PNF is an excellent choice for anyone looking to improve their flexibility and performance. By lengthening the muscles and stretching the Golgi tendon organs, PNF helps maximize your range of motion, giving you a competitive edge. Incorporating PNF into your training two to three times a week can significantly improve your overall performance, whether you're recovering from an injury or looking to push your limits.

3

Integrating Somatic Exercises Into Daily Life

IN THIS CHAPTER

» **Using the power of shaking to release tension and calm your nervous system**

» **Learning simple techniques to release built-up tension throughout your day**

» **Incorporating somatic dance for stress relief**

» **Creating a personalized de-stress plan to manage stress triggers effectively**

» **Using somatics to increase your mental focus**

» **Exploring self-hugging techniques for comfort, self-compassion, and relaxation**

Chapter **7**

Using Somatic Solutions for Stress Relief

Everyone is stressed out these days. From a never-ending to-do list, to taking care of yourself and others, to holding down a job and staying healthy, there is always so much on your mind. A little stress here and there is okay — it's something you can use to your advantage to get things done, stay out of danger, and just stay alive! But chronic stress isn't good for your immune system. Over time, you can start to feel its effects, such as poor sleep, anxiety, weight gain or extreme weight loss, lack of focus, and feeling irritable. If you don't find an outlet to manage your stress, it can be detrimental to your health and to your relationships with others. I know I am a much better mother when I have taken time to let go of my stress and relax. It's easier said than done, but somatic exercises can provide that much-needed movement that benefits the brain and the body.

Shaking It Off

Shaking therapy, also known as *therapeutic* or *neurogenic tremoring,* involves deliberately shaking your body to release tension and trauma, helping to regulate your nervous system. You may have noticed this in animals — have you ever seen your pet shake? My cat does this sometimes, and I remember my childhood dog doing it, too. It's a natural way to release stress. Competitive athletes often use this natural technique to relieve muscular tension before key moments, such as during pivotal moments in a game or a stressful shot. Shaking helps release built-up tension, burn excess adrenaline, and return your nervous system to a balanced, neutral state.

Your autonomic nervous system regulates many bodily processes, from blood pressure to body temperature, through *upregulation* (increasing available energy) and *downregulation* (decreasing energy). When stressed, your body triggers the fight-or-flight response, releasing adrenaline and cortisol. Your body does this to help you escape physical dangers, but modern stressors — like work pressure — can activate the same response, without actually using any of the adrenaline and cortisol. Shaking provides a way to help down-regulate your nervous system, lower your heart rate, and bring your body back to calm.

TIP

Incorporating regular shaking into your routine can prevent long-term emotional stress from building up and turning into deeper issues, like anxiety or depression. It's a simple yet effective way to release the stress your body doesn't need to hold on to. For more information on how the nervous system functions, see Chapter 4.

You can practice shaking therapy either seated or standing. Start with these steps:

1. **Start with your feet and hands.**

   Begin by gently shaking your feet and hands, which may feel less awkward. Let the movement flow naturally.

2. **Focus on your breath.**

   As you shake, pay attention to your breath. Occasionally pause, take a deep breath, and check in with how your body feels.

3. **Shake one side at a time.**

If you prefer, shake everything on one side of your body first, then switch to the other. Finish by shaking your head and neck gently.

4. **Stay curious.**

Don't look for any specific outcomes. Instead, stay curious about what comes up. Ask yourself how your body feels, how you felt before you started, and how you feel afterward.

5. **Start small.**

If you're new to shaking, start with 10 to 30 seconds. Even that short amount of time can begin to change your nervous system's state. As you get more comfortable, build up to two or three minutes, either in the morning, the evening, or whenever you're feeling stressed.

6. **Use shaking when needed.**

Feel free to shake anytime you need to release stress. I remember a particularly difficult time in my life when I was in an unhealthy relationship, constantly stressed, and walking on eggshells. I had a two-year-old son at the time, and we'd jump and shake to "Shake It Off" by Taylor Swift on his Thomas the Train bed every night. That simple act of shaking made a huge difference.

7. **Consider professional support for deep trauma.**

If you feel you have deep trauma, you might want to find a professional trained in trauma release therapies. Always be mindful of your limitations, and start small. Shaking it off can help regulate your nervous system, but it obviously doesn't address the root of any chronic stress.

Taming Your Tension

You can use somatic exercises anytime to release tension. For instance, as you read this, check in with your body. Are your shoulders tense? Are you clenching your jaw? You might be subconsciously holding onto tension somewhere. When you stop, take a deep breath and do a quick body scan.

REMEMBER

You have countless opportunities to relieve tension throughout the day. It doesn't always have to be a formal time for movement. I often do small things throughout the day. When I'm at my computer, I pause and relax my facial muscles. When I'm waiting to pick up my kids from school, I might tense and release my shoulders a few times.

Stress-relieving exercises can take many forms, from breathing exercises and physical movements to meditations, body scans, or simple tense-and-release techniques. The key is to stay mindful and incorporate these practices whenever you need them, so you don't let stress build up throughout the day.

Simple techniques to release built-up tension

Here are a few simple exercises you can use anytime to release tension:

>> **Deep breathing:** Sit or stand comfortably with your spine long. Take a deep breath, expanding your stomach and lungs, while keeping your shoulders relaxed. Slowly exhale. Repeat this two or three more times and notice how you feel. Deep breathing helps release physical tension and increase oxygen intake, which can induce a sense of calm.

>> **Facial tension release:** Tense your face as tightly as you can, then release everything. Stick out your tongue or let out a roar like a lion if it helps. You may not realize how much tension you hold in your face — releasing it regularly can make a big difference.

>> **Jaw unclenching:** To release jaw tension, gently slide your bottom jaw over the top a few times. Notice how it loosens the front of your neck. You can also brush your hands up the front of your neck, then flick them toward the sky for added release.

>> **Chest opener at your desk:** If you're sitting at a desk, clasp your hands behind your back, open your chest, and look up toward the ceiling. Take a deep breath, then release.

>> **Neck stretch:** Drape one arm over the opposite ear, letting your head fall gently toward your shoulder. Hold for three to five seconds, then switch to the other side.

>> **Seated Cat-Cow stretch:** While seated, arch your spine on an inhalation and round your spine on an exhalation. Let your upper back and head follow the movement of your spine, coordinating your breath with each motion.

>> **Grounding walk:** When possible, get outside and walk slowly, paying attention to how your feet connect with the ground. Feel the roll from the ball to the arch to the heel of each foot. If possible, take off your shoes and walk in the grass.

>> **Water therapy:** Run warm or cool water over your hands and focus on the sensation. Just like a shower relaxes you, this small act can mimic that calming effect when you can't take a full shower.

>> **Wrap up in a blanket:** Use a grounding or weighted blanket to feel more connected. In yoga, sandbags are often used for grounding, and they give the same sense of relaxation and rootedness.

>> **Pet therapy:** If you have a pet, run your fingers through their fur and focus on how it feels. This is a great way to de-stress. When I stroke my cat Lucky, I always feel better.

>> **Tense-and-release exercise:** Start by tensing and releasing each part of your body, moving from your feet to your head. You can also keep a stress ball nearby to squeeze whenever you feel anxious.

>> **Music therapy:** Calm music is excellent for lowering cortisol levels. I love to unwind with classical music or find some calm music while doing household chores. When you move mindfully, even vacuuming can become a somatic movement.

Incorporating tension release into your daily routine

You can incorporate these tension-release techniques throughout your day to keep stress at bay.

>> Morning routine:

- **Stretch in bed:** Start your day with a big stretch from your fingertips to your toes while you're still in bed. Roll to your side, sit up, and raise your arms overhead. Clasp your hands together and invert your palms toward the ceiling. Release and relax your shoulders with a few shrugs.

- **Facial tension release while brushing your teeth:** As you brush your teeth, take a moment to tense and release the muscles in your face. Laugh if it feels silly — this will help you de-stress even more!

- **Shake it off:** After brushing your teeth, do a quick shake to release any lingering nighttime energy.

>> During the day:

- **Mindful walking:** As you get ready for your day, pay attention to how your feet feel as they touch the floor. Notice the sensations with each step.

- **Desk stretches:** While seated, do some seated Cat-Cow stretches, neck stretches, and tense-and-release exercises for your feet, legs, shoulders, hands, and face.

- **Jaw massage:** Massage your jaw, cheeks, temples, and forehead if you feel tension building.

- **Afternoon walk:** Take a short walk in the afternoon. Focus on how your feet connect with the Earth.

» Evening routine:

- **End-of-day unwinding:** As you transition into the evening, turn on some calming music. If you have more energy, choose upbeat music and dance around the room.

- **Gentle stretches:** After dinner, do some light stretching or a Yoga *Nidra* practice (a deeply restorative and guided meditation practice that brings you into a state between sleep and wakefulness). You can also wrap yourself in a blanket and try some breathing exercises.

- **Shower mindfulness:** As you prepare for bed, run your hands under warm water or take a shower. Or mindfully wash your face with warm water. Focus on how the water feels against your skin.

- **Gratitude meditation:** Before sleep, go through a gratitude list in your head or do a short meditation to relax your mind.

De-Stressing Daily

As you grow more comfortable with incorporating somatic movements into your daily life, you might find that they become a non-negotiable part of your routine. The benefits are undeniable: Better sleep, lower anxiety levels, increased focus, and a deeper connection with your body. To maintain this balance, it helps to create a daily de-stress routine that works for you.

Think about how you want to begin your day — with intention. I like to begin my day with meditation. This morning ritual clears my mind, helps me focus on my breath, and connects me to a sense of calm before the day starts. You can try the same or start smaller — even a few minutes of deep breathing works wonders.

Throughout the day, consider integrating somatic movements whenever you can. Movement breaks are essential. Somatic practices don't need to be formal — sometimes my kids and I have mini dance parties after school. A quick shake, a stretch, or even turning on some upbeat music can shift your energy. If you prefer, a midday walk or gentle stretching can help you reset.

In the evening, focus on winding down. Restorative yoga postures or Yoga *Nidra* can relax your body and mind. Even a few minutes of self-massage or time with a weighted blanket can work wonders in easing deeper tensions. Before bed, check in with yourself — how do you feel? Try the practice of gratitude, which can help shift into a more restful state of mind.

Quick stress-relief practices for everyday use

There are countless somatic (and somatic-adjacent) techniques that can help you relieve stress throughout your day. Some of my go-to practices include somatic dance (covered in a later section in this chapter), mantra meditations, yoga postures, breathwork, progressive tense-and-release, mindful walks, chair yoga, somatic dance, face yoga, and Restorative yoga poses. The following sections explore some of these practices in more detail.

Mantras

Mantras are powerful affirmations or phrases that help you focus and relax. One of the reasons I love mantras is that they work almost instantly to shift my mindset. Some of my favorites start with "I am":

>> I am calm.

>> I am relaxed.

>> I am happy.

>> I am loved.

You can use these or any other phrase that resonates with you. I often share these "I am" affirmations with my kids when they're feeling upset or anxious. Another mantra I love is "ebb and flow, come and go" — it reminds me that everything is temporary, and we don't have to get attached to outcomes beyond our control.

REMEMBER

Feelings aren't good or bad — they're just passing experiences. It's how you react to your feelings that can get you into trouble. By repeating mantras, you can process your emotions without reacting impulsively.

Yoga postures

As Chapter 5 explained, certain yoga postures are ideal for moments of stress. One of my favorites is the Lion's Roar Breath (see Figure 7-1), where you inhale deeply while rounding your back and pulling your hands into your stomach. Follow these steps to perform this exercise:

1. **Start on your shins, sitting upright.**

2. **Inhale deeply, rounding your back and pulling your hands into your stomach.**

3. **Exhale forcefully, extending your arms out to the sides and opening your mouth.**

4. **Let out a loud "roar" as you exhale.**

   You may want to save this one for home!

5. **Repeat as needed until you feel a release of tension.**

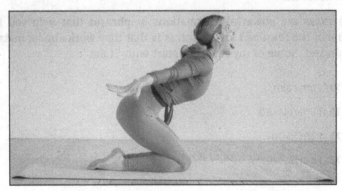

FIGURE 7-1:
Lion's Roar
Breath helps
release built-up
tension with
a powerful
exhalation.

Photograph by Guen Egan

You can also try the Tree Pose, which requires balance and focus to ground yourself. As you see in Figure 7-2, this pose brings your body and mind into alignment, making it difficult to feel scattered. To try the Tree Pose, follow these steps:

1. **Stand with your feet together and your arms by your sides.**

2. **Shift your weight onto your left foot and bring your right foot to rest on your inner left thigh (or calf if that's more comfortable).**

   If balance is an issue, you can modify this pose by placing a chair next to you and holding it with your right hand.

3. Bring your hands together in front of your chest or extend your arms overhead.

4. Hold the pose, focusing on your balance and breath, for five to ten breaths.

5. Repeat on the opposite side.

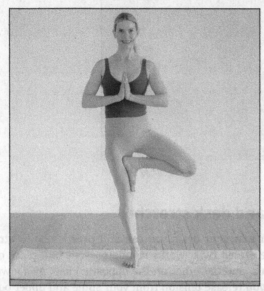

FIGURE 7-2:
The Tree Pose grounds your body and mind through balance and focus.

Photograph by Guen Egan

Another simple but powerful posture is the Mountain Pose, which was introduced in Chapter 5. Stand tall with your feet together and your head aligned over your shoulders (see Figure 7-3). Five deep breaths in this pose will help you feel strong, secure, and much more centered:

1. Stand tall with your feet together, toes pointing forward.

2. Align your head over your shoulders and your shoulders over your hips.

3. Ground through your feet, feeling them press into the Earth.

4. Lengthen through the crown of your head as you breathe in deeply.

5. Hold the pose for five to ten breaths, focusing on being stable and relaxed.

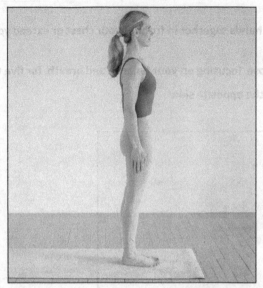

FIGURE 7-3:
The Mountain Pose builds stability and calm with a strong, centered stance.

Photograph by Guen Egan

Chair yoga and desk stretches

When you're stuck at your desk, you can still practice quick stress-relief techniques. A simple seated twist works wonders — sit tall, place one hand on the back of your chair, and the other on the opposite knee. As shown in Figure 7-4, this twist helps you release tension from your spine and upper body:

1. Sit tall at the edge of your seat with your feet flat on the floor.

2. Place your right hand on the back of your chair and your left hand on your right knee.

3. Inhale to lengthen your spine, then exhale and gently twist to the right.

4. Hold for five breaths, then return to center.

5. Repeat on the other side.

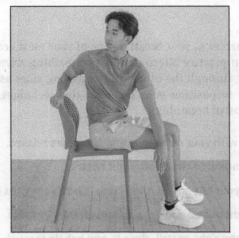

FIGURE 7-4:
A Seated Twist offers a simple way to release tension at your desk.

Photograph by Guen Egan

Another favorite is Cat–Cow at your desk, which allows you to move through your spine while seated. As you can see in Figure 7-5, inhaling as you arch your lower back and open your chest, and exhaling as you round your spine creates a calming flow of movement and breath:

1. Sit tall with your feet on the floor and your hands resting on your knees.

2. Inhale as you arch your back, lift your chest, and gaze upward (Cow Pose, as shown in Figure 7-5a).

3. Exhale as you round your spine, tucking your chin and drawing your belly button in (Cat Pose, as shown in Figure 7-5b).

4. Alternate between these movements for five to ten breaths.

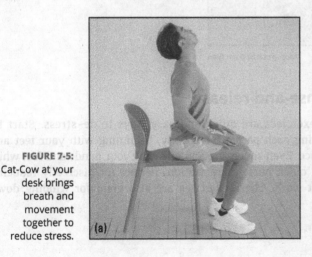

FIGURE 7-5:
Cat-Cow at your desk brings breath and movement together to reduce stress.

(a)   (b)

Photograph by Guen Egan

Breathwork

As you learned in Chapter 4, your breath is one of your most accessible tools for stress relief. You can practice alternate nostril breathing anywhere by closing one nostril, inhaling through the other, and switching sides as you exhale. See Figure 7-6 for how to position your hand for this technique. Here's how to perform alternate nostril breathing:

1. **Sit comfortably with your spine long and shoulders relaxed.**

2. **Use your right thumb to close your right nostril.**

3. **Inhale through your left nostril, then close it with your right index finger.**

4. **Release your right nostril and exhale through the right side.**

5. **Inhale through the right nostril, close it, and exhale through the left.**

6. **Continue alternating for five to ten breaths.**

FIGURE 7-6:
Alternate nostril breathing promotes calm through breath control and focus.

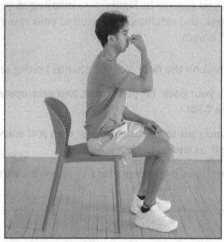

Photograph by Guen Egan

Progressive tense-and-release

Tense-and-release exercises are quick and easy ways to de-stress. Start by squeezing and releasing each part of your body, beginning with your feet and working up to your face. Even squeezing and releasing your hands and feet while seated can provide a quick burst of relaxation, perfect for discreetly reducing stress in public or at work. These exercises are also great for winding down before bed.

Mindful walks

Walking, especially outside, can do wonders for your nervous system. Even a five-minute mindful walk, where you focus on your footfalls and the sensation of the ground beneath you, can help you get unstuck and relieve stress. Even a brief walk indoors can be enough to reset your system and bring you back to the present moment.

Face yoga

Face yoga focuses on releasing tension in your facial muscles. Try making a fishy face with your mouth, then letting it go. You can also relax your jaw by letting it hang slack, moving it from side to side, or massaging your cheeks, forehead, and temples. These small exercises can have a big impact, especially if you've been staring at screens for too long.

Restorative yoga

As explained in Chapter 5, Restorative yoga involves long-held postures supported by props like bolsters, blocks, and blankets. You don't need a full hour-long class to experience its benefits.

Try this quick supported Goddess Pose by placing a bolster at an incline and resting your torso on it, with your legs in a butterfly shape (see Figure 7-7):

1. **Place a bolster on two blocks — one flat and one tall to create a slant.**

   You can use a large firm couch cushion, a firm pillow, or a few blankets folded and stacked on each other for a bolster.

2. **Sit with your lower back against the base of the bolster.**

3. **Lie back with your torso supported by the bolster and your legs resting in front of you or in a butterfly position (soles of the feet together, knees apart).**

4. **Breathe deeply and relax into the posture for two to three minutes.**

FIGURE 7-7: This supported Goddess Pose opens the chest and releases tension with gentle support.

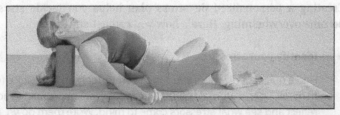

Photograph by Guen Egan

Another favorite is Legs-Up-The-Wall Pose, where you lie on your back with your legs propped against the wall. This pose is a perfect wind-down for the end of the day:

1. **Sit sideways next to a wall, with your hips as close to the wall as possible.**

2. **Bring your legs up onto the wall as you lie down on your back.**

3. **Rest your arms by your sides, palms facing up, and close your eyes.**

4. **Stay in the pose for five to ten minutes, breathing deeply.**
   See Figure 7-8.

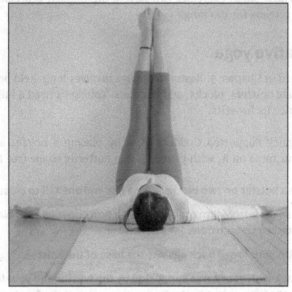

FIGURE 7-8: Legs-Up-The-Wall Pose is a calming, restorative posture that can help you unwind.

Photograph by Guen Egan

Creating a personalized de-stress plan

Creating a personalized de-stress plan helps you tackle stressors before they become overwhelming. Here's how you can get started:

1. **Identify your stressors.**

   Find a quiet space where you can sit comfortably and meditate for a few minutes. Keep a journal nearby. After your meditation, take a moment to reflect and see what stressors come to mind. Write them down. Are you feeling anxious about work? Do you feel like you don't have enough time for yourself?

Are you overwhelmed by your to-do list? Get it all out on paper — this will help you clarify what's really affecting you.

2. **Create a game plan.** Now that you've identified your stressors, it's time to come up with a plan for handling them:

- **Work stress:** If work is one of your biggest stressors, schedule in regular breaks throughout your day. Take a walk, eat mindfully, or do some chair yoga or mindful stretching. These short moments of self-care can help reset your mind and body so you can handle your workload with less tension.

- **Not enough time for yourself:** If you feel like you never have time for yourself, look at your schedule and find moments when you can wake up a little earlier. Use this extra time to practice yoga, Tai Chi, or a mindful mat Pilates session. You can also integrate breathwork during the day to reconnect and calm your mind.

- **Overwhelmed by your to-do list:** If your to-do list seems never-ending, try incorporating meditation twice a day. There's a great quote that says, "If you don't have time to meditate for five minutes, then meditate for an hour." It may feel like you don't have time to sit and focus, but meditation is exactly what you need to clear your mind and calm your nervous system. By doing this, you'll tackle your tasks more efficiently and with greater awareness. You may also find that some of the "must-do" items on your list are actually self-imposed, and you can let go of things that aren't truly necessary.

Try breaking your routine down into three main parts:

» **Morning:** Begin your day with a simple meditation or deep breathing exercise, followed by yoga, stretching, or Tai Chi.

» **Midday reset:** Take a movement break by walking, shaking, dancing, or doing a quick tense-and-release exercise. Consider a second meditation session if it suits your schedule.

» **Evening wind-down:** Unwind after dinner with restorative movements, Yoga *Nidra*, or a self-massage session. End your day by checking in with yourself and practicing gratitude.

Keep experimenting with these practices, and you'll soon discover what works best for you. Once you find your groove, somatic movements will become a natural, stress-relieving part of your daily life.

Busting a Move: Somatic Dance

Somatic dance, introduced in Chapter 5, focuses on how you feel when you move, not how you look. It's not performance-based but rather a way of dancing from the inside out, connecting your mind and body.

TIP

Focusing on your felt experience helps you build trust and confidence. There's no need to judge how good or bad you are as a dancer — just let the movements be free. This practice helps you reconnect with your body and develop skills to process intense emotions or trauma held within.

REMEMBER

Somatic dance is for everyone — regardless of age, experience, or level of fitness. It's a physical expression similar to yoga that fosters a deeper mind-body connection. Somatic dance offers a sense of freedom: No pressure, no criticism, just pure movement. Whether you're dancing at a friend's wedding or in your own living room, it's a chance to embrace your body and let loose.

You don't need to be an experienced dancer. If you have a body, you can move. Dance is part of every culture and is often used to celebrate, heal, or release energy. Somatic dance gives you a way to release built-up tension, celebrate your body, and reconnect with yourself.

The benefits of somatic dance for stress relief

Dancing releases feel-good chemicals that regulate your nervous system. Somatic dance invites you to slow down and be present in your body, noticing where you might be holding tension or stress.

Somatic dance is a positive outlet for anxiety and a way to cope with intense emotions that may be difficult to verbalize. The more you practice, the more comfortable and safer you feel in your body. You also begin to replace self-criticism with compassion. When you constantly criticize yourself, you add stress to your life. But when you embrace your flaws and stop nitpicking every little thing, you create space for more joy and freedom.

TIP

Dance with the intention to celebrate yourself, not to judge your performance. Let go of any worries about what you look like — this is about feeling good. Experiment with different types of music and see how each one brings up different emotions. Somatic dance can also be joyful, uplifting your spirit when you need a boost.

REMEMBER

Focusing negatively on a specific part of your body only adds to your stress. Somatic dance allows you to step out of that cycle and embrace how your body moves.

Simple dance movements to reduce stress

Here are a few easy movements you can try to reduce stress and get into a flow:

>> **Bouncing:** Let your legs be buoyant, bouncing gently up and down. You can add small hops or jumps if it feels right — imagine you're on a trampoline.

>> **Grapevine:** Step out with one foot, step the other foot behind it, step out again, and tap the opposite foot. Repeat on the other side. The grapevine is a fun, simple move that anyone can do!

>> **Hip Circles:** Soften your legs and circle your hips clockwise, then counterclockwise. Feel the tension melt away with each rotation.

>> **Hip Sways:** Let your hips sway from side to side like you're doing a hula dance. Keep your movements loose and relaxed.

>> **Leg Lifts:** As you sway from side to side, lift one leg, then the other. You can lift it to the front, side, or back — whatever feels natural.

>> **Rib Cage Sides:** Keep your knees soft and move just your rib cage from side to side. This movement is great for loosening up your waist and torso.

>> **Shoulder Rolls and Shakes:** Stand with your feet hip-width apart and circle your shoulders forward and back. Shake out your arms, playing with different heights — low, high, one arm at a time. Let the movement spread through your whole body.

>> **Side Lift:** Build on the side-to-side swing by lifting your arms toward the sky with each swing. Let the movement expand and get bigger as you go.

>> **Side-to-Side Arm Swings:** Start rocking side to side and let your arms swing freely. Feel your torso loosen as you swing, allowing your arms to wrap around you.

>> **Step-Together Step Tap:** Step out with one foot, bring the other foot to meet it, then step out again and tap. Repeat on the other side, letting the movement flow.

>> **Torso Circles:** Circle your entire torso in one direction, then reverse. Let your arms move with the flow, sweeping up and around as your body moves.

TIP

Get creative! Shimmy, shake, bounce, or spin — there are no rules. Let your body be the guide and don't worry about how it looks. Focus on how it feels.

Consider these tips for getting the most out of somatic dancing:

>> Find a quiet space where you can move freely without distractions.

>> Make gentle, fluid movements and pay close attention to how your body feels.

>> Let your movements evolve naturally, following any impulses or sensations you experience.

>> Focus on the connection between your breath and movement and allow any emotions to surface and be expressed through your dance.

REMEMBER

The goal is to explore and enjoy the process rather than aiming for perfection. Let your body move however it wants. You can listen to music or move in silence, following the rhythm of your heartbeat.

Self-Hugging for Stress Relief

Self-hugs can build self-esteem and confidence while making you feel safe and secure. It's a simple yet powerful gesture to remind yourself that you have the ability to comfort and care for yourself anytime you need it. Self-hugs provide:

>> **Self-soothing:** When no one is around to give you a hug, you can always hug yourself. This self-soothing technique offers comfort and a sense of security.

>> **Stress relief:** Hugging yourself can reduce cortisol levels, which helps release stress and anxiety, bringing you back to a calm state.

>> **Empowerment:** Wrapping your arms around yourself reminds you that you control your own wellness. This empowers you to take charge of your emotions and well-being.

>> **Self-affirmation:** A self-hug affirms your worth and value. You are loved, and you deserve kindness, compassion, and empathy from yourself and others. With every self-hug, you reinforce how amazing you truly are.

Hugs, in general, provide comfort, and it's often said that you need eight to twelve hugs a day.

TIP

Each hug should last at least 20 seconds for optimal benefits. You may not always have someone nearby to hug, but you can give yourself that same level of care by hugging yourself.

Step-by-step guide to giving yourself a comforting hug

Hugging yourself may feel awkward at first, but with practice, you might find it comforting and soothing. Follow these steps to give yourself a satisfying self-hug:

1. **Wrap your arms around your body**.

   See what feels natural. You might prefer to hug yourself around the tummy or closer to your chest.

2. **Place your hands on your shoulders or upper arms**.

   If your arms are lower, try cupping your elbows with your hands.

3. **Adjust the pressure**.

   Find the level of pressure you want. You might opt for a big, tight bear hug or a gentler, soothing embrace.

4. **Hold for 20 seconds**.

5. **If you want to, add a gentle rock or stroke.**

   You can rock back and forth or gently stroke your forearms or shoulders for extra comfort.

Variations of self-hugging techniques

There are different variations of self-hugging techniques, each providing a unique experience:

>> **Havening Technique:** Wrap your arms around yourself and gently stroke your arms from shoulders to elbows. As you do this, you can breathe calmly and repeat soothing words in your mind like "calm" or "relax."

>> **Butterfly Hug:** Cross your arms so your hands touch opposite shoulders. Gently tap your shoulders in an alternating rhythm like butterfly wings flapping. For many, this technique is incredibly calming.

>> **Incorporate rocking or stroking:** As you hug yourself, try rocking side to side or stroking your arms, shoulders, or sides of your waist for extra comfort.

>> **Weighted blankets:** If you enjoy the sensation of a hug, invest in a weighted blanket. Wrap it around you for a calming, hugging sensation.

TIP

You can also combine a few techniques. Start with rocking, then squeeze, then brush. Or sway a bit then vary the intensity. You'll probably notice you have different hugs for different days and different emotions. You may give yourself a huge hug when you feel like you've accomplished something or a very tender hug when you're feeling lonely or sad. Play around with the intensity and types of hugs you give yourself. Try giving yourself at least one hug a day to start with and build up from there if it feels good.

Benefits of self-hugging

Self-hugging offers a range of benefits that enhance your mental, physical, and emotional well-being.

Pain relief

Hugging yourself can actually reduce physical pain. When you cross your arms over your body, it confuses the brain's perception of pain location. By distracting your brain with the new sensation of the hug, you feel less of the original pain. Self-hugs also stimulate the release of oxytocin, the "love hormone," which plays a significant role in pain management. Oxytocin reduces pain sensitivity and is naturally released during comforting activities like hugging and cuddling. It's the same hormone released during childbirth to help manage labor pain, and during intimate moments, like an orgasm, to promote relaxation.

Safety and security

Hugs provide a deep sense of safety and comfort. In moments of anxiety, fear, or stress, hugging yourself can help reduce those negative emotions and make you feel more grounded. Think of how a child feels when comforted by a parent's hug — the sense of security is immediate. While you may not always have someone around to offer that comfort, you can give yourself the same kind of supportive reassurance. Self-hugging allows you to take charge of your emotional state and reduce feelings of loneliness or isolation.

Improved mood

When you're feeling down or stuck in a bad mood, a simple self-hug can be just the thing to help lift your spirits. Physical touch, even when it's self-inflicted, promotes relaxation by releasing endorphins — your body's natural mood boosters. The act of hugging increases serotonin levels, the hormone that stabilizes your mood, which helps you feel happier and more balanced. Self-hugging may not solve all your problems, but it can offer an emotional lift in a moment when you need it most.

Increased self-compassion

Touch is incredibly important for fostering compassion — not just from others but from yourself. When you physically comfort yourself with a hug, you are practicing self-compassion. This gentle act encourages your body to produce oxytocin, which is linked to reducing stress and increasing feelings of love and empathy. It's a reminder to be kind to yourself, even when you make mistakes or feel down. In doing so, you naturally boost your self-esteem and start to treat yourself with the patience and understanding you offer others. Over time, this practice of self-compassion can reshape the way you view and treat yourself, leading to greater self-acceptance and emotional resilience.

Integrating self-hugging into your daily practice

Adding self-hugging to your daily routine is easier than you think — and it's a simple way to give yourself some extra care and comfort whenever you need it! Try any or all of these ideas:

>> **Morning hug:** Start your day by hugging yourself to remind yourself you're alive, capable, and ready to tackle the day.

>> **Mid-morning check-in:** Give yourself a gentle hug to check in on how you're feeling.

>> **Midday pep talk:** Hug yourself after lunch to refresh your energy and boost your mood.

>> **Afternoon relief:** Use a self-hug to relieve any built-up tension or stress as the day progresses.

>> **Evening hug:** Remind yourself of your accomplishments and how far you've come with an evening hug.

>> **End-of-day embrace:** Close the day by thanking yourself for everything you did, acknowledging that everything you need is inside of you.

Enhancing Your Mental Focus

You can enhance mental focus with grounding yoga poses, body scanning, diaphragmatic breathing, somatic yoga, breathwork, walking meditation, and even massage therapy. Massage therapy can also boost energy levels and concentration.

Try these somatic movement practices to boost your mental clarity:

>> **Body scans:** Increase awareness by focusing on each part of your body.

>> **Diaphragmatic breathing:** Deep breathing has shown to improve mental clarity.

>> **Grounding exercises:** Bring yourself into the present moment to reduce distractions.

>> **Paying attention to the five senses:** Engaging your senses promotes mindfulness.

>> **Pendulation:** Shift your focus between areas of tension and relaxation in your body.

>> **Shaking and stomping:** Physical movements like these can release tension and increase energy.

>> **Tensing and relaxing muscles:** Increase awareness and reduce tension through controlled muscle engagement.

>> **Yoga:** Somatic yoga practices encourage mindfulness and mental sharpness.

>> **Walking meditation:** Walk mindfully to stay grounded and centered.

You can integrate mind-body awareness through all these somatic exercises. As you continue to delve deeper into each type of somatic movement and exercise, you strengthen your connection to yourself and develop a deeper mind-body awareness. You'll take what you learn and discover on the mat, off the mat.

IN THIS CHAPTER

» Discovering all the ways good posture helps

» Busting myths about posture

» Staying conscious of your posture

» Using somatic exercises to improve your posture

» Improving your flexibility with somatic exercises

Chapter 8

Improving Your Posture and Flexibility with Somatic Exercises

You can improve your posture — the natural way you hold your body — with somatic exercises by becoming more aware of how your body moves and connecting your mind, body, and breath. Mindfulness is the first step to understanding how you hold yourself. It helps you notice where your head is in relation to your torso, whether you tend to slouch or lock your knees, and other habits that may impact your posture. Typically, posture is an automatic function, but with awareness, you can start to make improvements.

Good posture doesn't look the same for everyone, but in general, it means that your weight is evenly distributed and your body is aligned properly. When you have good posture, the three natural curves of your spine are in balance: The cervical curve in your neck, the thoracic curve in the middle of your back, and the lumbar curve in your lower back. These curves create a gentle "S" shape. Ideally, your posture should maintain this natural alignment without any exaggerated curves.

Many of the habits you've built over the years can affect your posture. Sitting for long periods, spending hours on devices, and long periods of driving often lead to slouching and poor posture. Pregnancy can also affect how you hold yourself. Plus, stiff or tight muscles can further impact your alignment.

In this chapter, I take you through how to assess your posture, improve your awareness, and correct misalignments with somatic exercises. You'll discover how to strengthen your core, stretch for better alignment, and develop daily habits that will support healthy posture in the long run.

Knowing the Value of Good Posture

Good posture does more than just make you look confident — it has a direct impact on your overall well-being. When you allow yourself to slouch or hunch forward, your back becomes overstretched, and your front compresses. This leads to tension and imbalances. Good posture, on the other hand, helps you achieve a healthy balance by keeping you centered and aligned, so you feel strong, open, and in control of your body.

REMEMBER

When your body is properly aligned, you can experience benefits like improved mood, reduced headaches, better digestion, and less strain on your joints. Proper posture also helps you move with ease and supports your self-esteem by making you feel more open and stronger.

Maintaining good posture means keeping the natural curves of your spine in balance and distributing your weight evenly. This alignment allows your muscles and joints to work together efficiently, preventing unnecessary strain and discomfort.

TIP

One way to improve posture is through mindful movement. In yoga, instructors often call backbends the "antidepressants" of the practice because they counteract the forward-hunching positions most people adopt throughout the day. Backbends strengthen your back, open your chest, and help you move toward healthier alignment.

Health benefits of good posture

Maintaining proper alignment supports your body's natural functions, from improving your breathing and digestion to reducing pain and stress. Good posture is the foundation for better movement, greater energy, and long-term joint health. Good posture can lead to:

>> **Fewer injuries:** Good posture is key to preventing injuries, especially during physical activities. Whether you're lifting weights, practicing yoga, or engaging in sports like golf or tennis, proper alignment reduces the risk of straining muscles or joints.

Even everyday tasks like bending over to pick up your child or pushing a stroller can strain your back if they're done with poor posture. Office workers are also prone to issues like carpal tunnel syndrome or forward head syndrome when sitting with poor posture all day (see Figure 8-1).

>> **Improved breathing:** Good posture allows your lungs to fully expand, making it easier to breathe deeply. When you slouch, your lungs compress, limiting your oxygen intake. Breathing deeply helps fill your body with vital energy, improving how you feel and function.

Shallow breathing, often linked with poor posture, can contribute to lethargy and even depression. Standing tall with an open chest encourages deeper breaths, which calms your parasympathetic nervous system and boosts your mood. When you inhale deeply, you feel more energized, and when you exhale fully, you feel calmer.

>> **Improved mood:** Posture and breathing are closely tied to mood. When you carry yourself with good posture, you project confidence, which naturally improves your self-esteem. Standing tall and opening your chest can make you feel more positive and empowered.

Shallow breathing and poor posture, on the other hand, can make you feel sluggish and stressed. By improving your posture, you not only reduce negative emotions but also create space for positive emotions. Lifting your chest and spreading your collarbone reminds you that you're alive, capable, and ready to face the world with positivity (see Figure 8-2).

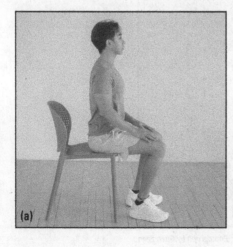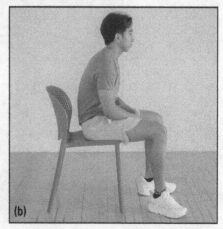

FIGURE 8-1: Example of good (a) and poor (b) posture while sitting at a desk, showing the impact on shoulder and neck alignment.

Photograph by Guen Egan

» **Fewer stress headaches:** Poor posture can create shoulder tension, which often leads to headaches (see Figure 8-3). If you find yourself hunching with your shoulders up by your ears, good posture helps by lengthening your neck and relaxing your shoulders. This release reduces tension in your neck and jaw, decreasing the chances of tension-related headaches.

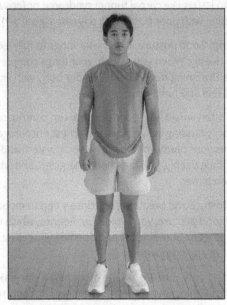

FIGURE 8-2:
Demonstration of a person standing tall, with an open chest and proper posture, ready to take deep breaths.

Photograph by Guen Egan

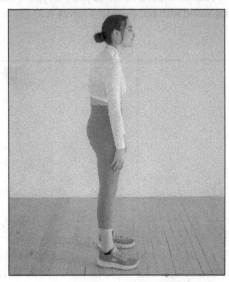

FIGURE 8-3:
Example of shoulder tension caused by poor posture.

Photograph by Guen Egan

>> **Better digestion:** Another benefit of good posture is improved digestion. When you sit or stand with proper alignment, your organs have the space they need to function properly. Slouching compresses your organs, leading to issues like bloating, constipation, and acid reflux. The fascia around your organs can also tighten due to poor posture, contributing to pain and digestive discomfort.

>> **Reduced fatigue:** Good posture helps you breathe deeper, delivering more oxygen to your body and brain. With more oxygen comes increased energy and better focus. Poor posture, on the other hand, leads to muscular imbalances and shallow breathing, which can leave you feeling drained. Correcting these imbalances through good posture can improve your efficiency and boost your energy level.

>> **Healthier joints:** Proper posture puts less stress on your joints, particularly your spine. If you hunch forward all day, you're compressing your spine, which can lead to discomfort or even injury. Good posture creates length in your spine and space between the vertebrae, alleviating pressure on the joints. Your shoulders, knees, and hips also benefit from better posture.

WARNING

Women, especially after pregnancy, often experience misalignment in their hips and back, which can be worsened by activities like nursing or bending over a child. Restoring good posture after pregnancy is essential to reducing strain and protecting your joints.

Debunking the posture myth

A common misconception about posture is the idea that you need to be rigid or stick-straight to have good alignment. In reality, your spine has natural curves, and it's important to maintain this curve while finding balance in your body. Good posture isn't about forcing your body into a certain position — it's about allowing your body to fall into alignment naturally. You don't need to grip your shoulder blades together or hold yourself at attention. Instead, let your shoulders naturally fall down your back.

REMEMBER

There isn't one "right" way to have good posture. Everybody is different, and what feels good for one person may not work for you. Through somatic movement, you get to know yourself better, allowing you to improve your posture without overthinking or becoming too tense. It's about working with your body, not against it.

Another common mistake is trying to muscle your way into good posture. While certain muscles, especially your core, need to be engaged, proper posture should feel more like ease than effort. When your bones are stacked properly, one on top of another, you need less muscular tension to hold yourself up.

Over time, as you work with your body's natural curves, good posture becomes second nature. It's not about staying rigid but being fluid enough to adapt to different environments.

Practicing Posture Awareness

To improve your posture, the first step is to become aware of how you naturally carry yourself. Start by closing your eyes and doing a body scan. This technique focuses on feeling your alignment from the inside. As you scan your body, pay attention to how your weight is distributed and any tension you might feel:

>> **Feet:** Do you feel your weight evenly distributed between both feet, or is more weight on one side?

>> **Knees:** Are your knees soft with a slight bend, or do they feel locked and rigid?

>> **Hips:** Do your hips feel tucked under, tilted forward, or are they neutral?

>> **Back and shoulders:** Is your spine naturally curved, or do you feel rounded forward or overly arched in your lower back? Are your shoulders relaxed, or are they tense and raised?

>> **Head and neck:** Is your head balanced above your shoulders, or does it feel like it's falling forward?

TIP

One of the best ways to practice posture awareness is to stand in front of a mirror. Look at yourself from both the front and the side to get a clear idea of your usual posture. You can also have a friend or loved one assess your alignment from different angles. Another effective method is taking photographs of yourself from the front, both sides, and the back. These photos will give you a clear visual of how you hold your body throughout the day. When reviewing your body, look at the following:

>> **Head and neck:** Is your head aligned over your shoulders, or does it jut forward?

>> **Shoulders:** Are your shoulders level, or is one higher than the other? Do they round forward or look slouched?

>> **Spine:** Do you see the natural curves of your spine (cervical, thoracic, and lumbar), or is there exaggerated curvature or hunching?

>> **Hips:** Are your hips level, or does one side sit higher? Is there any tilting forward or backward?

>> **Knees:** Are your knees straight, or do they lock back?

>> **Feet:** Do your feet point straight forward, or does one foot turn outward more than the other?

Regularly assessing your posture with these techniques can help you make small adjustments to bring your body into natural alignment.

Identifying poor posture

You can often identify poor posture based on how your body feels throughout the day. If you experience aches and pains in your shoulders, neck, jaw, back, or hips, it may be time to check in on your posture. Although soreness can come from other sources, poor posture frequently leads to joint and muscle discomfort. Your posture might need improvement if you have any of the following:

>> **Tight shoulders** at the end of the day may indicate you're holding them up or slouching forward, putting strain on your upper back.

>> **Hip or lower back pain** can suggest that you're letting your pelvis tuck under or sway backward.

>> **Locked knees** can create excess pressure on your lower back.

>> **Frequent headaches or a tight jaw** may result from letting your head hang forward of your spine.

TIP

To further assess your posture, check yourself in the mirror. If your head isn't over your heart and your heart isn't over your hips, you're likely falling out of good alignment. A simple way to correct this is to gently press your chin back in space until your head is aligned over your chest.

Another method is to stand against a wall. Ideally, your heels, buttocks, shoulder blades, and the back of your skull should all touch the wall, while the natural curves of your spine stay clear. Or, you can lie down on the floor and feel what parts of your body naturally rest against it. If your head cranes backward or looks up too much, your posture may need adjustment.

Mindfulness practices to enhance posture awareness

Mindfulness practices can help you become more aware of how you sit, stand, and walk. These small check-ins throughout the day make it easier for you to maintain good posture without overthinking it. Rather than focusing on your posture all day, try setting aside time for brief moments of awareness:

>> **Engage your core:** Lift your lower abs in and up while softening your ribs. This activates your deep abdominal muscles to help support your posture.

>> **Use mindful breathing:** Sit or stand tall and take a deep breath. Try expanding your lungs in all directions, focusing on your back and the sides of your waist. As you breathe, lengthen your spine and picture a string pulling your head toward the sky.

>> **Choose comfortable clothes and shoes:** Wearing clothes that allow you to move and breathe freely helps you maintain good posture. Avoid shoes that throw you off balance or cause strain. Your toes should feel free to spread and anchor down for stability.

>> **Eat mindfully:** Pay attention to your posture when eating, as sitting up straight can aid digestion. Slow down and enjoy your meal while maintaining proper alignment. Don't multitask when you eat — be aware and in the moment when eating.

Daily habits to maintain good posture

Good posture is something you build with small, daily habits. Here are a few easy ways to incorporate posture awareness into your routine:

>> **Stretch every morning:** Focus on opening your shoulders and rolling your head to each shoulder and slightly back (don't overdo the head dropping back as you make gentle neck circles). Try the chin press-back test to keep your head aligned over your shoulders.

>> **Exercise regularly:** Strengthening your muscles and joints, especially your core, will help support good posture.

>> **Check your reflection:** Look in the mirror in the morning and at night to adjust your posture from both the front and the side.

>> **Walk with awareness:** As you move throughout your day, focus on maintaining proper alignment while walking or running errands.

>> **Optimize your workspace:** Use ergonomic tools to promote good posture while working. Set up your desk to minimize strain on your neck, back, and shoulders.

>> **Soften your knees:** When standing, avoid locking your knees to prevent putting stress on your joints.

>> **Switch up your routine:** Try brushing your teeth or doing simple tasks with your non-dominant hand to prevent overuse on one side of your body.

>> **Mind your posture while sleeping:** Sleeping posture is just as important. Try sleeping on your back with your pillow at the correct height, or on your side with a pillow between your knees. Avoid sleeping on your stomach, as it puts strain on your neck.

TIP

For extra help with maintaining proper alignment throughout your day, try using props like a supportive chair at work or lumbar support while driving.

FINDING THE CORRECT PILLOW HEIGHT

The correct pillow height depends on your sleeping position and the natural curve of your neck and spine. A pillow that's too high or too low can throw your body out of alignment and cause strain on your neck and back.

For back sleepers, your pillow should support the natural curve of your neck so your head isn't tilted too far forward or backward. Choose a medium-height pillow that fills the space between the back of your head and your shoulders. Your goal is to keep your head, neck, and spine aligned in a straight line.

Side sleepers need a pillow that's high enough to keep the head aligned with the spine. Look for a pillow that fills the space between your ear and the surface of the bed, ensuring your neck doesn't tilt up or down. A thicker pillow is usually best for maintaining alignment.

It's best to avoid sleeping on your stomach because it puts unnecessary strain on the neck. If you can't break the habit, use a very thin pillow — or none at all — to reduce neck strain. You can also place a pillow under your pelvis to take pressure off your lower back.

No matter what position you sleep in, the pillow height should keep your head, neck, and spine in neutral alignment for optimal support and comfort.

Correcting Your Posture with Somatic Exercise

There are many exercises you can do to correct your posture. Focus on aligning your head over your shoulders and your shoulders over your hips. To do this, work on releasing tight muscles that pull your spine out of alignment, like those in your hips, shoulders, thighs, chest, and back. Then, strengthen the muscles needed to maintain good posture, such as your rear deltoids, abdominals, glutes, and pelvic floor.

Stretching for proper alignment

Stretching is essential for improving posture because tight muscles can pull your body out of alignment. The muscles of your chest, upper and lower back, hips, and legs, when tight, can make it difficult to maintain proper posture. Regular stretching helps release tension, increases flexibility, and strengthens the muscles needed for good alignment. Incorporating these stretches into your routine will help correct tight areas that contribute to poor posture:

» **Chest Opener at the Wall:** Your chest can become tight from sitting or hunching forward, which affects your shoulder alignment. Stand next to a wall with your right arm in a goalpost position against the wall and slowly turn your torso to the left to stretch the chest. You can also extend your arm straight to feel a deeper stretch. Hold for five breaths, then repeat on your left side.

» **Cobra Pose:** Cobra strengthens your back while stretching your chest. Lie on your stomach with your arms bent and your hands near your shoulders (see Figure 8-4a). Engage your core and lift your chest. Keep your lower back long and your abdominals active to support your spine (see Figure 8-4b). Hold for five breaths, lower, and repeat two more times.

» **Pigeon Pose:** Tight hips can cause lower back tension, so the Pigeon Pose is great for opening the hips and relieving back strain. From all fours, slide your right shin forward so your knee is on the outside and your foot is angled under your torso. Slide your left leg back and lower your hips toward the mat. Hold for eight breaths, then switch sides (see Figure 8-5). (If you have knee pain, try the Supine Figure Four Pose instead.)

» **Figure Four Pose:** Similar to the Pigeon Pose, this stretch works the piriformis and outer hips. Lie on your back with knees bent, placing your right ankle above your left knee. Reach through and grab your left thigh, drawing your legs toward you. Hold for five breaths, then switch sides. This can also be done seated in a chair.

>> **Standing Hip Flexor Stretch:** Tight hip flexors can pull your lower back out of alignment. Stand tall and bend your right knee back, catching your ankle with your hand. Pull your heel toward your rear, while lengthening the front of your thigh toward the ground. Hold for five breaths, then switch sides. This stretch is simple and can be done anywhere to counteract tightness in your hips (see Figure 8-6).

>> **Wall Angels:** Wall Angels help with shoulder retraction and chest opening. Stand with your back against a wall, feet slightly away from the wall, and your arms in a goalpost position, with your elbows at shoulder height (see Figure 8-7a). Try to keep the back of your wrists and arms pressed against the wall as you glide your arms up and down, like making a snow angel (see Figure 8-7b). This stretches your chest while strengthening the muscles that help prevent slouching.

>> **Windshield Wipers:** Tight hip flexors, quads, and psoas muscles can put strain on your spine. Lie on your back, knees bent, and feet flat. Then drop your knees side to side in a windshield wiper motion to release tension in the hips and front of the thighs.

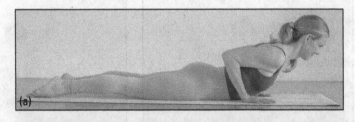

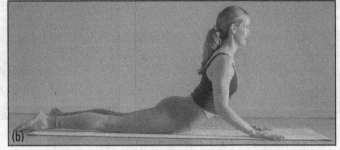

FIGURE 8-4: The Cobra Pose strengthens your back and stretches your chest.

Photograph by Guen Egan

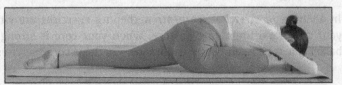

FIGURE 8-5: Tight back or hips? Try the Pigeon Pose.

Photograph by Guen Egan

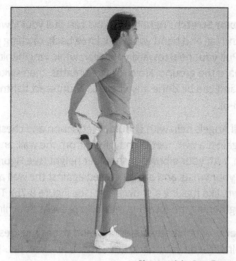

Photograph by Guen Egan

FIGURE 8-6:
Try stretching
your hip flexors
regularly to help
with alignment.

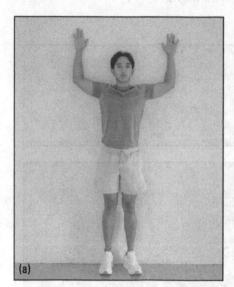

(a)   (b)

Photograph by Guen Egan

FIGURE 8-7:
Sure, you've
heard of snow
angels, but have
you heard of
Wall Angels?

Strengthening core muscles

In addition to stretches, core-strengthening exercises are vital for supporting your spine and improving posture. When your core is strong, you have better balance, less pain, and more endurance. Try these core exercises:

>> **Bird Dog:** From all fours, extend your right arm and left leg while engaging your core. Hold for a few seconds, then switch sides. This helps strengthen your back and core, improving posture and balance. Keep your pelvis steady the entire time, as if you were balancing a cup of water on your lower back. See Figure 8-8.

>> **Chin Tuck:** One simple yet effective exercise is the chin tuck, which helps align your head over your shoulders and strengthens the muscles that keep your neck in a neutral position. Sit in a chair with your feet flat on the floor or stand with feet hip-width apart. Relax your shoulders and look straight ahead. Gently pull your chin back without looking up or down, creating a "double chin" effect. Hold for five seconds. Relax and repeat five to six times, making sure not to hunch your shoulders or arch your back.

>> **Dead Bug:** Start on your back with your knees and feet at 90 degrees (as if your shins were resting on a tabletop) and your arms reaching up to the ceiling with the palms facing each other. Extend your right arm and left leg simultaneously, keeping your core engaged. Make sure to keep your pelvis level the entire time, as if you were balancing a marble between your pubic bone and belly button. Return to center and switch sides. This move strengthens both your core and stabilizers.

>> **Glute Bridge:** Lie on your back with your feet flat. Press through your heels, engage your glutes, and lift your hips toward the ceiling. This exercise strengthens your core and lower body, both of which are important for posture. See Figure 8-9.

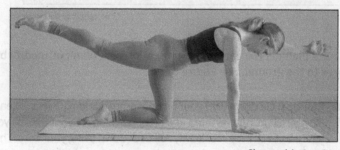

FIGURE 8-8: The Bird Dog helps strengthen your core muscles.

Photograph by Guen Egan

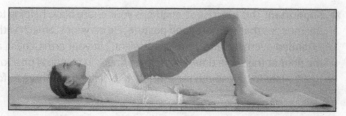

FIGURE 8-9: Glute Bridges are great for your core and lower body.

Photograph by Guen Egan

>> **Knee Folds/Toe Taps:** Lie on your back with your feet flat, making sure your pelvis is neutral, not tucked or tilted. Lift one leg into a tabletop position while keeping the pelvis neutral. Lower and repeat on the other leg. To make this harder, lift both legs into tabletop and tap your toes down, using your core to lift them back up. See Figure 8-10.

>> **Planks:** Planks are fantastic for building core strength, which is essential for maintaining good posture. A strong core supports your spine and keeps your body aligned. Start on all fours with your hands under your shoulders and your knees on the ground. Walk your feet back, straightening your legs until your body forms a straight line from head to heels. Engage your core, making sure not to let your hips sag or your back arch. Your body should be in a straight line. Hold for 30 to 60 seconds, then rest. Repeat for two more sets.

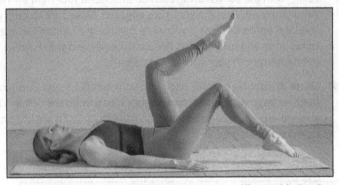

FIGURE 8-10:
Toe Taps may look simple, but they are effective.

Photograph by Guen Egan

TIP

If a full plank is too challenging, try a forearm plank or modify by dropping your knees to the ground. See Figure 8–11.

>> **Roll-Ups:** Lie down with your arms overhead and your legs extended long. Slowly roll up, one vertebra at a time, reaching for your toes as you scoop your abs back in space. Slowly roll back down using your core. This move challenges your entire abdominal region, helping build strength for better posture.

>> **Superman:** This exercise strengthens your entire back, helping to balance the muscles that support good posture. Lie on your stomach with your arms extended overhead and your legs straight. Lift your arms, chest, and legs off the floor at the same time, keeping your neck in a neutral position (think "chin tuck"). Hold for five to ten seconds, then lower. Repeat three to four times.

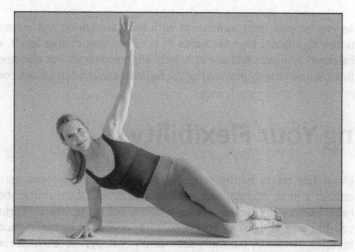

FIGURE 8-11:
You can modify the side plank by dropping your knees to the ground.

Photograph by Guen Egan

Creating a balanced stretching and strengthening routine

To maintain good posture, create a balanced routine that targets all the major muscle groups that affect alignment, including the hips, back, chest, shoulders, and core:

>> **Upper body:** Focus on opening the chest, stretching the shoulders, and relieving tension in the neck. Exercises like the Cobra, Wall Chest Openers, Shoulder Retractions, and Chin Tucks help with both flexibility and strength in this area.

>> **Lower body:** Incorporate stretches for the hips, hamstrings, quads, and lower back. Pigeon Pose, Figure Four, and Standing Hip Flexor Stretches work well for flexibility, while exercises like Glute Bridge and Bird Dog help strengthen key stabilizers.

>> **Core:** Combine stretching with core-strengthening exercises like planks, Superman, and Dead Bugs. These moves will support your spine, improve alignment, and help prevent injuries.

>> **Full-body:** Alternate between upper- and lower-body routines to hit all the major areas of tension. Focus equally on both sides of the body to maintain symmetry in your posture.

TIP

Aim to incorporate both stretching and strengthening exercises three to four times per week, dedicating 15–20 minutes per session, or try to add 10 percent every week to your time.

As you become more consistent with both stretching and strengthening, you'll notice significant improvements in your posture, energy levels, and mood. This balanced approach will not only help align your body but also keep your muscles flexible and strong, preventing the tightness that often causes poor posture.

Improving Your Flexibility

Flexibility refers to the range of motion of muscles and connective tissues around a joint. Maintaining flexibility is essential for overall health because it helps prevent injuries, improves posture, enhances athletic performance, allows you to move with ease, boosts balance, and even increases blood flow to your muscles. Flexibility naturally decreases as you age, so it's important to keep it up throughout your life.

REMEMBER

I love the saying, "I bend so I don't break." Flexibility not only supports physical health but also promotes mental openness. When your body is flexible, your mind tends to be more adaptable and at ease, helping you feel less stressed and more resilient.

Effective stretching routines

A daily full-body stretch routine can benefit your physical and mental well-being. Stretching improves flexibility, reduces muscle tension, and helps you feel more relaxed. You can incorporate *static stretches*, where you hold a position, and *dynamic stretches*, where you move continuously through the stretch.

REMEMBER

Keep in mind that stretching should feel slightly uncomfortable but never painful. Over time, a consistent routine will help your muscles loosen up and adapt to the activity.

Here's an example of a stretching routine that helps you improve flexibility throughout your whole body. Hold each stretch for 10 to 60 seconds, gradually working up to longer holds as your flexibility improves:

1. **Neck Rolls:** Slowly roll your head in a circle, moving gently in each direction to release tension in the neck.

2. **Shoulder Rolls:** Roll your shoulders backward a few times, then switch to rolling them forward. This helps relieve tension in the upper back and shoulders. Chapter 13 has lots more on shoulder mobility if you're interested.

3. **Overhead Triceps Stretch:** Extend one arm overhead, bend it at the elbow, and gently press on the elbow with the opposite hand. Hold for 30 seconds, then switch sides.

4. **Standing Hip Rotation:** Stand with feet hip-width apart and make large circles with your hips, rotating in each direction to loosen your hip joints.

5. **Standing Hamstring Stretch:** Extend one leg straight in front of you, keeping the back knee slightly bent, and lean forward over the extended leg. Hold for 30-60 seconds, then switch sides.

6. **Quad Stretch:** Stand tall, bend one knee, and hold the top of your foot behind you, aligning your knees. Hold for 30-60 seconds on each side to stretch the front of the thigh.

7. **Inner Thigh Stretch:** Stand with your legs wide apart, bend one knee and sit back toward the heel while keeping the opposite leg straight. Hold for 30-60 seconds, then switch sides.

8. **Calf Stretch:** Lie on your back and extend one leg toward the ceiling. Flex your toes back until you feel a stretch in the calf. Hold for 30-60 seconds, then switch sides.

9. **Ankle Circles:** While lying on your back, lift one leg toward the ceiling and circle the ankle in both directions. Repeat on the other side to improve ankle mobility.

10. **Child's Pose:** End in Child's Pose by sitting back on your heels with your arms extended forward. Hold for 30-60 seconds to release the lower back and relax the whole body. You can find more information on this pose in Chapter 5.

TIP

Include stretches for each major body part or muscle group to ensure you have a well-rounded routine or pick and choose certain areas of the body to address specific needs or sports.

Combining flexibility with strength training

Combining strength and flexibility training can enhance your overall physical well-being, boost sports performance, speed up recovery, and create a more balanced fitness routine. One option is to alternate strength days with stretching days. I strength train twice a week, practice Pilates 1-2 times a week, and do yoga 3-4 times a week. You can incorporate flexibility training in a multitude of ways: As part of your warm-up, between sets of strength exercises, or as a cool-down:

>> **Warm-up:** Before strength training, perform dynamic stretches that target the muscles you'll be using. Examples include plank to Downward Dog, walking lunges, knee swings, trunk rotations, or side-to-side lunges.

» **Stretching between sets:** While strength training, add flexibility exercises between sets. For example, after an overhead triceps exercise, follow with a triceps stretch before moving on to the next strength exercise. Or, combine flexibility with a strength move, like holding a strap overhead while doing squats to open your upper body while strengthening your lower body.

» **Cool-down:** After strength training, incorporate static stretches or use a foam roller to help your muscles recover.

REMEMBER

Flexibility training improves your range of motion, reduces muscle soreness, lowers your risk of injury, and enhances performance in both strength and cardio exercises.

Chapter **9**

Enhancing Your Sleep with Somatic Techniques

How great is that feeling when you wake up refreshed, energized, and ready to tackle the day? Amazing, right? Unfortunately, many of us know the opposite feeling too — grogginess, foggy thinking, and that heavy, sluggish feeling that comes from a bad night's sleep. Maybe your mood is low, or your body feels stiff and weird. Everything is off.

Sleep isn't just about getting enough rest — it's about getting the *right* kind of rest. Sleep impacts everything, from how your mind functions to how your body feels. The good news is, there's a lot you can do to take control of your sleep and get it working for you.

In this chapter, you discover some practical tricks to improve your sleep using somatic techniques. Somatic practices focus on tuning into your body, listening to its signals, and responding with mindful movements and relaxation. Whether you struggle with getting consistent, restful sleep or just want to elevate your nighttime routine, these techniques offer simple but effective ways to help you feel more grounded and relaxed.

I break it all down. You learn how sleep cycles work, why they're crucial for your health, and how to recognize when you're not getting enough rest. From there, you learn about setting up a solid sleep routine, mastering pre-sleep relaxation, and addressing your sleep issues — all using somatic exercises. By the end of the chapter, you have a toolkit of easy-to-use techniques to help you sleep better and wake up refreshed.

Discovering the Value of Sleep

Ah, sleep — the magical time when your body and brain get to hit the reset button. You know you need sleep, but somehow it always seems to be just out of reach — kind of like trying to catch that last bite of dessert on a plate that keeps sliding away. Whether you've spent the day running a marathon or just binge-watching your favorite show, sleep lets you recharge and tackle whatever tomorrow throws your way. So let's stop treating it like an optional bonus and give it the VIP status it deserves!

Sleep isn't just a nice-to-have; it's as essential to your health as food and water. Think of sleep as your body's overnight maintenance crew. While you're tucked in bed, your brain is busy filing away memories, processing what you've learned, and taking out the mental trash by clearing out toxins and waste. Without enough sleep, your body doesn't get the chance to repair itself — it's like skipping a vital tune-up for your car and expecting it to run smoothly.

REMEMBER

Sleep is the chance your body gets to grow, rejuvenate, and recover. That's why kids — who are practically growth machines — need even more sleep than adults. But even for us grown-ups, sleep is crucial for keeping everything in balance.

Understanding sleep cycles

As you sleep, your body cycles between different stages of *non-REM (NREM)* and *rapid eye movement (REM)* sleep. A full sleep cycle lasts about 90 to 110 minutes, and throughout the night, you typically go through four to six cycles. Each stage serves a purpose in helping you wake up refreshed and ready for the day (see Figure 9-1):

>> **Stage 1 (NREM):** This is your lightest sleep, the "dipping your toe in the water" phase. It lasts only a few minutes but helps ease you into deeper sleep.

» Stage 2 (NREM): Your heart rate slows, your body temperature drops, and you start to relax even further. This stage accounts for about half of your total sleep time and gets your body ready for the heavy lifting of deep sleep.

» Stage 3 (NREM): This stage involves deep, slow-wave sleep. Your body is in full recovery mode, repairing tissues, building muscle, and giving your immune system a boost. This is the sleep you need to feel truly rested.

» REM Sleep: As you move into REM sleep, your brain becomes as active as when you're awake. This is where dreaming happens, and your body temporarily paralyzes itself to prevent you from acting out those dreams. REM is crucial for emotional processing, memory consolidation, and cognitive function.

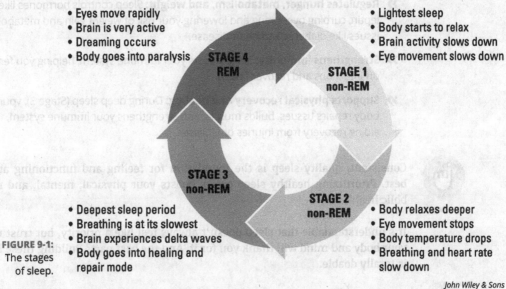

- Eyes move rapidly
- Brain is very active
- Dreaming occurs
- Body goes into paralysis

STAGE 4 REM

STAGE 1 non-REM
- Lightest sleep
- Body starts to relax
- Brain activity slows down
- Eye movement slows down

STAGE 3 non-REM
- Deepest sleep period
- Breathing is at its slowest
- Brain experiences delta waves
- Body goes into healing and repair mode

STAGE 2 non-REM
- Body relaxes deeper
- Eye movement stops
- Body temperature drops
- Breathing and heart rate slow down

FIGURE 9-1: The stages of sleep.

John Wiley & Sons

REMEMBER

Each stage serves a unique purpose, and skipping any one of them can leave you feeling groggy and unrefreshed — even if you technically "got enough sleep."

Learning how sleep cycles affect your health

I get it — some people treat sleepless nights like a badge of honor, as if burning the midnight oil means they're getting more done. But honestly? That's not helping you in the long run. Your body needs rest — plain and simple. When you skip out on sleep, you're not doing yourself any favors, and it catches up with you in more ways than one.

The good news? It's entirely within your power to build healthy sleep habits, and the benefits are huge. Sleep isn't just about feeling rested — it's about helping your body and mind function at their best. Let's take a closer look at all the ways sleep plays a role in your health:

>> **Boosts mood, reduces stress, and sharpens your mind:** A good night's sleep regulates your emotions, keeps stress in check, and improves decision-making, mental clarity, and focus.

>> **Promotes heart health:** Sleep helps regulate your blood pressure and heart rate, both essential for long-term cardiovascular health.

>> **Regulates hunger, metabolism, and weight:** Sleep controls hormones like leptin, curbing overeating and lowering your risk of weight gain and metabolic issues like diabetes and heart disease.

>> **Strengthens immunity:** Sleep boosts your immune system, helping you fend off infections and recover faster.

>> **Supports physical recovery and healing:** During deep sleep (Stage 3), your body repairs tissues, builds muscle, and strengthens your immune system, aiding recovery from injuries or illnesses.

Consistent, quality sleep is the foundation for feeling and functioning at your best. Prioritizing healthy sleep cycles boosts your physical, mental, and metabolic health.

It's understandable that sleep doesn't always feel like a priority, but trust me — your body and mind will thank you for it. And the best part? Building these habits is totally doable.

Somatic exercises can help you relax both mentally and physically, setting the stage for deeper, more restful sleep night after night.

Recognizing Symptoms of Sleep Deprivation

We live in a world that glorifies burning the candle at both ends, right? Whether it's staying up late to finish that project or scrolling through your phone long past bedtime (guilty!), sleep deprivation has become almost socially acceptable.

But here's the deal: Your body doesn't care about deadlines or social media. It *needs* sleep, and it's pretty good at throwing up red flags when it's running low. The tricky part? Sleep deprivation is sneaky — it creeps up on you, and before you know it, you're feeling foggy, snappy, and just *off*. While it might seem like no big deal to skimp on sleep here and there, those sleepless nights add up, impacting everything from your mood to your immune system. The sooner you recognize the signs and take action, the better you'll feel — not just tomorrow, but in the long run.

REMEMBER

Sleep deprivation isn't always a loud, obvious "I'm exhausted" feeling. Sometimes it's subtle, showing up in ways you might not even link to sleep.

Common signs of poor sleep

Here's what to watch for:

>> **You're nodding off during the day:** Even if you've had a full night's sleep, feeling drowsy during work meetings or while driving is a big clue your sleep quality isn't cutting it.

>> **You can't focus or retain information:** Struggling to concentrate, forgetting simple things, or feeling like your brain's in a fog? Your mind needs rest to function properly.

>> **You're hungrier than usual, especially for junk food:** Sleep deprivation messes with hormones like leptin and ghrelin, which regulate hunger. So, if you're suddenly craving chips and cookies more often, it could be because you're running low on sleep.

>> **You're more clumsy or accident-prone:** Bumping into furniture, dropping things, or making silly mistakes could be signs that your motor skills and coordination are suffering from fatigue.

>> **Your mood is all over the place:** Feeling irritable, moody, or snapping at loved ones over small things is your body's way of saying, "Hey, I need some rest!"

>> **Your sex drive has taken a nosedive:** Yep, sleep plays a role here too. When you're exhausted, your interest in intimacy may take a hit.

Long-term effects of sleep deprivation

We all know that a bad night's sleep can leave you feeling cranky, unfocused, and maybe a little off. But what happens when those sleepless nights stack up over time? Unfortunately, long-term sleep deprivation isn't just about feeling tired — it can lead to a host of serious health problems, both physical and mental.

The truth is, your body and brain need sleep to function properly, and when they don't get it, the consequences can be significant.

The following sections break down some of the long-term risks associated with sleep deprivation. And yes, there are quite a few!

Physical health risks

When you don't get enough sleep over a prolonged period, your body starts to suffer in more ways than one. Sleep is the time when your body repairs itself — without it, you're at greater risk for developing chronic health conditions, some of which may surprise you:

>> **Cancer:** According to a study by Johns Hopkins, among others, long-term sleep deprivation has been linked to an increased risk of breast, ovarian, and prostate cancers.

>> **Cardiovascular disease:** Sleep deprivation raises your risk of heart disease, high blood pressure, and stroke.

>> **Diabetes:** Your body's ability to regulate blood sugar is thrown off by lack of sleep, increasing your risk of developing type 2 diabetes.

>> **Hormonal imbalances:** Sleep deprivation can cause a drop in testosterone and growth hormone production, affecting libido and muscle growth. Athletes and bodybuilders know how crucial sleep is for recovery and performance.

>> **Impaired immunity:** Sleep deprivation weakens your immune system, reducing natural killer cells and antibody production, which makes you more vulnerable to infections.

>> **Kidney disease:** Prolonged lack of sleep can also affect kidney function, leading to long-term health issues.

>> **Obesity:** Sleep impacts hunger-regulating hormones like leptin and ghrelin. When you're sleep-deprived, your body craves more food, often high in calories, leading to weight gain.

Mental health and cognitive decline

Your brain needs rest just as much as your body does, and long-term sleep deprivation can take a serious toll on your mental well-being. Here's how sleep deprivation impacts your mind over time:

>> **Anxiety and depression:** Chronic sleep deprivation can make you more vulnerable to mental health issues like anxiety, depression, and even suicidal thoughts.

>> **Cognitive decline:** You might notice a decline in your ability to learn, concentrate, and think clearly. Long-term sleep deprivation has even been linked to an increased risk of dementia.

>> **Memory issues:** Sleep is critical for memory consolidation. Without it, you'll find yourself forgetting things more often.

>> **Mood changes:** Sleep-deprived people tend to be more irritable, emotionally reactive, and prone to negative interactions with others. This isn't just about having a short fuse — sleep impacts how you process emotions.

REMEMBER

Your mental health is just as important as your physical health. If you're feeling more stressed, anxious, or moody than usual, take a look at your sleep habits. It might be time to prioritize rest.

Decreased quality of life and increased injury risk

When your body and brain aren't functioning at their best, your quality of life takes a hit. Sleep deprivation can make you more prone to accidents and injuries:

>> **Car accidents:** Drowsy driving is dangerous. You're more likely to fall asleep at the wheel or make poor decisions when you're sleep-deprived.

>> **Falls:** Sleep deprivation affects your coordination and balance, making you more likely to experience falls or other accidents.

>> **Workplace accidents:** Reduced alertness and slower reaction times make you more prone to accidents on the job.

WARNING

Sleep deprivation can make you a danger to yourself and others. Think of it like this: If you're sleep-deprived, you're operating at less than full capacity, and that affects everything from your reaction times to your emotional regulation.

Common symptoms of long-term sleep deprivation

When sleep deprivation stretches out over weeks or months, the effects go beyond just feeling tired. Long-term sleep loss takes a significant toll on your overall health, especially in ways that aren't always obvious at first.

>> **Avolition (lack of motivation):** Over time, your drive and energy can plummet, making it harder to stay on top of daily responsibilities.

>> **Feeling cold:** Sleep plays a role in regulating body temperature. With long-term deprivation, you may notice feeling unusually cold, even when it's warm.

>> **Hallucinations:** Severe sleep deprivation can cause you to see or hear things that aren't really there, especially after multiple days of poor sleep.

>> **Hyperactivity:** For some people, chronic sleep deprivation triggers bursts of energy or jitteriness, followed by a crash. It's your body's last-ditch effort to keep going.

These are just a few of the more extreme symptoms that emerge with prolonged sleep deprivation. The longer you go without quality sleep, the more likely you are to experience these more unusual effects.

WARNING

If you've been dealing with long-term sleep deprivation, your body may be trying to send you messages through some of these signs. Don't ignore them — prioritize rest before the symptoms worsen.

Setting Yourself Up for Great Sleep

Let's be real — life gets busy. We've all had those nights where sleep is the last thing on the agenda. But here's the thing: No amount of caffeine or a long nap on the weekend can truly replace the benefits of regular, quality sleep. It's about building long-term habits that set you up for success, night after night.

The good news? Improving your sleep isn't about an extreme overhaul. You can start with small changes that have a big impact, like creating a simple bedtime routine, setting consistent sleep and wake times, and adjusting your environment so it encourages rest. When you make sleep a priority, your mind and body will thank you. And once you find a routine that works, it becomes second nature, leaving you feeling more relaxed and confident about bedtime.

REMEMBER

Life will throw curveballs — whether it's an all-night work deadline, a sick kid, or jet lag. And that's okay. Just like with healthy eating, one bad night doesn't undo all your progress. The key is sticking to your routine in the long run for lasting results.

Creating a sleep routine

You know how kids have those bedtime rituals, like a bath, a bedtime story, and a kiss goodnight? These routines signal to their brains that it's time to sleep. And guess what? Adults aren't all that different. Establishing a consistent, calming routine tells your body that it's time to wind down. The trick is to keep it simple and something you can do no matter where you are.

Think about two or three calming activities that help you transition into sleep mode. Maybe it's a warm shower, 15 minutes of reading, or a few minutes of meditation. If you're someone who likes structure, jot down your routine and stick it to your mirror as a reminder. You could even create a calming playlist or make a cup of herbal tea that you sip every night. The key is consistency.

And don't forget — make your routine adaptable. For instance, while lighting a favorite candle might be relaxing, it's not practical if you're traveling. Instead, pack a sleep mask or your favorite calming essential oils that you can use anywhere. Flexibility is just as important as consistency.

TIP

You don't need to make bedtime a two-hour production. A manageable 10 to 20 minute wind-down is all it takes. If you have longer routines, like a long yoga session, try doing them earlier in the evening so you can still keep your bedtime routine simple and stress-free. Bedtime should feel like a relaxing wind-down, not another chore on your to-do list.

Establishing a consistent bedtime and wake time

Let's talk about something your body *loves*: Consistency. Your body's internal clock, also known as the *circadian rhythm*, thrives on routine. By going to bed and waking up at the same time every day (yes, even on weekends), you keep your internal clock in sync, making it easier to fall asleep and wake up feeling refreshed.

Think about it like eating meals at the same time every day. When you stick to a schedule, your body knows when to expect breakfast, lunch, and dinner, and you feel more energized. The same goes for sleep. The more consistent your sleep schedule is, the easier it is to fall asleep and wake up naturally.

I'm personally in bed by 10 p.m. and awake by 5:45 a.m. most days. I give myself a half-hour window, which ensures I'm generally well-rested. If you're not a morning person, that's okay!

TIP

You can ease into a new routine by shifting your sleep and wake times by 15–30 minutes each day until you find a schedule that works for you. And yes, this even applies on weekends. While the temptation to sleep in might be strong, sticking to your schedule will keep your internal clock on track.

If life gets in the way and you have a late night, don't panic. Just get back on track the next day. A little disruption won't throw off your routine if you stay consistent over time. Think of your sleep schedule as a long-term investment in your health.

Pre-sleep relaxation techniques

Once you have a routine and sleep schedule down, the next step is to focus on your relaxation game. The goal is to calm your body and mind before bed, so you can fall asleep faster and sleep more soundly. Even if you have a basic routine like shower, brush teeth, and sleep, adding a few more relaxation techniques can take your bedtime to the next level:

» **Breathwork:** Deep, slow breathing can lower your heart rate and engage your parasympathetic nervous system (the part of your brain that helps you relax). Even just five minutes of focused breathing before bed can make a huge difference.

» **Cool your room:** There's a reason it's hard to sleep in a hot room — your body temperature naturally drops at night, signaling that it's time for sleep. Try lowering the thermostat or cracking open a window. A fan can also cool the room and provide a soothing background noise.

» **Essential oils:** Scents like lavender, ylang-ylang, or chamomile are known for their calming properties. Use a diffuser or spritz a little on your pillow to help set a relaxing mood.

» **Foot massage:** Giving yourself a gentle foot rub can relieve tension, improve circulation, and lower your heart rate, making it easier to drift off to sleep. Or better yet, have your friend or partner give the rub.

» **Gentle yoga:** Restorative yoga poses, like Child's Pose or Supine Twists, can help relax your muscles and quiet your mind. Stick to relaxing stretches instead of more intense moves that accelerate your heart rate.

» **Gratitude reflection:** Spend a few minutes reflecting on the positives in your day. Writing down three things you're grateful for can help quiet your mind and end the day on a peaceful note.

» **Progressive muscle relaxation**: Starting at your toes and moving up your body, slowly tense and release each muscle group. This method helps you notice where you're holding tension and allows your body to relax fully.

>> **Take a warm bath:** A warm bath can lower your core temperature, signaling to your body that it's time for bed. Plus, it's a great way to relax your muscles after a long day.

Foods, lights, and other habits

What you eat and drink during the day — and especially before bed — can have a big impact on your sleep. Maintaining a balanced diet rich in whole foods and low in processed junk can set you up for better rest. And while you don't want to go to bed on a full stomach, a small snack before bedtime can actually help you sleep better. Try these foods to give your sleep a little boost:

>> **Bananas:** These are packed with potassium, which helps regulate your sleep-wake cycle.

>> **Chamomile tea:** Caffeine-free and soothing, chamomile is a great pre-bedtime beverage.

>> **Cherries:** These contain melatonin, a hormone that supports your body's sleep cycle.

>> **Kiwis:** Some studies suggest that eating two kiwis before bed can help you fall asleep faster.

>> **Oatmeal:** This comforting snack contains tryptophan, which promotes the production of serotonin and melatonin.

>> **Oily fish:** Salmon and other fatty fish are rich in omega-3 fatty acids, which can improve serotonin levels.

>> **Nuts:** Pistachios, walnuts, and almonds are high in melatonin and make a great pre-sleep snack.

While food can help, light is another critical factor in your body's sleep cycle. Exposure to bright lights — especially blue light from screens — before bed can trick your brain into thinking it's still daytime, delaying the release of melatonin. This can make it harder for you to fall asleep. So, as bedtime approaches, dim the lights and avoid screens for at least an hour before bed. Also try to stay away from these pitfalls:

>> **Alcohol:** It may make you drowsy, but alcohol disrupts REM sleep, making your rest less restorative.

>> **Caffeine:** Stick to decaf after 1 p.m. Caffeine has a sneaky way of lingering in your system, making it harder to fall asleep. In some cultures, this is not the

case and people drink coffee long into the evening. As always, listen to what your body tells you!

>> **Exercise:** While working out is great for sleep, doing it too close to bedtime can sometimes boost your adrenaline and make it harder to wind down.

>> **Heavy or spicy meals:** Eating a big meal (or a spicy one if you're not accustomed to them) close to bedtime can lead to indigestion and make it difficult to fall asleep.

>> **Napping:** While a short power nap is fine, long or late naps can throw off your nighttime sleep schedule.

Using Somatic Techniques Before Bed

If you've ever felt like your body is still holding onto the day's tension as you lie in bed, you're not alone. That's where somatic techniques come in. These gentle movements and exercises help you release physical and mental stress, making it easier to fall asleep or start the day feeling refreshed. Whether you're preparing for sleep or just waking up, somatic movements offer a calming way to unwind or ease into the morning. Think of them as a gentle reset button for your body and mind.

Somatic techniques focus on connecting your body's sensations with mindful movements. These include restorative postures, breathing exercises, self-hugging, meditation, and visualization, all of which help promote restful sleep and a more relaxed state as you incorporate them into your bedtime (or morning) routine.

Gentle movements to relax your body

If you're feeling physically tense before bed, try the following somatic exercises. Each movement can help you release tension, calm your nervous system, and prepare your body for a deeper, more restorative sleep.

Articulating Bridge

The Articulating Bridge helps release tension in your spine and hips while gently engaging your core.

1. **Lie on your back on a firm surface, with your knees bent and feet flat, hip-width apart, as shown in Figure 9-2a.**

2. **Slowly lift your pelvis toward the ceiling, one vertebra at a time, until your body forms a bridge position, as shown in Figure 9-2b.**

3. **Pause at the top, then lower yourself back down, again one vertebra at a time, until your spine returns to the floor.**

4. **Repeat this motion three to five times, focusing on the fluidity of the movement and your breath.**

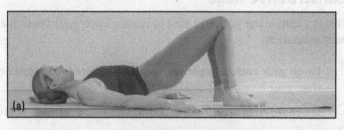
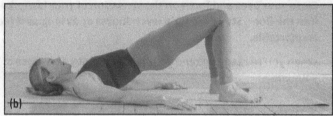

FIGURE 9-2:
The Articulating Bridge helps release back and hip tightness.

Photograph by Guen Egan

Banana Pose

This stretch is great for releasing side-body tension and lengthening the muscles along your spine. Follow these steps to try it:

1. **Lie on your back with your legs extended.**

2. **Cross one ankle over the other, then take the same arm as your top foot and reach overhead.**

3. **Gently shift your upper body and legs to the opposite side, creating a curved "banana" shape, as shown in Figure 9-3.**

4. **Hold this position for five to eight breaths, feeling the stretch along your side. Then switch sides.**

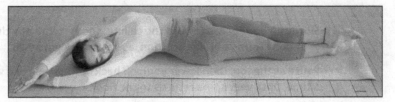

FIGURE 9-3:
Monkey around
with the Banana
Pose to loosen
tension in
your sides.

Photograph by Guen Egan

Constructive Rest

This is a simple but powerful pose to release lower back tension and promote full-body relaxation.

1. **Lie on your back with your knees bent and your feet positioned wider than your hips.**

2. **Let your knees drop inward, resting them against each other.**

3. **Close your eyes and focus on the sensation of your lower back softening into the floor. Stay here for a few minutes or as long as it feels comfortable.**

4. **When you're ready, extend your legs and enjoy the sense of ease in your body.**

Pose Butterfly

This posture opens up the hips and chest, encouraging deep, calming breaths.

1. **Sit up straight and bring the soles of your feet together, letting your knees fall open to the sides like butterfly wings.**

   See Figure 9-4a.

2. **Stay in this pose for several minutes, breathing slowly and deeply.**

   See Figure 9-4b.

3. **To come out, gently bring your knees together and extend your legs.**

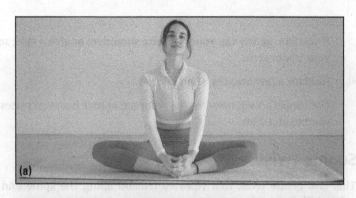

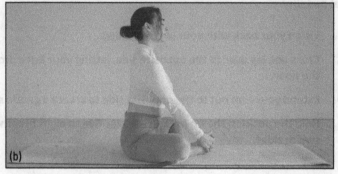

FIGURE 9-4:
Quiet your mind and muscles with the Butterfly Pose.

Photograph by Guen Egan

Knee-to-Chest Pose

This movement gently stretches the lower back and relaxes the hip flexors, which often carry tension.

1. **While lying on your back, draw one knee to your chest and gently hug it.**

2. **Relax your hip flexor as you hold this pose for several breaths.**

3. **Switch sides and repeat, feeling the release in your lower back and hips.**

Self-Hug

This is a comforting movement that encourages self-compassion while releasing shoulder tension. See Chapter 7 for lots more about the benefits and techniques for self-hugging.

1. **Sit on the edge of your bed or lie down.**

2. **Wrap your arms around yourself and give yourself a gentle hug.**

3. If you like, gently tap your opposite shoulders or give a light squeeze to your upper arms.

4. Hold for a few breaths, then release.

This simple act not only stretches your upper back but also creates a sense of warmth and calm.

Supine Twist

This is a gentle twist that releases tension along the spine and improves spinal mobility.

1. Lie on your back with your legs extended.

2. Cross one leg over to the opposite side, letting your knee drop toward the floor.

3. Extend your arm out to the opposite side to create a gentle spinal twist.

4. Hold the position shown in Figure 9-5 for five to eight breaths, then switch sides.

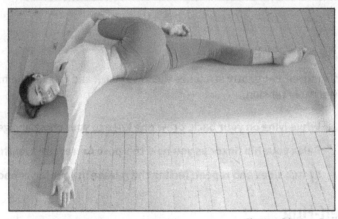

FIGURE 9-5:
When done correctly, Supine Twists feel sublime.

Photograph by Guen Egan

Breathing exercises to calm your mind

Incorporating breathing exercises into your bedtime routine can be a powerful way to calm your mind and prepare for sleep:

>> **4-7-8 breath:** Inhale for a count of four, hold for a count of seven, and exhale for a count of eight. Repeat this breath cycle as much as you need. It helps

activate the parasympathetic nervous system to reduce anxiety and promote sleep. Adjust the counts if needed to match your natural breath rhythm.

WARNING

A long breath hold can induce anxiety in certain people. Take this approach slowly and with caution, especially if you're prone to anxiety.

» **Equal breathing (*Sama Vritti*):** Inhale and exhale for the same length of time (for example, four counts in, four counts out). This creates a balanced, rhythmic breath that calms the mind and prepares your body for sleep.

» **Pause breathing:** Inhale fully, pause at the top, exhale fully, and pause at the bottom. This technique creates space between each breath, allowing for deeper relaxation. After a few minutes, return to normal breathing and notice how you feel.

» ***Viloma* breathing:** Break your breath into parts. Inhale partially, pause, inhale more, pause again, then fill your lungs completely. Exhale in one long breath. After a few cycles, reverse the process by exhaling in segments. This breathwork helps reduce anxiety and tension, balancing your energy.

Visualization techniques for deeper relaxation

Visualization is a powerful tool to calm your mind and ease your body into a restful state. By focusing your imagination on peaceful or positive images, you create mental "scenes" that help quiet racing thoughts, release physical tension, and prepare you for sleep. Think of it as guided daydreaming, but with the purpose of relaxation and mental clarity. The beauty of visualization is that it doesn't require any equipment — just your mind and a little focus.

Each technique invites you to fully engage your senses, which helps distract you from any lingering worries or stresses from the day.

Body scan

A body scan is a simple yet effective way to release physical tension and promote relaxation. By mentally scanning your body from head to toe, you not only bring awareness to each part, but also send a signal to those areas to relax and let go of any built-up stress. The key here is to move slowly and deliberately, giving each body part your full attention.

1. Lie in bed in a comfortable position, closing your eyes and taking a few deep breaths.

2. Begin with your toes and feet. Imagine them softening, releasing any tightness or tension.

3. Gradually work your way up through your legs, allowing the muscles to relax, then move to your hips, lower back, and abdomen.

4. Visualize each muscle group softening as you continue scanning upward through your chest, shoulders, arms, hands, neck, and finally the top of your head.

As you complete the scan, you may notice a sense of lightness or stillness in your body, as though all tension has melted away. This technique not only relaxes your body, but also helps focus your mind, bringing your attention fully into the present moment.

Color breathing

Color breathing combines deep breathing with visualization, creating a powerful tool for releasing stress. The practice involves imagining that each breath you take fills your body with a soothing color, while each exhale releases tension in the form of a darker, more negative hue.

1. Close your eyes and settle into your breath.

2. As you inhale, imagine you're breathing in a soft, calming color — maybe a light blue, pink, or green — something that represents peace and relaxation for you.

3. Visualize this color flowing through your body, filling every cell with calm energy.

4. As you exhale, imagine breathing out a darker color — something that represents stress, tension, or negativity. Visualize the darker color leaving your body with each breath, making space for more relaxation.

5. Continue this pattern, letting your mind settle into the rhythm of the breath and colors.

    The goal is that, over time, your body will feel lighter and your mind will become more tranquil.

Color breathing is a gentle yet powerful way to cleanse your body of any stress and prepare for deep rest.

Guided imagery

Guided imagery takes you on a mental journey to a place that makes you feel calm, safe, and at ease. Whether it's a beach, a mountain, or your favorite childhood spot, guided imagery immerses your mind in positive, soothing experiences, which can help shift your focus away from daily worries and into a more peaceful state.

1. **Close your eyes and take a few deep breaths.**

2. **Imagine a scene that makes you feel relaxed and happy. It could be a sunny beach with the sound of gentle waves, a quiet forest with birds chirping, or a peaceful meadow bathed in golden light.**

3. **Engage all your senses in this visualization.**

   What do you see? What can you hear? Feel the warmth of the sun on your skin or the cool breeze on your face. Smell the fresh air or flowers around you. The more vivid your mental image, the more effectively it will soothe your mind.

4. **You can listen to a guided meditation that walks you through peaceful imagery if it's hard to conjure a scene on your own.**

   These audio guides can be found online or via meditation apps, and they provide step-by-step cues for visualizing your happy place.

As your mind becomes fully immersed in this mental journey, your body will follow, relaxing and preparing for sleep.

Lovingkindness meditation (*Metta*)

Lovingkindness meditation, also known as *Metta*, is a heart-centered practice that involves sending positive thoughts and wishes to yourself and others. It's not just about feeling good — it's about fostering compassion and emotional connection, which can reduce stress and improve overall well-being.

1. **Begin by closing your eyes and taking a few deep breaths.**

2. **Picture someone you care about deeply — maybe a family member, friend, or even a pet.**

3. **In your mind, repeat the mantra: "May you be safe. May you be happy. May you be healthy. May you be at ease." As you say these words, imagine sending love and kindness to that person.**

4. **After a few repetitions, shift your focus to yourself. Say the same mantra: "May *I* be safe. May *I* be happy. May *I* be healthy. May *I* be at ease."**

5. **Lastly, extend this lovingkindness to all beings, known and unknown, across the world.**

You can spend as much or as little time on each part as you like. This practice not only helps relax your mind before bed, but it can also cultivate a deeper sense of peace and connection.

Addressing Sleep Issues Somatically

Somatic movement and exercises can help you address sleep issues by targeting the physical manifestations of tension, stress, and anxiety in your body. Gentle stretching and yoga help release the tightness in your muscles, while mindfulness, breathing exercises, and meditation calm your mind. When you combine these practices, you can tackle the root causes of your sleep problems holistically.

WARNING

If you only focus on your thoughts, it can feel impossible to "think your way out" of a restless night. Addressing what's held in your body is key to a more restful sleep.

As you begin to slow down and tune into your body's needs, you'll start recognizing patterns and triggers that may be contributing to your sleep troubles. Maybe you're not moving enough during the day, leading to restlessness at night. Or perhaps you're holding tension in your muscles, making it difficult to get comfortable. Gentle yoga and stretching can help release these tight spots, preparing your body for relaxation. Or you may have a racing mind, which can be calmed through meditation and breathing practices, so that bedtime feels more peaceful.

By tapping into somatic practices, you become more in tune with your body. This increased awareness will not only help you establish better sleep hygiene but will also allow you to create a nighttime routine that supports relaxation and restful sleep.

Techniques for overcoming insomnia

Insomnia isn't just about feeling restless at night — it's often tied to how your mind and body handle stress and anxiety. Trying to force yourself to sleep by "willing" it often backfires, especially when your body is tense or your mind is racing. That's where somatic techniques come in. They help shift your focus from thinking about sleep to connecting with your body, which naturally calms your nervous system and promotes relaxation.

Instead of focusing only on routines, let's explore how these body-centered practices can tackle insomnia at its root:

>> **Shift your focus from thoughts to body sensations:** Insomnia often comes with overthinking and mental chatter. When you're lying in bed, unable to sleep, one of the most effective ways to counter this is to shift your focus to your body. Notice the sensation of your breath, the way your back feels against the mattress, or the warmth of your blankets. Redirecting attention

from your thoughts to your physical body helps interrupt the mental loop of insomnia.

>> **Somatic breathing for insomnia:** Deep breathing exercises, like 4-7-8 breathing, can soothe an overactive nervous system. These techniques engage your parasympathetic system, which helps lower your heart rate and reduce anxiety — key elements in fighting insomnia. By slowing your breath, you signal to your body that it's time to rest, rather than fight or stay alert.

>> **Body-based mindfulness:** Mindfulness practices centered on body awareness, like body scans, are particularly effective for insomnia. As you lie in bed, mentally scan your body from head to toe. Rather than rushing through, pause at each part — your toes, feet, calves, and hips — giving it permission to relax. This body-mind connection helps release the built-up tension that contributes to sleeplessness.

>> **Release physical tension with somatic movement:** Insomnia is often worsened by physical tension in your muscles. Try gentle movements like Supine Twists or Knee-to-Chest poses to release tightness in the lower back and hips, areas that tend to hold tension. Even a simple shoulder roll or neck stretch can make a big difference if you're feeling physically "stuck" in bed. These movements not only relax your body but also offer a meditative experience, shifting the focus away from mental strain.

>> **Overcome the fear of not sleeping:** One of the major struggles with insomnia is the anxiety about not being able to sleep. This anxiety, in itself, can prevent sleep from happening. Practicing acceptance — acknowledging that it's okay not to fall asleep right away — can reduce this pressure. Use your breath and somatic movements to ground yourself in the present moment, releasing the fear that often accompanies insomnia.

Unlike general sleep strategies, these somatic techniques work directly with your body's natural relaxation mechanisms. They can interrupt the cycle of insomnia by helping you cultivate a sense of calm that begins in your physical body and extends to your mind.

WARNING

Insomnia can be a serious medical condition. If you continue to struggle with insomnia on a regular basis, see your physician for help in addressing this life-threatening issue.

Managing sleep-related anxiety

If you've ever experienced sleep anxiety, you know how overwhelming it can be. It's that feeling of dread as bedtime approaches, worrying about whether you'll be able to fall asleep — or stay asleep. The more you stress about it, the harder it becomes to relax and drift off.

Sleep-related anxiety often stems from a cycle of sleeplessness, where insomnia leads to more worry, and the worry, in turn, leads to more insomnia. Breaking this cycle is crucial. Start by focusing on the same healthy sleep habits covered in earlier sections of this chapter:

» **Practice relaxation techniques:** Guided meditation, visualization, and breathing exercises can help quiet anxious thoughts and bring your focus back to your body.

» **Reserve your bedroom for sleep:** Make your room a sanctuary for sleep by keeping it cool, dark, and clutter-free. Try keeping work materials or anything anxiety-inducing out of sight.

» **Stick to a bedtime routine:** Avoid screens (including the TV), create a calm environment, and wind down with a book or some gentle stretching.

TIP

If your anxiety persists, consider journaling before bed. Write down your worries and let them go. You might also find it helpful to consult with a therapist to explore further strategies for managing sleep-related anxiety.

Using somatic practices to combat restlessness

Restlessness can keep you tossing and turning all night, but somatic practices offer an excellent way to calm your body and mind. When you focus on your body's sensations in the present moment, you ground yourself, releasing the physical tension that often contributes to restless nights:

» **Body scans:** Take a mental tour of your body, bringing awareness to any areas of tightness or discomfort, and imagine releasing that tension as you exhale.

» **Breathwork:** Slow, deep breathing can shift your body into its "rest and digest" mode, signaling to your nervous system that it's time to unwind.

» **Mindful movement:** Gentle exercises like yoga, dancing, or even mindful walking can help release pent-up tension and leave you feeling grounded.

» **Progressive muscle relaxation:** Focus on tensing and then relaxing each muscle group in your body, starting from your toes and working your way up. This helps activate your body's relaxation response.

These techniques are simple but powerful ways to quiet your restlessness and help you drift off more peacefully.

Tips for dealing with frequent awakenings

Waking up multiple times during the night can leave you feeling frustrated and exhausted. But there are a few things you can do to minimize these nighttime disruptions:

» **Create the perfect sleep environment:** Keep your bedroom cool, quiet, and dark. Blackout curtains or a white noise machine can work wonders if noise or light is waking you up.

» **Limit water intake before bed:** Drinking too much fluid close to bedtime can wake you up for bathroom trips in the middle of the night.

» **Monitor your diet:** Eating a large meal too close to bedtime can lead to discomfort and wakefulness. Alcohol, spicy food, and caffeine are also known to cause sleep disturbances.

» **Stick to a consistent sleep schedule:** Keeping your body on a regular rhythm can reduce nighttime awakenings.

TIP

If you do wake up and can't fall back asleep, try not to stress about it. Try a calming activity like reading or listening to soft music until you feel sleepy again. Although you might be tempted to do so, don't turn on the TV or look at your phone.

4

Taking Your Somatic Practice to the Next Level

Taking Your

Somatic Practice

to the Next Level

IN THIS PART . . .

Incorporating meditation into your somatics practice.

Uncovering advanced somatic techniques for additional benefit.

Adopting somatic flow sequences into your practice.

IN THIS CHAPTER

» **Understanding how well meditation fits with somatic exercise**

» **Cultivating a practice space that works for you**

» **Using meditation while you move**

» **Discovering the hows and whys of grounding**

» **Practicing walking mindfully**

» **Nurturing your inner peace**

Chapter **10**

Incorporating Meditation

Meditation is a timeless practice people have used for thousands of years to bring clarity, peace, and focus to their minds. Whether you're a seasoned practitioner or just beginning your journey, incorporating meditation into your daily routine provides profound benefits for both your mental and physical well-being. Meditation quiets the noise of daily life and allows you to connect with the present moment.

In addition to enhancing mental clarity, meditation pairs beautifully with somatic practices, deepening your awareness of the mind-body connection. Through mindful breathing, visualization, and grounding techniques, you can boost your physical and emotional resilience.

In this chapter, I show you how to create a balanced meditation practice that fits seamlessly into your lifestyle and explain how combining movement with mindfulness can elevate both your meditation and somatic exercises.

Understanding Meditation at a Glance

I've been practicing and leading meditation for over 20 years now, and I honestly feel like I can't live without it. Meditation is a practice thousands of years old, with many different forms and styles, both sitting or lying down. At its core, meditation is about creating space in your mind and anchoring yourself in the moment using different techniques.

What is meditation?

Contrary to popular belief, the goal of meditation isn't to completely empty your mind. One of my favorite teachers used to say that it's okay to "get *LIT*" (Lost in Thought) — what matters is that you guide your mind back to your mantra, breath, or whatever anchor you've chosen to stay present. It's natural to have thoughts during meditation; sometimes, these thoughts carry you away to the past or the future. Meditation is a practice that teaches you to come back to the present moment without judgment.

REMEMBER

When you become more mindful in your meditation practice, you also become more mindful in your daily life. You get better at responding to situations instead of reacting impulsively. The benefits of meditation are wide-ranging:

>> **Connects you to yourself:** Meditation allows you to reflect, understand, and be more in tune with your feelings and motivations.

>> **Enhances sleep quality:** A regular meditation practice can help you fall asleep more easily.

>> **Fosters a sense of peace:** As your practice deepens, you cultivate a feeling of inner calm.

>> **Reduces anxiety:** Staying present reduces worries about the future or the past.

>> **Relieves stress:** By creating mental space, meditation helps you calm your mind and body.

Self-guided meditation

If you want to experiment with setting up your own meditation practice, you can absolutely do it on your own. The key is to keep it simple and flexible. Start by setting aside time each day — staying consistent is helpful, but don't worry if it varies. You also need to prepare a space that feels welcoming and comfortable.

I meditate on my own twice a day, usually on my bed with my back against the headboard, although I used to do it on the couch in my living room.

REMEMBER

Your meditation space can be anywhere that works for you. You don't have to sit with perfect posture; you just need to be comfortable. You can lie down if you like. Feel free to shift your position during practice, scratch your nose, or do whatever you need to stay comfortable. You're still human — the goal is relaxation, not perfection.

As you practice, you may notice that over time, it becomes easier to "drop in" quickly (settle into your meditation). But every day is different, and there's no judgment here. There's no right or wrong way to meditate, just a daily practice of getting to know yourself better and giving yourself the space to be present. You're a human *being*, not a human *doing*.

With so many different styles of meditation available, it's helpful to try a few and see which ones feel most comfortable to you:

» **Breath meditation:** You use your breath as an anchor. Follow each inhalation and exhalation, or use breath counts like the 4-7-8 technique (inhale for four counts, hold for seven, exhale for eight). Breath-based meditation can be as simple or structured as you need it to be. Experiment to see what works best for you. See Chapter 4 for much more about breathwork.

» **Body scanning:** A body scan involves breathing deeply and guiding your mind's eye through each part of your body, feeling it relax and release. This technique is particularly good for bringing more somatic awareness into your meditation. See Chapter 6 for step-by-step guidance on body scanning.

» **Mantra meditation:** You can use a mantra to focus your mind. A mantra is a word or phrase that you repeat over and over in your head. I was given a mantra by my *Vedic* meditation teacher, and I use it every time to help me settle in. Vedic meditation originated over 5,000 years ago in India and involves the silent repetition of a mantra given to you by a trained teacher. The mantra is kept secret and doesn't have an attached meaning. If you're interested in Vedic meditation, you can receive a mantra from a teacher, but you can also choose your own. See Chapter 7 for more about using mantras.

» **Sound meditation:** If you find it helpful, you can add sound to your meditation practice. Play sound bath music or meditative tunes to help you center. Binaural beats or solfeggio tones can enhance focus, reduce stress, and increase mindfulness. Natural sounds — like ocean waves, a bubbling stream, or birds chirping — can also be very soothing. Choose something that resonates with you.

- » **Transcendental meditation (TM):** Similar to Vedic meditation, TM involves sitting quietly with your eyes closed, taking deep breaths to relax your mind and body, and silently repeating your mantra. This can be a Sanskrit sound or a word/phrase of your choice.

- » **Yogic mantras and affirmations:** Another option is the "so hum" mantra, which reflects the breath and loosely translates to "I am that." As you inhale, silently say "so," and as you exhale, say "hum." You can also use positive affirmations like "I am calm," "I am brave," "I am free," or "let go." These affirmations can help cultivate specific feelings you want to bring into your life, such as courage, healing, or patience.

TIP

Over time, you'll discover which style feels most natural. Experiment with several styles until you find the one that works for you.

Classes and teachers

If working with a teacher or attending a class feels right for you, many options are available. Meditation centers and individual instructors often offer specific styles, such as Vedic meditation or TM. In both practices, a teacher provides you with a personal mantra. After receiving this instruction, you meditate under the guidance of your teacher before transitioning to practicing on your own. When I learned Vedic meditation, my training took three days to complete. Similarly, TM typically involves about three sessions with a teacher.

REMEMBER

Strive to connect with a teacher or class that feels right. Avoid anyone who makes you feel insecure or negative about yourself. Meditation is personal, and finding the right guide makes a significant difference in creating a lasting practice. Find an open space that resonates with you.

Explore different types of classes:

- » **In-person classes** offer live instruction from experienced teachers. You can find a variety of meditation styles, including mantra-based sessions, breathing exercises, guided visualizations, or body-scan meditations. In-person settings provide the added benefit of real-time feedback and a sense of community. See Figure 10-1.

- » **Online courses and apps** provide flexibility, allowing you to practice at your convenience. Platforms like Headspace and Insight Timer offer guided meditations for everything from stress relief to enhancing focus. Many teachers also offer live-streamed or pre-recorded sessions that you can follow from home.

>> **Retreats and workshops** provide an immersive experience, perfect for those looking to deepen their practice. These often combine seated meditation, mindful movement, and group discussions in a multi-day format, giving you focused time to learn and grow with the support of expert teachers.

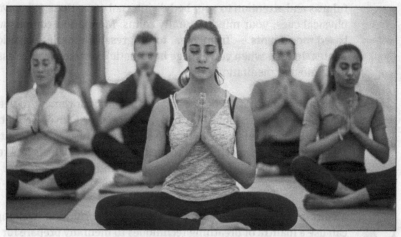

FIGURE 10-1: Group meditation can build community and camaraderie.

Working with a teacher can have many benefits:

>> **Accountability and motivation:** Regular sessions provide structure that keeps you showing up even on tough days, building a stronger, more consistent routine.

>> **Community and support:** Meditation classes often create a sense of community. Practicing alongside others enhances your motivation and provides a space to share experiences and learn from different perspectives.

>> **Personalized guidance:** The teacher can adjust the practice based on your needs. They help you explore different meditation styles, offering suggestions that reflect your personal preferences.

>> **Structured learning:** Structured learning helps you develop a consistent practice. Teachers guide you step by step, ensuring you learn proper techniques while avoiding common challenges.

TIP

Starting with a teacher or class provides valuable support, but eventually feeling comfortable with meditating on your own is important. Over time, you should develop the ability to guide yourself into relaxation and mindfulness. Balancing self-guided practice with occasional teacher-led sessions or group classes deepens your practice. For instance, attending a guided class weekly can keep your meditation routine fresh and engaging.

Connecting Meditation with Somatic Practices

Somatic practices already contain a meditative component, as they require mindfulness and attention to your body's internal sensations. When you focus on these physical cues, your mind naturally calms. Meditation complements all somatic-based movements — from yoga, to progressive muscle relaxation, to Tai Chi, to Pilates. In fact, when you engage in somatic exercises, you're essentially practicing a moving meditation.

You can use meditation before or after somatic movement to deepen the connection between your mind and body. Personally, I love meditating after a yoga session. Yoga opens your body, loosens your muscles and joints, and helps you relax. By the time you sit down to meditate, your body feels less restricted, making it easier to stay still for 5, 15, or even 20 minutes — however long you choose to meditate.

TIP

Meditation also pairs beautifully with mindful running, walking, or hiking. You can use a mantra or breathing techniques to mentally prepare for physical activity. During movement, continue to meditate by syncing your breath with your strides, using a mantra to keep you motivated, or focusing on staying present during a mindful walk. Breath counts, such as inhaling for four steps and exhaling for four steps, help maintain this connection.

The synergy between meditation and somatic exercise

Somatic movement and meditation both emphasize paying attention to your body's sensations. This heightened awareness allows you to become more in tune with the signals your body sends, deepening your understanding of how your mind and body interact. As you calm your mind, your body follows, and vice versa. Studies show that long-term meditators experience benefits like lower heart rates and increased brain size in the prefrontal cortex — evidence that both your brain and body can change for the better through these practices.

Meditation and somatic exercises complement each other by reinforcing the mind-body connection in different but deeply supportive ways. While somatic exercises encourage you to tune into your body's sensations and movements, meditation brings your focus to the mind, helping you become more aware of your thoughts and emotions. When combined, they allow you to balance physical and mental awareness, creating a holistic practice that benefits your overall well-being.

REMEMBER

The mindfulness you cultivate through somatic exercises transfers directly into your meditation practice. For example, during somatic movement, you already pay close attention to how your body feels. Meditation amplifies this by calming the mind, making it easier to notice subtle sensations and changes within your body. This heightened awareness allows you to adjust your movements, improve alignment, and respond to your body's needs more effectively.

On the flip side, the focus and clarity you develop in meditation can deepen your experience of somatic exercises. As your meditation practice strengthens your ability to stay present, you'll find it easier to maintain focus and stay grounded throughout your movements. Whether you're practicing yoga, Pilates, or even mindful walking, your mind becomes more attuned to how your body moves, creating a fluid connection between mental focus and physical action.

How meditation enhances the benefits of somatic practices

Meditation takes your somatic practice to the next level by sharpening your body awareness and helping you engage with your physical sensations in a more mindful way. As you practice somatic exercises, you'll notice a reduction in physical pain, improved energy levels, and the release of stored tension or trauma in your muscles. Meditation enhances this process by helping you:

>> **Process discomfort:** Rather than reacting to physical discomfort, meditation teaches you to observe it, allowing you to modify your movements mindfully.

>> **Improve focus and intentionality:** Meditation trains your mind to stay present, making it easier to focus on each movement and adjust your posture or alignment as needed.

>> **Increase body awareness:** Meditation improves your connection to physical sensations, allowing you to tune in to how your body feels during movement.

>> **Reduce tension and fatigue:** The calm mental space created through meditation allows you to relax your body more fully, helping you release tension and feel more energized.

>> **Release emotions:** As you release physical tension, meditation gives you the space to process and let go of any emotions that arise, leading to a more balanced mind and body.

TIP

Use meditation as a tool to process the sensations and emotions that surface during somatic exercises. By combining these practices, you'll develop a deeper connection to your body and mind, making your overall routine more effective and rewarding.

Start with your breath awareness to center yourself before you exercise. Keep focusing on your breath to bring yourself back to the moment or each movement as you exercise. Listen to your body and take breaks as you need to or adjust your movements according to how your body feels. Trust yourself so that you know you are the one in control of your movements and as you keep developing your connection between your mind and body you can trust what feels right. Listen to your body so you can also know when you may need to take a rest day. Practice gratitude for your body's abilities and be thankful for the opportunity to move. As you cultivate a mindset of gratitude, you'll keep tapping into the mindfulness aspect of your movements.

Incorporating meditation into your overall somatic routine

You can easily integrate meditation into your daily somatic routine. A simple way to start is by meditating at least once a day, as a stand-alone practice, and then incorporating shorter meditation sessions before or after your somatic exercises. The goal is to stay grounded and mindful throughout your day.

Personally, I meditate twice a day — once in the early morning when I wake up, and again in the afternoon as a mental reset. You can do something similar by finding a time that works for you, even if it's just for a few minutes.

REMEMBER

Consistency is key, so even a brief moment of meditation before or after your workout can make a difference.

Try incorporating meditation into your somatic routine at different points:

>> **Pre-workout meditation:** Take a few minutes to check in with your body and your breath before starting your workout. This helps you center yourself and prepare mentally for the movements ahead.

>> **Post-workout meditation:** After completing your somatic exercises, sit for a quick meditation. This seals in the benefits of your practice, giving you a moment to reflect on how your body feels and to calm your mind.

>> **During movement:** Meditate as you move! Whether you're walking mindfully, flowing through yoga, or doing Pilates, staying connected to your breath and your body helps you stay present in the moment.

REMEMBER

Meditation doesn't have to be complicated. You can keep it simple by incorporating these small moments of mindfulness throughout your day. For instance, before going for a mindful walk, close your eyes and do a quick body scan. After a yoga session, sit comfortably and breathe deeply for a few minutes to deepen the relaxation.

Meditation allows you to disconnect from the outer world and reconnect with yourself. By adding it to your routine — before, during, or after somatic exercises — you can enhance your mental and physical awareness, ensuring you get the most out of your practice.

Creating a balanced practice

Creating a balanced meditation practice means aligning your sessions with your energy and priorities. When you view meditation as a tool to support your well-being, you'll see how even brief, intentional sessions bring mental clarity and calm into your day.

TIP

Rather than focusing on the length of your sessions, focus on maintaining a rhythm that feels realistic and adaptable. Studies have shown that even just ten minutes of meditation per day can have real health benefits.

Meditation can be a grounding morning routine, a midday reset, or an evening wind-down, depending on your schedule — and body needs. As you practice regularly, you'll find that meditation becomes a source of balance, helping you navigate challenges with greater ease.

To balance your meditation practice, try these tips:

>> **Combine meditation with movement:** On especially busy days, try combining meditation with a walk or stretching session to keep your mind engaged while moving your body.

>> **Integrate meditation into key transitions:** Use meditation to transition between different parts of your day, such as after work or before meals, to keep yourself balanced and centered.

>> **Tune into your energy levels:** Adapt your meditation length and style to match your energy. For instance, a short, energizing breathwork session might fit well in the morning, while a calming body scan can help you unwind at night.

With time, your meditation practice will support not only your well-being but also your productivity and mental clarity. You'll approach each day with more presence and feel more balanced across all aspects of life.

REMEMBER

Meditation doesn't have to look the same every day. By being mindful of your needs, you can create a practice that feels balanced and sustainable.

Adapting your practice to fit your lifestyle and goals

You might be preparing for a race, gearing up for finals as a student, running a Fortune 500 company, or balancing life as a busy stay-at-home parent. Whatever your lifestyle, you can find a way to fit meditation into your schedule and make it work for you. Meditation isn't a one-size-fits-all practice — you get to shape it in a way that aligns with your goals.

Take a moment right now to close your eyes and connect with your breath. What do you notice? What do you feel? Breathe deeply and start to envision where you want to be and what you want to accomplish. This little check-in helps you align with what's most important in your life. What are your values? How do you want to show up in the world? How do you see meditation fitting into that?

Next, think about the times when you feel most stressed. See if you can create a schedule that includes moments to check in with yourself again — finding peace and calm throughout your day. Maybe you want to meditate before a big exam or meeting. Maybe, as a parent, you want to wake up a bit earlier than your kids to connect with yourself first, so you can be fully present for them. If you're a runner preparing for a marathon, you might schedule a fitness-focused meditation before your runs. Or, if you're a busy executive, meditating before bed helps you unwind from the day.

REMEMBER

Your meditation practice is for you, but it also impacts everyone around you. When you show up for yourself, you show up better for your loved ones, colleagues, employees, students — you name it. Meditation helps you be the best version of yourself, and that ripple effect spreads to everyone in your life.

To tailor your practice, try these tips:

>> **Define your goals:** Get clear on what you need from your practice. Are you looking to improve focus, cultivate patience, or simply find a moment of calm in a busy day? Your goals will guide the way you meditate.

>> **Choose the best timing:** Experiment with different times of day to see when meditation feels most beneficial. Morning sessions help start your day mindfully, while evening sessions can help you unwind.

>> **Adjust to your daily needs:** Your practice can be as flexible as your life. On busy days, a quick five-minute check-in might be enough, while quieter days offer the chance to deepen your practice.

Setting Up Your Space

I truly love my meditation space — and guess what? It's my bed! I wake up, grab a glass of water, and settle in with my back against the headboard, hands resting on or under a pillow in my lap, depending on how I feel that day. Your meditation space doesn't have to be fancy or formal. It just needs to feel comfortable and inviting.

You don't need to sit like a statue on a meditation cushion unless that feels right for you. You can rest against something for back support, sit cross-legged on the floor, or even lie down if that's what works best. The key is to find what feels good for you — there are no rules here. My bedroom feels like my sanctuary, and meditating there is my way of getting closer to myself. But you can meditate anywhere that feels peaceful, whether that's a corner of your living room, a favorite chair, or even your backyard. Your space can be as cozy and simple as you'd like. See Figure 10-2.

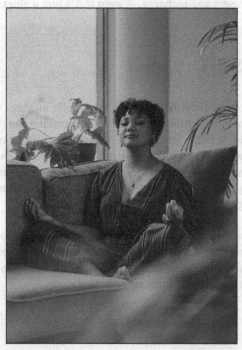

FIGURE 10-2:
Your meditation space can be anywhere you feel comfortable and at peace.

Delmaine Donson/Getty Images

To set up your meditation space, follow these tips:

>> **Choose a comfortable spot:** Find a location that feels supportive, whether that's a cushion on the floor, a chair, or even your bed. Make sure your body feels relaxed and supported.

>> **Limit distractions:** Try to pick a place that's relatively quiet and free from interruptions. While complete silence isn't necessary, a peaceful environment can help you focus.

>> **Add personal touches:** If it enhances your experience, bring in objects that bring you calm, like a candle, a plant, or soft lighting. These elements create a sensory connection to your practice. However, keep it simple. It's less about the objects around you and more about creating an environment that feels calming and welcoming.

>> **Stay flexible:** Sometimes, you'll need to meditate on the go — in a doctor's office, on the subway, or while waiting for an appointment. Knowing you have a consistent "home base" to return to makes it easier to meditate anywhere, while your dedicated spot at home adds a special sense of comfort.

Once you've set up your space, you'll find it easier to settle into your practice and look forward to meditation each day. Your meditation space can serve as a sanctuary, a place to reconnect and recharge — even if it's just a quiet corner of a room.

Grounding Yourself

Grounding is one of my favorite practices, especially on days when I'm feeling scattered or overwhelmed. Think of grounding as pressing the "reset" button for your mind and body. It helps you reconnect with the present moment, bringing you back down to earth — literally! Whether you've been rushing through your day, bouncing between tasks, or just feeling out of sync, grounding helps you find your center through simple breathing exercises, visualizations, or even quick stretches that bring your awareness back to your body.

Grounding isn't just a mental exercise; it's a full-body reset. Even when you don't have time for a long meditation session, a quick grounding exercise can bring immediate benefits to both your mind and body. Grounding is a technique that keeps you rooted in the present moment.

TIP

When you feel more grounded, you naturally feel less stressed. There are many ways to ground yourself — from connecting to nature by walking barefoot on grass or sand, to focusing on your breath. Grounding might even involve listening to music or calling a friend. It's a technique you can use to stay connected to the here and now.

Benefits of grounding for mental and physical health

Grounding offers benefits that go beyond just making you feel more present — it can have a profound impact on your mental and physical health. By taking a moment to reconnect with the earth and your body, you can

>> **Boost immune function:** Some studies suggest that grounding — especially physical contact with the Earth — can improve your immune function by reducing inflammation and lowering stress.

>> **Improve focus and clarity:** When your mind is all over the place, grounding helps you center your thoughts. It clears mental fog, allowing you to focus better and think more clearly.

>> **Increase physical relaxation:** As you ground yourself, your muscles naturally relax. It's like your body gets the memo from your mind that everything's okay, and suddenly you can breathe a little easier.

>> **Reduce stress and anxiety:** Grounding immediately calms your nervous system. By bringing your attention back to the present moment and connecting with the Earth beneath you, grounding can lower your stress levels and help ease anxiety.

Simple grounding exercises to start your practice

Grounding exercises are incredibly simple, and you can do them anytime, anywhere. To get grounded, start by finding a stable seat, tapping into your breath, and focusing on something that anchors your thoughts. The very first step is to connect to whatever is physically supporting you. Feel the floor, your mattress, a cushion — whatever is beneath you, holding you up. Notice how it feels and the texture of the surface, and allow your body to surrender into what's beneath it. If you're walking, feel the earth under your feet. Notice how you move through the ball of each foot and the heel.

You can also use your surroundings and nature to help ground yourself. One of my favorite grounding techniques is called 5-4-3-2-1. Here's how it works: Identify five things you can see, four things you can touch, three things you can hear, two things you can smell, and one thing you can taste. This exercise shifts your focus from whatever may be distressing you to your immediate environment. I especially love doing this grounding technique with my boys! Here are a few more easy grounding exercises to get you started:

>> **Barefoot walking:** This is one of the easiest and most effective ways to ground yourself. Find a patch of grass, dirt, or even sand, and walk barefoot. As you walk, focus on how the ground feels beneath your feet — the texture, the temperature, the sensation of each step. This physical connection to the earth immediately helps you feel more centered.

>> **Body scan:** You can do this sitting or lying down. Close your eyes and take a few deep breaths. Then, slowly bring your attention to different parts of your body, starting from your feet and moving upward. Notice how each part of your body feels — heavy, light, tense, or relaxed — and consciously release any tension as you breathe out.

>> **Breathing with intention:** Stand or sit comfortably, close your eyes, and take slow, deep breaths. With each exhale, imagine any stress or tension leaving your body and sinking into the earth. With each inhale, feel the stability and calm of the ground rising up through your body. Continue for a few minutes, breathing in strength and breathing out tension.

>> **Seated grounding:** Sit in a comfortable chair with your feet flat on the floor. Close your eyes and take a deep breath. As you exhale, imagine your feet sinking into the ground, connecting with the Earth beneath you. Let the weight of your body rest fully in your seat, feeling the support beneath you. Stay here for a few moments, breathing deeply and feeling your connection to the ground.

>> **Tree visualization:** Stand tall and close your eyes. Imagine yourself as a tree, with roots growing down from the soles of your feet into the Earth. With each breath, visualize those roots growing deeper, anchoring you firmly in the ground. This visualization not only helps you feel stable and grounded, but it also brings a sense of calm and focus.

TIP

Anytime you feel stressed, scattered, or unbalanced, take a moment to ground yourself. It only takes a minute, but it can make a world of difference for your mind and body.

Combining Meditation with Movement

Combining meditation and movement is a favorite! I love to be very mindful of my breath as I move through poses in my yoga practice. I love to stay very focused on engaging the correct muscles when I lift weights or do Pilates. I love to tap into my form when I'm running. Mindful movement is good for your heart and soul. When you combine meditation with movement, you are much less likely to injure yourself. You're tapping into to what your body needs and listening to it. You also get more joy out of your movement because you're fully experiencing it.

Meditative movement differs from mindlessly going through the motions or distracting yourself with a screen or music. Instead, you become deeply engaged with each movement, enhancing your mental focus and your physical experience.

TIP

To meditate while moving, try these suggestions:

>> **Mindful running or walking:** Sync your breath with your steps, like inhaling for four steps and exhaling for four. Use a mantra or focus on the rhythm of your body to keep yourself present. The next section ("Practicing Mindful Walking") delves more deeply into mindful walking.

>> **Pre-movement meditation:** Before you start any activity, close your eyes and take a few deep breaths to check in with your body. Visualize the workout ahead and set an intention, such as staying present or listening to your body's signals.

>> **Yoga and Pilates:** As you move through poses or exercises, stay aware of your breath and body alignment. This focus keeps you connected and helps you get the most from each movement.

Practicing Mindful Walking

Mindful walking is a wonderful way to turn something as simple as walking into a grounding, meditative experience. Unlike regular walking, mindful walking invites you to bring your full awareness to each step, helping you connect with the present moment and leave distractions behind. This practice can be done anywhere — indoors or outdoors — and doesn't require any special setup or equipment.

Basic principles of mindful walking

Mindful walking transforms walking from a routine activity into a conscious, grounding practice. You can turn any walk into a meditation that calms your mind and centers your body by following several core principles to help you stay fully present as you walk:

>> **Engage your senses:** Be aware of what's around you without getting caught up in it. Notice the sounds, smells, and colors in your environment. Allow your senses to take in everything without needing to label or analyze it.

>> **Feel each step:** Each step matters. Pay attention to how your feet make contact with the ground, how your body shifts with each step, and the sensations that arise. This physical awareness helps you stay rooted in the present.

>> **Observe without judgment:** Thoughts will come and go as you walk, and that's perfectly okay. Instead of judging or reacting to each thought, gently bring your attention back to your steps and breath.

>> **Slow down:** Mindful walking isn't about reaching a destination quickly. Instead, slow your pace so you can focus on each step. Moving at a relaxed, comfortable speed makes it easier to tune in to your body and surroundings.

>> **Stay connected to your breath:** Your breath anchors you to the present moment. Syncing your breath with your steps — like inhaling for two steps, exhaling for two — creates a steady rhythm and keeps your focus from drifting.

Practicing these principles not only makes walking more meditative, but it also helps you build mindfulness skills you can carry into other areas of life. As you develop a mindful walking practice, you may find yourself feeling more grounded and at ease, even on the busiest days.

Mindful walking doesn't need a special time or place. Try bringing these principles into your regular walks, whether it's around your neighborhood or on your way to work. Each step is an opportunity to reconnect with yourself.

Follow these steps to practice mindful walking:

1. **Start with your posture**.

   Stand tall, with your shoulders relaxed and your head balanced above your spine. Take a deep breath and feel your connection to the ground through your feet.

2. **Focus on your steps**.

   As you begin walking slowly, notice each step. Feel the sensation of your heel touching the ground, the roll of your foot, and the push-off with your toes. Pay attention to how each step feels — the pressure, balance, and subtle movements involved.

3. **Coordinate your breath**.

   Try to match your breathing with your steps. For example, you can inhale for two steps and exhale for two. This rhythm helps you stay focused and creates a steady, calming pattern as you walk.

4. **Engage your senses**.

   Notice what's around you without getting caught up in it. Observe the sounds, sights, and smells, and allow yourself to be fully present in the environment. If you're outdoors, feel the air on your skin or the sun's warmth (or the chill in the air).

5. **Refocus when needed**.

   If your mind wanders, gently bring your attention back to your steps and breathing. As with any meditation practice, mindful walking doesn't require perfection; it's normal for thoughts to come and go. Each time you refocus, you strengthen your ability to stay present.

Practicing mindful walking is a way to bring meditation into motion. Instead of rushing from point A to point B, you create space to simply *be*, even while moving. This can be a particularly helpful practice on busy days, allowing you to slow down, re-center, and reconnect with yourself.

TIP

Although staying present while you walk can be a refreshing way to clear your mind and connect with yourself, your thoughts can easily drift to your to-do list or yesterday's worries. Sometimes, a simple mantra can help you stay in the moment. You might silently say "Here" as you step with one foot and "Now" as you step with the other. This reinforces your intention to stay present.

REMEMBER

Don't worry if your thoughts wander — that's natural! Each time you return to the present, you strengthen your mindfulness. Over time, staying present during walking becomes easier.

Integrating mindful walking into your daily life

Mindful walking is something you can practice anytime you're heading somewhere on foot. It's a chance to really pay attention to what's happening inside you while staying present with your environment. You can also set aside dedicated time for an intentional, mindful walk. Maybe take a walk right after dinner to relax and unwind, or, if possible, walk home from work to let go of the day's stress before you step into your home. If your schedule allows, try a midday lunch break walk to recharge.

TIP

Leave your cell phone at home or in your car to avoid the tempting distractions of technology.

Discovering Sitting Meditation

Sitting meditation can be challenging for many people. It may feel uncomfortable to sit for a period of time, or you might be tempted to give up the moment you start "overthinking." But once you realize that there's no right or wrong way to meditate, you can take the pressure off yourself.

TIP

Start small, maybe sitting for just five minutes a day, and allow your mind to fill with thoughts — it's completely natural. Over time, as you keep practicing, you'll start to notice that you feel less attached to these thoughts. With even more time, you may find that there's more space between them.

Steps for sitting meditation

You can engage in sitting mediation by following just a few steps:

1. **Find a quiet space.**

   Choose a space free from distractions if possible. This will help you focus and settle into your practice.

2. **Sit comfortably.**

   Find a seat that you can maintain, but remember that it's okay to shift if you need to. Many people like to sit cross-legged, but you can also extend your legs out in front of you, or sit in a chair. Support your back unless you can sit upright comfortably.

3. **Align your posture.**

   You don't need to sit perfectly straight, but aim to keep your head aligned over your heart, and your heart over your hips. This helps keep your breath full and flowing. Let your natural curves guide your posture; there's no need to be rigid.

4. **Set a timer.**

   Use a timer or casually check the time every so often. Maintain a consistent practice to build a habit. Experiment with different times of the day to see what feels best, but eventually aim to stick with a regular time. I meditate first thing in the morning, around 6 a.m., and again around 2 p.m. My morning meditation is almost always right after I wake up.

5. **Focus on your breath.**

   With each out-breath, consciously release any mental and physical tension. This will help you settle deeper into the meditation.

Techniques for maintaining focus and posture

You don't need to sit rigidly when meditating. Find a posture that feels relaxed and supportive. Many people mistakenly think they need to be super straight and still, but the goal is to be comfortable and at ease while sitting.

If you don't typically sit cross-legged, you might prefer sitting in a chair or on your couch. Let your feet relax on the floor, with your legs uncrossed, and rest your hands in your lap or by your sides. A blanket under your hips or behind your back can add extra support.

If you're sitting on the floor, feel free to rest against a wall for support. And remember, you can even lie down for meditation if that feels best.

TIP

If you start to doze off or feel your head dropping forward, gently bring your head back and reconnect with your breath to refresh yourself. Focus will naturally come and go; the more you try to control it, the harder it becomes to stay present. Return to your breath, your mantra, or whatever technique you're using, and stay nonchalant about it. The more easygoing you can be, the more likely you are to stick with your practice and go deeper in your meditations.

How sitting meditation complements other somatic exercises

Sitting meditation pairs beautifully with other somatic exercises. When you establish a regular meditation practice, you start to develop a deeper awareness of your body and mind and how they relate to each other. This heightened awareness carries over into your somatic movement, helping you stay present and attuned.

You can start or end a somatic session with meditation. Meditation can also help you focus before you begin moving or serve as a check-in with yourself after you've finished. This heightened awareness isn't limited to your meditation — it carries over into your somatic movement, helping you stay present, centered, and fully engaged with each motion.

You can integrate sitting meditation into other somatic exercises at various points in your movement:

>> **Use meditation to set an intention:** Before starting a somatic session, spend a few minutes in meditation to center yourself and set an intention. This intention could be something as simple as staying present, moving with awareness, or listening to your body's signals. By focusing on your intention, you give your practice a sense of purpose.

>> **Check in with your body:** After meditating, take a moment to scan your body and notice how it feels. Are there areas of tension, fatigue, or ease? This check-in can guide you to adjust your somatic practice based on what your body needs most that day.

>> **Combine breath awareness with movement:** During somatic exercises like yoga or Pilates, bring the breath awareness from your meditation into each movement. Matching your breath with each motion helps you stay present and connected, enhancing the mind-body connection.

>> **End with meditation to absorb the benefits:** After finishing a somatic session, sit for a few minutes in meditation to absorb the effects of your movement. Reflect on how your body feels now compared to before and allow yourself to fully rest in that relaxed, post-exercise state.

Using Meditation for Mindfulness and Focus

Meditation is also an incredible tool for improving focus. Through daily meditation, you train your mind to stay focused on a single point of concentration. Each time you meditate, you're strengthening your brain's ability to stay present, letting go of distractions, and focusing on the task at hand. Meditation reminds you to live fully in each moment, helping you appreciate what's happening right now. After all, if you miss this moment, you're missing out on your life.

I'll admit that I still get easily distracted, even after 20-plus years of meditating. We live in a world full of distractions. You can open endless tabs on your computer or scroll through social media, jumping from cooking videos to cute cats in seconds. Meditation offers a calm space amid all this digital chaos. It helps you become more intentional, so even if you do get pulled into a cute animal video, you're aware of what you're doing and (hopefully) set a time limit. As you learn to focus in your daily meditation, that focus becomes easier to find in your daily life.

TIP

Give it at least two months of daily practice, ideally 5 to 20 minutes a day, to start seeing real changes. After 45-60 days, you may notice measurable effects on your focus and attention.

Developing concentration through meditation

Research on meditation shows that it can actually change your brain, affecting both its structure and function. Meditation increases tissue in the anterior cingulate cortex, an area involved in attention and impulse control. It also strengthens the brain's neural circuitry for concentration and focus, and increases stability in the *ventral posteromedial cortex* (vPMC) — the part of the brain linked to mind-wandering. With time, this stability helps rein in wandering thoughts, leading to better focus.

In yoga, we often talk about *ekagrata*, or "one-pointed concentration," which means focusing on a single point or object. This skill is useful in balancing postures like Tree Pose or Crow Pose, and it's just as valuable in meditation. By focusing on your breath or a mantra, you train your mind to quickly return to that anchor. With practice, your ability to concentrate sharpens.

Enhancing mindfulness in daily activities

Mindfulness doesn't have to stay on the meditation cushion; there are many ways to bring it into your daily life. Here are some simple techniques:

>> **Active listening:** When talking with someone, focus fully on what they're saying without planning your next response. Active listening anchors you in the moment and strengthens connections.

>> **Gratitude practice:** Reflect on what you're grateful for each day. Practicing gratitude can improve happiness, sleep, and even support your immune system, all while keeping you connected to the present moment.

» **Heartbeat awareness:** Place your hand on your heart, close your eyes, and feel its steady rhythm. This gentle focus brings you into the moment and soothes your nervous system.

» **Mindful breaks:** Build mini mindful breaks into your day. Check in with your posture, your breathing, or how you feel before and after meals. These quick pauses help you reset and reconnect with your body.

» **Mindful eating:** Try eating with your non-dominant hand. This small adjustment forces you to slow down and pay attention, making each bite more mindful.

» **Mindful technology use:** Be intentional with your screen time. Set do-not-disturb on your phone, limit social media to specific times, and create device-free zones in your home. Staying off devices while eating or spending time with loved ones can help you feel more connected. Try setting a timer to limit your time on devices.

» **Observing your surroundings:** See your daily life as an art gallery. Notice the details wherever you are, whether you're navigating without Google Maps or simply looking around. This fresh perspective brings a sense of curiosity and presence to everyday moments.

» **Pay attention to your thoughts:** Take moments to sit with your thoughts instead of zoning out with a screen. Be mindful of what comes up without trying to push it away. This practice enhances creativity, reduces stress, and deepens self-awareness.

» **Single-tasking:** Focus on one thing at a time. Avoid multitasking by closing unnecessary tabs or apps, and work through tasks step by step. You'll feel more productive and centered when you're fully engaged in one activity.

Feeling Calm and Collected: Inner Peace Practices

Inner peace may seem elusive in today's busy world, but with intentional practices, you can cultivate a sense of calm and balance within yourself. Inner peace doesn't come from avoiding life's challenges; it comes from learning to face them with resilience and grace. Through meditation, visualization, self-care, and mindfulness, you can train your mind to remain calm and collected, even in difficult moments. This section explores simple yet powerful techniques that can help you build a foundation of inner peace, so you feel more centered, clear-headed, and connected to yourself. Each of these practices is somatic in nature.

Meditation practices for cultivating inner peace

There are many meditation practices that can help you cultivate inner peace. As with all the techniques mentioned in this book, try several to find the ones that benefit you the most:

>> **Diaphragmatic breathing** is a powerful tool for activating your body's relaxation response. When you take a full inhalation, your body sends a signal to your brain to calm down. Then, with each exhalation, you release more tension, relaxing your nervous system. A long, complete exhale also reminds you to let go of stress and worries, leaving more room for inner peace. Turn to Chapter 4 to read more about how to perform diaphragmatic breathing.

>> **Gratitude** does wonders for calming the nervous system and releases dopamine and serotonin, two feel-good brain chemicals. For a simple gratitude meditation, close your eyes, focus on your breath, and think of something or someone you're grateful for. Silently say "thank you" as you bring these things to mind. You may even begin to feel grateful for yourself and the qualities you appreciate within.

>> *Metta* **meditation,** also called "lovingkindness meditation," is another powerful way to foster compassion and peacefulness. You start by thinking of someone you love, then someone neutral, then someone with whom you have difficulty, and finally, yourself. Silently repeat: "May you be safe, may you be happy, may you be healthy, may you be at ease." Then, extend the same wishes to yourself: "May I be safe, may I be happy, may I be healthy, may I be at ease."

>> **Peaceful fingers** is one of my favorites. Sit comfortably with your hands resting in your lap. Close your eyes or soften your gaze. Tap your thumb to the tip of your index (pointer) finger. As you tap, silently say the word "peace." Tap your thumb to your middle finger and say "begins." Tap your thumb to your ring finger and say "with." Finally, tap your thumb to your pinky and say "me." Together, the phrase becomes "Peace begins with me." I find myself tapping my fingers this way at random times throughout the day to feel calmer and to stay peaceful with myself and others.

>> **Self-care rituals** can also be grounding. Take time to care for yourself — soak in a warm bath, give yourself a foot rub, or set aside a few moments each day for a practice that brings you joy and relaxation. Self-love practices support peace and inner calm. See Figure 10-3.

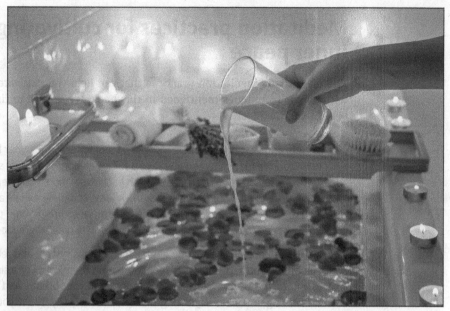

FIGURE 10-3:
Your self-care ritual may be simple or quite involved — whatever works!

Visualization techniques to reduce stress

Visualization is an effective way to reduce stress, alleviate anxiety, and boost your mood. Here are several visualization techniques to try:

» **Alleviating stress in the moment:** When stress flares up, close your eyes, take a few deep breaths, and imagine a calming scene. This could be anything that brings you peace — maybe you're lying in a field of flowers, watching a sunset, or floating on a pool raft. Envision the colors, sounds, and sensations around you to feel transported to that peaceful place.

» **Combining visualization with deep breathing:** Use deep breathing to enhance relaxation. As you inhale, imagine the breath entering through the soles of your feet, moving to the crown of your head. As you exhale, see the breath exiting from the crown back down through your feet. You might also visualize your breath as a color: Inhale a calming blue, exhale a stressful red.

» **Creating a favorable outcome:** Close your eyes and take a few deep breaths. Imagine the issue that's bothering you, but picture it as already resolved. Don't worry about how it was fixed; focus on how it feels now that it's done. Visualize the details — where you are, who's with you, and what you're doing as you feel the relief of resolution.

» **Guided imagery:** Guided imagery is especially useful for reducing your heart rate and stress. Listen to a guided visualization on YouTube or a meditation app. Often, you'll start with a blank slate and gradually build a calming scene. Relaxing your body and softening your eyes prepares you for the experience.

>> **Happy memory recall:** For a quick pick-me-up, close your eyes and bring a happy memory to mind. Focus on every detail: The sights, sounds, and feelings of that moment. You can stay with one memory or go through several. Recalling happy memories can be grounding and lift your mood immediately.

>> **Healing light visualization:** If you're feeling physical discomfort, close your eyes and visualize a healing light entering your body. Imagine it moving slowly, soothing and releasing any pain as it passes. Let the light linger over any areas that need extra care, and see the discomfort gradually leaving your body.

>> **Motivational visualization:** If you're feeling low-energy or overwhelmed, visualize yourself accomplishing a task with ease. Picture the space you're in, what you're doing, and how good you feel completing it. This visualization can be especially helpful before a somatic exercise or when you're tackling a challenging day.

>> **Sensory visualization:** Visualize a peaceful place you love. Close your eyes and think of five things you see, four things you hear, three things you can feel, two things you can smell, and one thing you can taste. For instance, if you're visualizing a park, imagine the trees swaying, birds chirping, the wind in your hair, the fresh smell of grass, and the taste of warm tea.

Throughout your day, build in small moments of mindfulness, such as practicing active listening at lunchtime or doing a quick body scan. In the evening, reflect on what you're grateful for, and consider winding down with a peaceful meditation, warm bath, or gentle yoga postures.

Progressive muscle relaxation

Progressive muscle relaxation (PMR) involves tensing and then releasing your muscles to relieve stress and anxiety. This practice increases awareness of where you hold tension, helping you recognize the contrast between tightness and relaxation. I prefer doing it while lying down, especially before final relaxation in yoga practice or before bedtime to alleviate stress, but PMR is a great way to relax before seated meditation, helping you let go of "the wiggles" and settle into stillness.

To practice PMR, follow these steps:

1. **Lie or sit down comfortably.**

2. **Start by tensing your feet for a few seconds, then release.**

3. **Gradually move upward, tensing each muscle group for a few seconds before releasing.**

4. **Finish with your face and take a moment to notice the overall sense of relaxation.**

5. **After you've finished with each muscle group, allow yourself a few moments of stillness to enjoy the calm.**

TIP

For added variety, try PMR in different ways: Start with the right side of your body, then move to the left. Or, focus on the front of your body first, then the back. As you tense each muscle, don't strain; think of it like squeezing a stress ball and then letting go. Be sure to focus on the release, noticing how the tension melts away each time you relax.

IN THIS CHAPTER

» **Using the Alexander Technique to keep your body balanced**

» **Examining how small movements matter with Body-Mind Centering**

» **Discovering the value of gentle motion with the Feldenkrais Method**

» **Categorizing movement with Laban Movement Analysis**

» **Leveraging light touch with the Trager Approach**

» **Growing with Continuum Movement**

Chapter **11**

Uncovering Advanced Techniques

A dvanced doesn't mean complicated here — it means refined and focused. Some techniques use hands-on guidance to help you feel subtle shifts in posture and alignment. Others invite you to play with movement through different intensities and flows, exploring contrasts like the difference between a whisper and a shout, or between floating and grounding.

Keeping an open mind is key as you explore these techniques. Some may feel like a perfect fit; others might challenge you in new ways. That's all part of the journey! Whether you're aiming for improved flexibility, effortless movement, or simply a deeper connection with your body, each of these advanced practices offers something valuable. Each approach opens a unique "entry point" into your body's wisdom and potential, letting you go beyond the basics and discover what it truly means to move with awareness and ease.

All of the practices covered in this chapter help you unlock new layers of aware-ness and freedom in your body. Somatic practices are about so much more than just physical exercise — they're tools for self-discovery, growth, and a little self-care along the way.

The Alexander Technique

I start this chapter with the Alexander Technique (AT) — a method I first encoun-tered as an acting major at New York University. My fabulous teacher, Joanne, used vivid imagery, like "hot honey melting down our spine or legs," to help us let go of tension and feel our muscles soften. She had us work in pairs, one of us lying on our back while the other gently repositioned our bones, finding that sweet spot of alignment. The Alexander Technique opens the door to lighter, more mindful movement, where each gesture feels effortless and intentional.

Frederick Matthias Alexander, a Shakespearean actor who lost his voice while performing, created this technique. He discovered that his voice loss was due to poor posture, which caused him to contract his neck muscles too much. As an act-ing student, my classmates and I studied the Alexander Technique to help us stop tensing our muscles and relax more on stage, making us more available for movement and speech.

AT involves gentle hands-on contact as well as spoken guidance. In my classes, we would listen to our teacher guiding us in how to move, while a fellow student gently manipulated us into proper alignment without any tension. You'll also learn to move your body lightly and economically. Often, you tense more muscles than you need to perform a simple task. Try picking up a spoon without tensing your shoulder or clenching your jaw, for example. I remember practicing getting up out of a chair repeatedly, trying to use as little muscle as needed to stand.

Through AT, you also learn to minimize interference between your neck, head, and back, and to recognize and change habits that impact your movement and posture. Practicing AT can help alleviate back pain, neck aches, sore shoulders, repetitive strain injuries, breathing problems, voice loss, and even sleep disorders.

Principles of the Alexander Technique

The main principle of AT is to allow your skeleton to rest in its natural position, whether you're standing, sitting, or lying down. When your skeleton is in its nat-ural alignment, your muscles can do their job more efficiently. AT principles guide you toward greater physical performance and well-being by re-educating your movement patterns and increasing mindfulness through:

» **Awareness:** You develop a refined awareness of your body and your environment, noticing subtle movements and shifts.

» **Direction:** You practice sending clear messages from your brain to your body, making movement intentional and efficient.

» **End-gaining:** Instead of pushing for results, you learn to take a balanced, reasonable approach, using only the necessary amount of effort.

» **Habitual tension:** Over time, you become more aware of patterns of tension and misuse that interfere with natural movement.

» **Inhibition:** AT helps you recognize habitual movements and teaches you how to change them consciously.

» **Mind-body connection:** AT emphasizes that your mind and body are deeply connected, each influencing the other.

Benefits for posture and movement efficiency

AT offers a range of benefits for your posture and movement efficiency, including:

» **Enhanced coordination and balance:** Proper alignment improves your stability and coordination.

» **Efficient movement patterns:** You learn to move with greater awareness and minimal effort, bringing grace and fluidity to daily tasks.

» **Hands-on guidance:** Working with a professional AT teacher provides hands-on corrections, allowing you to feel and embody proper alignment.

» **Improved postural awareness:** By focusing on the head-neck relationship, you recognize and adjust habits like slouching, forward head posture, and neck strain.

» **Mental repatterning:** As you reinforce the mind-body connection, you start to address harmful habits and repattern your movement in meaningful ways.

» **Pain management:** Addressing postural imbalances helps alleviate discomfort in areas like the head, neck, and shoulders.

» **Proprioceptive awareness:** AT sharpens your sense of where your body is in space, helping you better recognize tension and movement.

» **Reduced muscle tension:** Releasing unnecessary tension, especially in your neck and shoulders, leads to a more balanced, relaxed posture.

Integrating AT exercises into your daily life

This section explains some simple yet powerful exercises to incorporate AT principles into your everyday routine.

REMEMBER

With the Alexander Technique, you focus on economical movement, using only the energy and effort required to accomplish each task. As you practice these exercises, you'll notice a shift in your postural habits and a greater sense of ease and efficiency in your movements.

Constructive Rest

Constructive Rest is ideal for tuning into your body and creating a sense of ease before or after any physical activity. It's also a great way to reset during the day, giving your body a break from habitual tension patterns. Follow these steps:

1. **Lie down on the floor with a stack of books or a yoga block under your head.**

2. **Bend your knees and place your feet flat and wider than hip-width.**

3. **Let your knees drop gently toward each other.**

4. **Rest your hands on your abdomen or by your sides, palms facing up.**

5. **Breathe naturally, allowing your body to settle into the floor.**

    See Figure 11-1.

6. **Notice any areas of tension or discomfort and imagine releasing those points of tightness at each exhale.**

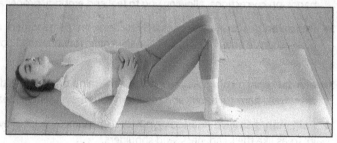

FIGURE 11-1:
The Constructive Rest position.

Photograph by Guen Egan

TIP

Use this position as a mini-meditation. Close your eyes and focus on your breath for five minutes to relieve stress and center yourself.

Standing up

This simple exercise can transform how you approach everyday movements. Practicing mindful standing helps you learn to rely on the right muscles and reduces strain, especially if you're prone to tensing unnecessarily when standing up. Practice this exercise every time you stand to become more mindful of your movements:

1. **Start from a seated position.**

2. **Release any tension in your neck and shoulders with shoulder or neck rolls.**

3. **Move your feet back slightly, hinge forward from your hips, and then stand up using only the muscle effort you truly need.**

4. **Feel the strength in your legs and the balance as you rise. Avoid clenching your jaw or tensing your upper body.**

TIP

Each time you stand up, imagine you're balancing something fragile on your head. This visualization helps you keep your spine aligned and rise gracefully without unnecessary muscle strain.

Fingertips rule

You can use this technique throughout the day to release hand tension and improve your posture, especially during activities that require repetitive hand movements, like typing, playing an instrument, or using a phone. The fingertips rule helps you stay aware of any unnecessary strain you might be holding in your hands, wrists, and arms, and reminds you to keep those areas relaxed as you work. Follow these steps:

1. **Stand with your hands at your side, keeping your shoulders and chest relaxed.**

2. **Imagine lifting only your fingertips without engaging your shoulders, chest, or back.**

3. **Focus on the sensation of lifting from the bones in your fingers and hands, rather than involving larger muscles.**

4. **As you lift, notice how your posture aligns naturally when you engage your fingers delicately instead of tightening your upper body.**

TIP

Try this exercise before starting any activity that requires fine motor skills or hand precision. You may find that keeping your fingers relaxed enhances your focus and dexterity.

Whispered "ahh"

The whispered "ahh" can be a quick reset whenever you feel stressed or tense. It's especially helpful if you tend to hold tension in your voice or throat. As you practice this, notice if the sound helps you feel more present and calm. Repeat a few times until you feel a noticeable release:

1. Sit comfortably, keeping your back straight but relaxed.

2. Gently inhale through your nose, filling your lungs without strain.

3. On the exhale, release a soft, whispered "ahh" sound, letting your breath flow out slowly and steadily.

4. Imagine that you're letting go of any tension with each "ahh," allowing your jaw, neck, and shoulders to relax further.

TIP Use this exercise before any activity that requires focus or calm, like giving a presentation, practicing yoga, or simply unwinding at the end of a long day.

Body-Mind Centering

Body-Mind Centering (BMC) is similar to the Alexander Technique in that it helps you improve your movement and body awareness. BMC deepens your understanding of how the body's smallest movements connect to their larger expression through movement, voice, touch, and consciousness. This approach promotes a greater sense of balance, coordination, and ease in all kinds of movement, from yoga and dance to everyday activities.

Bonnie Bainbridge Cohen, a renowned movement educator, occupational therapist, and pioneer of somatic movement, created Body-Mind Centering by developing a process of repatterning the body through a unique language that describes the connection between body and mind.

Exploring the body-mind connection

BMC explores the mind-body connection by bringing awareness to different tissues, breathing, vocalization, and embodiment:

>> **Breathing:** BMC emphasizes the influence of both physiological and psychological states on your breath. As you become more aware of your breath, you can begin to deepen it, exploring the impact on your behavior and physical functioning. To connect with your breath, focus on each inhale and exhale,

feel your breath moving from your center, and notice the way it influences your entire body.

>> **Embodiment:** In BMC, embodiment is the process of experiencing your body's systems from the inside out. You move beyond thinking about your body and simply allow yourself to "be" in your body. Imagine your head softening, your heart listening, and your entire being grounded in presence.

>> **Identifying Tissues:** BMC explores how different types of tissues contribute to movement and mind-body connection. There are four primary types of tissues:

- **Epithelial:** Covers surfaces in your body, including skin. Focus on sensations of touch, texture, and boundaries.

- **Connective:** Includes bone, cartilage, tendons, and ligaments. Explore qualities of flexibility and stability within these structures.

- **Muscular:** Comprises skeletal, smooth, and cardiac muscles. Experiment with different types of muscle contractions and their impact on movement.

- **Nervous:** Forms the brain, spinal cord, and nerves. Notice how the nervous system affects movement patterns in your body.

>> **Voice:** BMC uses the qualities of your voice as a channel between your conscious and subconscious. Try becoming more aware of your vocal structures and how they resonate through your body. Explore connections like the link between your pelvis and vocal mechanisms, which can empower your voice, or the way your hands move as you speak.

Techniques to enhance body awareness

To develop body awareness in BMC, you can practice a variety of techniques:

>> **Body scanning:** Lie down or sit comfortably. Close your eyes and mentally scan your body, noticing each part in sequence from head to toe. Observe sensations like warmth, tension, or lightness, without judgment. This helps you connect with each part of your body and brings attention to any areas of tension or relaxation.

>> **Mindful movement:** Move with intention, keeping your attention focused on each action. For example, if you're walking, notice the sensation of each foot touching the ground, the movement of your legs, and the balance of your body. This technique cultivates a heightened awareness of how each part of your body interacts with the world.

>> **Proprioceptive exercises:** Practice exercises that heighten your sense of where your body is in space. For instance, close your eyes and slowly lift one arm, sensing its position without looking. This builds spatial awareness and helps refine coordination.

>> **Revisiting developmental movements:** Explore movement patterns from infancy to adulthood, such as rolling, crawling, and walking. These foundational movements remind your body of its natural developmental pathways and increase ease in movement.

>> **Voice exploration:** Experiment with vocal sounds, noticing how different tones resonate through your body. For example, try making a deep "mmm" sound and feeling the vibration in your chest, or a higher "eee" sound and noticing its impact on your head and neck. This exploration enhances awareness of how your voice is linked to your physical and emotional state.

Applications for improving coordination and balance

BMC offers practical ways to improve balance and coordination:

>> **Cultivating ease in movement:** BMC encourages you to let go of tension and release holding patterns in the body, which allows for greater freedom, especially in the spine. Releasing unnecessary holding improves balance and stability, letting your body move in a more integrated way.

>> **Developing touch awareness:** Touch plays a key role in BMC and can create trust and connection. Holding your own hand or having someone place a hand on your shoulder can provide immediate centering and comfort. Use touch to enhance your awareness of grounding and presence.

>> **Observing mind-body shifts:** Notice how mental states impact your body's movements. For example, balancing can feel more challenging when you're distracted, while focusing your mind often enhances stability. BMC helps you tune in to how your mind affects physical actions, so you can find ease in movement even during moments of mental stress.

The Feldenkrais Method

Developed by Moshé Feldenkrais, the Feldenkrais Method is a somatic practice that uses gentle movement and awareness to help you improve your movement and function. Through this method, you become more aware of habitual movement patterns and areas where you store tension, allowing you to develop new, healthier ways of moving.

Fundamentals of the Feldenkrais Method

The Feldenkrais Method is rooted in the idea that awareness and gentle, intentional movement can improve not only how you move but also how you think, feel, and function. Its core focus is on enhancing your self-awareness in order to replace habitual movement patterns with healthier, more efficient ones. Feldenkrais draws on principles of physics, biomechanics, motor development, psychology, and learning theory. This method has two primary approaches:

>> **Awareness Through Movement (ATM):** In a group setting, a teacher guides you through movements using verbal instructions.

>> **Functional Integration (FI):** In a one-on-one session, an instructor uses gentle, hands-on guidance along with verbal cues to help you experience more comfortable and efficient movement.

Feldenkrais also builds on several other key principles:

>> **Gentle, non-goal-oriented approach:** Unlike many forms of exercise, the Feldenkrais Method doesn't aim for specific fitness or flexibility goals. Instead, it focuses on learning and self-discovery. You aren't trying to "achieve" a certain range of motion or "correct" a posture. Instead, you're encouraged to notice what feels natural and how you can move with less effort.

>> **Small, gradual movements:** Feldenkrais emphasizes tiny, incremental movements to help you become more sensitive to subtle differences in muscle engagement and joint alignment. By moving slowly, you bypass habitual movement patterns and awaken your nervous system to new options for movement.

>> **Mind-body connection:** The Feldenkrais Method fosters a deep connection between mind and body. As you focus on the sensations of each movement, you create new neural pathways and expand your movement "vocabulary." Over time, this awareness transforms not only your movement but also your posture, balance, and emotional responses.

>> **Learning by exploration:** The Feldenkrais Method is built on curiosity and exploration rather than repetition or effort. By encouraging you to explore how you can move in ways that feel pleasant and unforced, Feldenkrais allows you to rediscover the joy of natural movement and deepen your connection with your body.

Benefits for flexibility and mobility

Practicing the Feldenkrais Method offers many benefits for flexibility, mobility, and overall well-being. By becoming more aware of how you move, you can open up tight areas and find a better balance in your musculature and experience other impacts:

>> **Enhanced breathing:** Feldenkrais helps you breathe more deeply and freely, creating more space and movement throughout your body. As you learn to relax into your breath, you may find that it brings more freedom and ease to your whole system.

>> **Improved posture:** With Feldenkrais, you retrain your nervous system to move more efficiently, which reduces strain and enhances your alignment. Over time, this method helps you carry yourself with less effort and greater ease.

>> **Increased coordination:** The slow, deliberate movements in Feldenkrais improve your coordination and allow you to move through daily tasks with more balance and control.

>> **Joint health:** The gentle approach of Feldenkrais minimizes strain on your joints and soft tissue. You get to explore your full range of motion without overstretching or risking injury, which helps keep your joints healthy.

>> **Pain management and faster recovery:** Feldenkrais can help you manage pain, reduce stress and anxiety, and support quicker recovery from injuries. By moving mindfully, you create a path to feeling better and bouncing back faster.

>> **Stress relief:** Engaging in these gentle, mindful movements can lower your stress levels, allowing your body and mind to relax more deeply. As you connect with your movements, you'll likely feel a sense of calm and centeredness that stays with you.

TIP

By connecting with subtle movements, you build a foundation for lasting change in your physical and mental well-being.

Sample exercises to incorporate into your routine

When you practice Feldenkrais movement lessons, remember to use slow and gentle movements, paying attention to how your body feels. Experiment with different variations and always listen to your body:

>> **Arm lifts with awareness:** Lie on your back and slowly lift one arm straight up toward the ceiling. Observe the movement in your shoulder and notice the subtle adjustments your body makes as you lift. Lower your arm down gently and repeat on the other side. Try this a few times, becoming more mindful of each lift.

>> **Head nods with subtle variations:** Gently nod your head forward and back, then side to side, exploring the range of motion in your neck. This is a simple exercise you can do throughout the day to release tension and improve neck mobility.

>> **Knee to chest with gentle rotation:** Lie on your back, bring one knee to your chest, and gently rotate your leg in and out. Explore the range of motion in your hip joint, then try making small circles with the leg. Repeat on the other side.

>> **Pelvic tilts with breath:** Sit comfortably on the floor or a stool. Slowly rock your pelvis back and forth, coordinating the movement with your breath — inhaling as you rock forward and exhaling as you rock back. Notice any sensations this creates and try to release tension as you move.

>> **Spinal undulations lying down:** Lie on your back and roll your spine gently from side to side, creating a wave-like motion. Feel the movement ripple through your spine and observe how your breath changes. Move slowly to keep your attention on each vertebra.

>> **Walking with focused steps:** As you walk, focus on each step, noticing how your feet connect with the ground and how your weight shifts. This exercise is similar to mindful walking and helps you stay attuned to subtle shifts in your body as you move.

REMEMBER

Each Feldenkrais movement is an opportunity to connect more deeply with yourself. Through these simple exercises, you may notice subtle changes in your physical and mental state, feeling more grounded and comfortable in your own body.

Laban Movement Analysis (LMA)

Another pioneer in the somatic movement world was Rudolf Laban, a choreographer and dance theorist known for creating Laban Movement Analysis (LMA). LMA is a comprehensive method for describing, interpreting, and documenting human movement. It breaks down movement into distinct categories to help people gain a deeper understanding of their physical expression, habitual patterns, and body mechanics. It's widely used in dance education, dance therapy, theater training, and even everyday movement analysis.

The beauty of LMA lies in its ability to break down movements into their simplest forms, helping performers and individuals explore these basic movements and connect with their inner impulses.

REMEMBER

This framework lets you better understand how you use your body and how you express emotions through movement — one reason it's so popular among dancers and actors.

Understanding the elements of LMA

LMA is based on four main categories, known as BESS:

>> **Body:** This category focuses on how different body parts connect and influence each other during movement. Body analysis describes the physical and structural characteristics of your body as it moves, considering which parts are active, how they move in relation to each other, and how each part contributes to the movement as a whole.

>> **Effort:** Effort describes the dynamic qualities of movement and can reflect texture, energy, and inner attitude. It's broken down into four elements, each with two opposing qualities:

- **Weight:** Strong or light

- **Time:** Sudden or sustained

- **Space:** Direct or indirect

- **Flow:** Bound or free

Combining these elements creates eight unique types of movement, such as "dab" (direct, quick, light, and bound), "float" (indirect, sustained, light, and free), "punch" (direct, quick, heavy, and bound), and more. Each type of effort brings out different qualities in movement, allowing you to explore a range of expressions, from fluid and graceful to sharp and intense.

>> **Shape:** Shape describes how your body forms and changes shape in space. It includes:

- **Shape forms:** The basic forms your body creates, whether stationary or in motion.

- **Shape qualities:** How your body changes shape over time.

- **Modes of shape change:** How your body interacts with the environment, adapting and flowing to support movement.

>> **Space:** Space is the dimension in which movement occurs and includes your relationship with the area around you. LMA divides the body's movement possibilities into 27 points and multiple zones for spatial exploration. It also incorporates directions (such as high/low, forward/back, and right/left) and pathways (such as curvy, straight, and circular) to describe where movement is happening. Words like "over," "under," "around," and "toward" also define how the body moves in space.

Using LMA to analyze and improve movement patterns

LMA provides a detailed approach to understanding and refining movement. By observing and analyzing the elements of Body, Effort, Shape, and Space, you gain a clearer picture of how you move and where improvements can be made.

TIP

For example, if you observe someone sitting down using LMA, you might examine how they position their body, the quality of their effort, their relationship to the space around them, and the shape they create as they sit. This analysis helps identify any tension or inefficiencies in movement. Through this kind of observation, you can adjust certain patterns to develop more balanced, coordinated, and intentional movements.

Practical applications for dance and physical therapy

Laban Movement Analysis is a valuable tool not only for dancers and performers but also for individuals in physical therapy and dance movement therapy.

>> **Dance and theater:** LMA enables dancers and actors to explore nuanced movement qualities, articulate emotions through movement, and express complex inner states physically. Dance therapists use LMA to observe how clients' movements reflect their emotional states, helping them track change and engage in non-verbal communication. By identifying subtle movement shifts, LMA supports emotional expression and therapeutic progress.

>> **Physical therapy:** In physical therapy, LMA can help you correct dysfunctional movement patterns by teaching you to move in functional and pain-free ways. For example, something as simple as lifting your arm can be analyzed to reduce strain or unnecessary tension, creating more ease in daily movements. Each person's movement patterns are unique, and LMA allows therapists to understand individual needs, helping clients develop more efficient, expressive, and sustainable ways of moving.

For more about Laban Movement Analysis, visit https://labaninternational.org/.

The Trager Approach

Somatic pioneer Milton Trager developed the Trager Approach, a physical therapy technique that uses gentle movements and light touch to support mental and physical health. Trager began exploring this approach when he was only 18 years old, starting by giving his boxing coach a massage and noticing how his touch could bring relief and relaxation. Over the next 65 years, he continued to evolve his method. The Trager Approach can help you:

>> Release tight muscles

>> Increase joint mobility

>> Let go of physical and mental patterns that no longer serve you

Trager based his approach on the idea that physical change follows a change in mindset. He believed that by shifting mental patterns, you could create physical change, allowing your body to move with more freedom and ease. Trager designed his approach to support natural, effortless movement.

The Trager Approach includes two main components: Tablework and Mentastics:

>> During *Tablework*, you lie on a padded table, and a practitioner guides your body through gentle compressions, rocking, swinging, and lifting movements. These rhythmic motions encourage your body to relax and feel lighter, often helping to reduce back pain, neck pain, and tension. Tablework sessions, which typically last 60-90 minutes, provide a passive experience, where you're moved and guided by a practitioner. You lie comfortably while gentle movements help you feel as though you can move freely without effort.

>> After Tablework, practitioners often teach *Mentastics* — simple, playful movements you perform on your own to carry the feeling of ease and freedom into your daily life. Mentastics can be done anytime and are adaptable to fit your needs, reinforcing the relaxation and mobility you experience during Tablework.

Principles of the Trager Approach

Whether you're lying passively on the table or practicing Mentastics on your own, the Trager Approach encourages you to release physical and mental patterns that may have developed from trauma, accidents, or illness, helping you feel more comfortable and at home in your body. The Trager Approach relies on several key principles that create a supportive, safe, and healing experience:

>> **Awareness:** Trager emphasizes awareness. You stay in tune with how each movement feels and communicate what you're experiencing in the moment. This awareness develops both during Tablework and Mentastics, helping you become more attuned to the sensations in your body.

>> **Client comfort:** Throughout your session, you should feel completely comfortable. Practitioners guide you through gentle, non-intrusive, and effortless movements, without any forced actions or strain. You stay fully clothed, and practitioners don't use any oils or lotions, allowing you to feel safe and at ease.

>> **Client involvement:** Even when you're lying on the table, you actively participate in the session. Practitioners move your body in ways that mimic natural movement, helping you experience the sensation of moving effortlessly and freely.

>> **Hook-up:** Before each session, the practitioner takes a moment to enter a meditative state known as "hook-up." This is a deep presence and awareness that the practitioner gets into before working with a client. In this meditative state, they can be more fully in tune with the client's body and connect with them in a calm, grounded way.

>> **Soft hands:** Practitioners use a soft, gentle touch to guide each movement. This touch communicates ease and release, without any sense of force or pressure. By using soft hands, they help you let go of deep-seated physical and mental patterns, allowing your body to relax fully.

>> **Subtle breaks in contact:** Practitioners periodically release contact, letting you feel the contrast between guided movement and your own sense of balance. This shift reinforces the benefits of the session and encourages you to experience independence in movement.

Techniques for releasing tension and improving movement

Milton Trager understood how gentle, rhythmic movement, performed with great sensitivity, could create positive, long-term changes. The Trager Approach has a

Zen-like quality, relying on soft, subtle movement that effectively releases tension and improves ease of movement. During a Trager session, you reeducate your nervous system to move with less effort while promoting a sense of playfulness in your body. By releasing tension in your muscles and joints, the Trager Approach increases your range of motion and guides you into a deeply relaxed state.

TIP

Use this method to gain better awareness of your movement patterns and identify and release tension with ease through techniques like the following:

>> **Compression and elongation:** The practitioner gently compresses and then elongates your muscles, releasing bound-up tension. This movement feels similar to kneading dough and creates a sense of spaciousness and relaxation.

>> **Gentle touch and pressure:** The practitioner uses mindful, light touch to locate areas of tension and applies pressure only as needed. Unlike deep tissue massage, which can be intense, Trager remains soft and comfortable throughout.

>> **Gravity-assisted movements:** Using your own bodyweight, these movements gently release tension and stretch muscles, allowing your body to relax and open up naturally.

>> **Rhythmic rocking and swaying:** Like the soothing motion used to calm a baby, these rhythmic, rocking movements help release deep-seated tension and stimulate the nervous system. The gentle swaying brings about a profound sense of relaxation.

>> **Shimmering:** This oscillating movement is applied to the skin, helping you feel more freedom and ease. Shimmering releases tension on a deeper level, allowing you to move with less restriction.

Incorporating Trager principles into your somatic practice

Building on the core principles of the Trager Approach, you can integrate these techniques into your own practice to enhance body awareness, ease, and fluidity in movement. By embracing Trager's playful, mindful exploration, you foster a deeper connection with your body and support lasting physical and mental relaxation.

Here are some ways to incorporate Trager principles into your routine:

>> **Engage in Mentastics exercises:** Mentastics are self-guided, playful movements that you can perform while sitting, standing, or lying down. These dance-like exercises help you cultivate awareness and grace, encouraging fluid, unrestricted movement.

>> **Experiment with light touch:** Following the principle of "soft hands," use a gentle, relaxed touch when moving your own body, such as your hands or shoulders. This playful contact helps you release tension without force, inviting a sense of lightness and relaxation.

>> **Practice body scans:** Periodically scan your body, noticing areas of tension and allowing yourself to release them. This gentle awareness encourages a calm, relaxed state and reinforces the Trager principle of moving with ease.

>> **Reconnect with your presence:** Like the practitioner's "hook-up" before a session, take a moment to ground yourself before any activity. A few deep breaths help you establish a calm, present state that enhances mindful, relaxed movement.

>> **Try gentle bouncing:** Stand comfortably and allow your body to perform a light bounce, feeling the up-and-down rhythm through your ankles, knees, hips, and shoulders. This rhythmic movement helps release tension and echoes the calming effects of the Trager Approach.

TIP

Integrate these principles into your life to help your body move with greater ease, less tension, and a natural sense of flow.

Continuum Movement

Continuum Movement is a somatic practice that uses breathwork, mindfulness, sensory awareness, and a range of fluid movements to promote healing, growth, and creativity. Emilie Conrad, the founder of Continuum, created this approach to help individuals improve their range of motion, sense of connection, well-being, and spiritual awareness. Continuum taps into the body's natural rhythms, inviting you to explore different states of being through what Conrad called "dives" — structured sequences that involve breath, sound, and spontaneous movement.

In Continuum, you work with three "anatomies" — primordial, cultural, and cosmic — which represent different lenses to explore states of being within yourself. You also practice two core concepts known as *baseline* and *open attention*. Baseline refers to a grounded, present state of awareness, while open attention is a nonjudgmental focus on sensory experiences.

TIP

Use these frameworks together to encourage yourself to slow down, connect with your breath, and release tension, allowing you to experience yourself as fluid and adaptable.

Fundamentals of Continuum Movement

You can practice Continuum solo or with a group. Dives often start with you lying down, focusing on your breath, and creating sound to stimulate movement from within. You pause frequently to let each sound and movement settle, allowing yourself to "be" rather than "do." As Emilie Conrad famously said, "Movement is not something we do; it is what we are."

Continuum Movement involves various techniques that connect you more deeply to your body:

» **Breath:** Breath serves as the origin of all movement in Continuum. By exploring different breathing techniques, you stimulate internal sensations and heighten your connection to your physical self.

» **Innovation:** Continuum encourages you to stay open to adaptability and creativity. You're constantly discovering new ways to move and experience your body's potential.

» **Movement:** Movements in Continuum are fluid and exploratory, designed to awaken your body's natural rhythms. This approach promotes flexibility, adaptability, and resilience.

» **Sensation:** Continuum helps you tune into subtle sensations, allowing you to "wake up" new areas of your body and tap into a sense of vitality and life force.

» **Sound:** Sound is a key component that eases mobility and releases stress. By vocalizing sounds that resonate through your body, you can access deeper levels of relaxation and self-awareness.

Benefits of fluidity and adaptability

Continuum Movement provides numerous benefits that enhance physical and emotional resilience:

» **Connection and well-being:** By tuning into your body through breath, sound, and movement, you build a stronger sense of trust in yourself. This practice encourages ongoing growth, learning, and emotional healing.

>> **Creativity and exploration:** Continuum invites you to explore new perspectives and embrace a sense of curiosity. The practice of open attention helps you approach life with adaptability and creativity.

>> **Deep relaxation:** Continuum's gentle, flowing movements support a state of relaxation, promoting ease in both body and mind. Practicing this flow encourages you to let go and adapt to life's natural rhythms.

>> **Fluidity in movement:** Through Continuum, you connect with the natural rhythms of your body, allowing you to experience movement as fluid, adaptable, and unrestricted.

>> **Spiritual and universal connection:** As you work with Continuum's principles, you may feel a greater sense of connection to all living things. Conrad likened Continuum's rhythms to the ebb and flow of ocean waves, encouraging you to feel your place within the larger universe.

Exercises to promote deeper body awareness

As you focus on sensation and movement, you may find that Continuum Movement fosters a deeper sense of ease, presence, and adaptability in all areas of your life. Practicing these exercises helps you connect with the fluidity of your body and brings you into a state of open awareness:

>> **Arm and Leg Waves:** Lie down and make slow, wave-like movements with your arms and legs, as though you're flowing through water. Pay attention to the sensations in your limbs, noticing any points of tension or ease.

>> **Body Scanning:** Tune into your body by mentally scanning from head to toe. Focus on sensations, paying attention to areas of tension, relaxation, or warmth, and allow yourself to experience each sensation fully without judgment.

>> **Joint Rotations:** Slowly rotate each joint, starting with your ankles and working up to your wrists, shoulders, and neck. Move in a way that feels natural and explore each joint's range of motion while noticing any restrictions or ease.

>> **Melting Exercises:** Practice letting gravity take over. Begin lying down and imagine your body gradually sinking into the ground, releasing any strain. This exercise helps you connect with the support of the Earth and encourages a deep release of tension.

>> **Pelvic Tilts:** Lie down with your knees bent and feet flat on the floor. Gently tilt your pelvis forward and backward, engaging your core muscles. Notice areas that feel stuck and those that feel more fluid. This movement can also be done seated or standing.

» **Spinal Undulations:** Roll through each vertebra of your spine in different directions. Try this movement standing, seated, or even in a Downward Dog position, paying attention to the sensations along your spine. See Figure 11-2.

» **Tensing and Releasing:** Begin by tensing one area of your body (for example, your feet), then release and notice the shift in sensation. Gradually work your way up the body, tensing and releasing different areas. You can do this exercise lying down, seated, or standing.

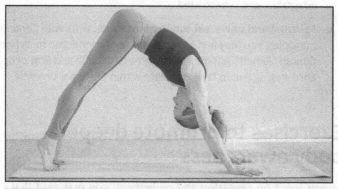

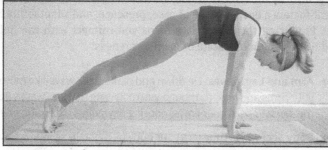

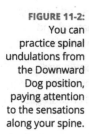

FIGURE 11-2:
You can practice spinal undulations from the Downward Dog position, paying attention to the sensations along your spine.

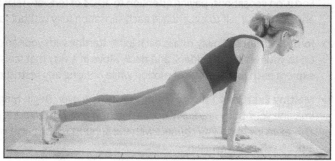

Photographs by Guen Egan

Staying Safe

Embarking on advanced somatic practices can be deeply rewarding, but it's essential to prioritize safety and listen to your body as you explore these techniques. It's important to set boundaries and listen to what your body is telling you in any atmosphere whether you're at home or working with a trained professional.

TIP

Before diving into these advanced practices, consider checking with your doctor. Creating a safe, supportive space allows you to move freely and feel prepared for any physical or emotional release that may arise as you explore deeper layers of your somatic journey.

Ensuring proper technique to prevent injury

When you begin somatic movement, understanding the correct technique is critical for preventing injury and making this a sustainable, lifelong practice. Begin with a trained instructor who can provide the knowledge and support you need, especially for advanced or nuanced movements. Professional guidance ensures you're building a solid foundation and allows you to gain the full benefit of each session. Once you feel more comfortable, try mixing instructor-led sessions with your own practice. For example, meeting with a professional once a week and supplementing with at-home practice a few more times each week is a great way to build confidence and skill.

Listening to your body's signals

Your body is your best guide. Pay close attention to sensations and signals that arise during somatic movement. If you're working with a professional, don't hesitate to communicate how you're feeling in the moment.

Somatic movement teaches you to tune into your body on a deeper level. This practice strengthens your intuition, enhances your ability to feel subtle cues, and promotes a sense of freedom and joy in movement. Remember, your body will always guide you in the right direction when you listen to what it's telling you.

TIP

Use advanced somatic practices to connect with your body's cues and responses and reach a deeper understanding of your needs.

Adjusting practices based on individual needs and limitations

Everybody is unique. Part of the journey in somatic movement is recognizing and honoring your individual needs and limitations. Keep these tips in mind:

>> **Focus on self-discovery, not results:** Somatic movement is a journey of self-discovery rather than a goal-oriented practice. Let go of the need to achieve specific outcomes, and instead focus on learning more about your body and its sensations. This awareness leads to a deeper, more fulfilling experience.

>> **Personalize your practice:** A trained instructor can adapt sessions to align with your unique profile, ensuring you're supported in a way that feels safe and beneficial. Adjustments may be necessary, and a good practitioner will help you modify movements to stay within your comfort zone.

Chapter **12**

Creating Somatic Flow Sequences

I magine moving through your day with a sense of ease, lightness, and connection to your body. Picture yourself feeling grounded in the morning, centered in the afternoon, and relaxed in the evening, with each part of your day anchored by a short, intentional sequence of somatic movements. Somatic flows are all about tuning in, letting go, and moving in ways that feel nourishing and natural for you.

But perhaps the most rewarding aspect of somatic flows is that they're a gift you give yourself — time to be present, to notice, and to connect. This practice is about honoring where you are right now and letting go of any expectations of "how it should look." Instead, you follow your body's signals and build flows that feel authentic and restorative. With time, you may even find yourself slipping into somatic flows throughout your day, bringing moments of calm and awareness to everyday routines.

Here, you get to play the role of both student and creator as you design your own somatic flows — gentle, purposeful movement sequences that can transform how you experience your body and mind. This isn't about rigid routines or strict exercise regimens; it's about exploring movements that feel good, support your intentions, and suit your unique needs. Whether you're looking for a quick energy boost, a moment of mindfulness, or a way to unwind, you'll learn how to build flows that meet you where you are.

In this chapter, you learn how to start from the basics: Setting your intentions, choosing movements that align with your goals, and sequencing exercises in a way that feels both logical and intuitive. You also explore how to adapt your flows for different times of day, experiment with various types of movement, and create smooth transitions that make each sequence feel cohesive and natural. Whether you're completely new to this practice or already familiar with its benefits, you're in the right place. This chapter guides you through each part of the process so you can confidently design flows that nurture your body, refresh your mind, and support your well-being.

Designing Your Own Flow

Creating your own flow sequences allows you to dive into your body's wisdom and creativity. As you experiment with movement, you'll discover how different flows can serve various purposes. Some flows might gently wake up your body in the morning, while others help you shake off tension after a long day. You may design short, simple flows to ground yourself before a busy meeting or flowing, expressive sequences that energize your entire body. The beauty of somatic flows is that they're fully customizable — designed by you, for you.

You are the creative director of your somatic experiences, able to design flows that feel right for you. Designing a somatic exercise flow starts with mindful awareness of your body.

REMEMBER

As you move, focus on how each part of your body feels, incorporating gentle, intentional movements. Breathwork plays a key role, helping you stay present and allowing each sensation to guide you in adapting the flow to meet your body's needs in the moment.

Think of somatic flows as a way to explore movements like contracting and relaxing muscles, rotating joints, and moving through different planes. Above all, listen to your body and move with ease. There's no need to push — this is about enjoying the process.

TIP

When designing your flow, keep these points in mind:

>> **Be patient with yourself:** Allow yourself to grow and learn through these practices. Somatic movement is an exploration — there's no right or wrong way to approach it.

>> **Choose an area to focus on:** Decide which area of your body to start with. Maybe your shoulders feel tight, or you'd like to begin with your spine. Choose a starting point that feels intuitive.

>> **Contract and release:** Engage in simple contractions and releases of your muscles. Notice the sensations as you tense and then relax each area.

>> **Explore micromovements:** Pay attention to the small, subtle movements in your joints. Try rolling your shoulders or circling your ankles, noticing each tiny shift.

>> **Flow between areas:** Move fluidly from one body part to another. Focus on smooth transitions and connect each movement with gentle intention.

>> **Get comfortable:** Find a space where you feel relaxed and consult a professional if you have any injuries or specific concerns.

>> **Integrate awareness:** Keep checking in with yourself as you move. Notice how each part of your body feels and how each movement affects the next.

>> **Link your breath with movement:** Coordinate each movement with your breath. This keeps you grounded and enhances the connection between your mind and body.

>> **Listen to your body:** If you feel any discomfort or strain, modify your movements. Use your breath to help you gauge if you're pushing too far.

>> **Scan your body:** Do a slow body scan from head to toe, noticing any areas of tension, discomfort, or pain. Let these observations guide you as you move.

>> **Start with grounding:** Begin by grounding yourself through deep breathing. Focus on your feet touching the floor or your seat connecting to the Earth below you. Notice the weight distribution and bring yourself fully into the present moment.

There are no rules to designing your flow — anything goes! Having that kind of freedom might inspire you, but it can also paralyze you. To get you started, try this simple flow as a warm-up or as a stand-alone practice:

1. **Ground yourself**.

   Stand with your feet hip-width apart. Feel your feet connecting with the ground. Notice your weight distribution and use your breath to anchor yourself.

2. **Begin with your neck and shoulders**.

   Let your head fall gently from side to side, then turn it right to left, and finally look up and down. Roll your shoulders back a few times, then forward. Pay attention to any tense spots and feel yourself relaxing.

3. **Move into your spine**.

   Rotate your trunk, keeping your hips stable. Try a few gentle twists in each direction. Then, move into a gentle arch and round of the spine, feeling each vertebra move. See Figure 12-1.

4. Engage your hips.

Make circular movements with your hips as if you're hula-hooping. Sway your hips from side to side, enjoying the sensation of releasing tension.

5. Focus on your legs.

Bend your knees slightly, as if taking mini squats. Then, roll each ankle in circles, tuning into any tension or tightness.

6. Finish with your arms.

Slowly raise your arms to the sides and up above your head. Notice any areas of tightness or ease. Lower your arms back to your sides and repeat a few times, moving slowly. See Figure 12-2.

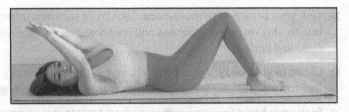

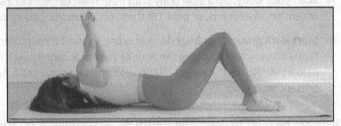

FIGURE 12-1: Gently rotate your trunk in both directions, keeping your hips stable.

Photograph by Guen Egan

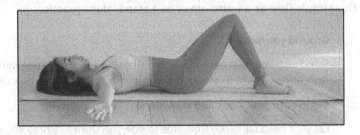

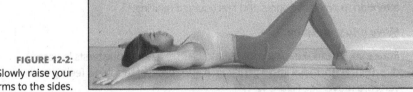

FIGURE 12-2: Slowly raise your arms to the sides.

Photograph by Guen Egan

Identifying personal goals and intentions

To identify your personal goals and intentions for somatic movement, begin by visualizing the life you desire. Close your eyes and create a vivid mental picture of your future self. This vision can be as near as a few months from now or as far as five years ahead. The key is to focus not on how you think you *should* be, but on how you *want* to feel in your body.

Try this visualization exercise:

1. **Imagine an ideal day in your future**.

   What does it look like? Are you moving freely, feeling strong and agile? Notice the activities that bring you joy and the people who surround you.

2. **Reflect on your values**.

   If time or money were no object, how would you spend your days? What activities or states of mind are most important to you?

3. **Identify your core feelings**.

   Do you want to feel more relaxed, energized, or resilient? Envision the sensations you want to cultivate in your body.

Allowing these questions to guide you can reveal meaningful personal goals and intentions for your somatic practice.

Setting realistic and achievable objectives

To transform your goals into tangible actions, consider using the SMART framework. This method ensures your goals are Specific, Measurable, Attainable, Realistic, and Time-bound:

>> **Be specific:** Avoid vague goals like "I want to be in shape." Instead, articulate exactly what you want to achieve. For instance, "I want to improve my flexibility to touch my toes" or "I want to carry my groceries with ease."

>> **Make it measurable:** Define how you'll track your progress. For example, instead of "I want to walk more," set a goal to walk 10,000 steps daily or take a 20-minute mindful walk three times a week.

>> **Set attainable goals:** Make sure your objectives are realistic for your current life and fitness level. If 4 a.m. workouts don't suit you, schedule a 15-minute somatic flow in the afternoon instead. Start small and build gradually.

>> **Stay realistic:** Avoid goals that require massive changes overnight. If pull-ups are a goal, set a gradual progression, like practicing strength exercises weekly, and give yourself several months.

>> **Keep goals time-bound:** Assign deadlines to your goals. For instance, "I will practice yoga three days a week and increase to hour-long sessions by the end of the summer." A timeframe adds motivation and keeps you focused.

The SMART approach can provide structure, but your goals are ultimately personal. Write them in a way that feels meaningful to you and review them regularly to stay inspired.

Staying motivated

Establishing a consistent somatic flow practice can help you stay motivated and committed, even during those lull times. By setting a routine and creating an environment that supports your practice, you build a strong foundation. Consider these tips to stay motivated and set yourself up for success:

>> **Establish a routine:** Having a routine when you begin practicing somatic flows helps you stick with it. Knowing when and where you'll practice can make it easier to show up consistently.

>> **Set aside dedicated time for practice:** Don't wait for the time to feel inspired; move first and the inspiration will arise. Mark your movement dates in your calendar, and show up as if they were appointments or work meetings. Remember, no one else can make this time for you. Showing up for yourself consistently can be a powerful form of self-care.

>> **Find a workout buddy:** Exercise with friends, family, or groups to add joy and accountability. If you've set plans with someone, you're less likely to skip your session.

>> **Follow positive influences:** Surround yourself with supportive, motivated people and look to role models who inspire you.

>> **Set goals and rewards:** Reward yourself for milestones, like new sneakers after completing a month of workouts or a massage after reaching a larger goal.

>> **Switch it up:** Avoid boredom and muscle overuse by trying new activities or classes. Variety keeps things exciting and supports a balanced routine.

>> **Create a conducive environment:** Find a space that makes you want to get on your mat, connect your mind and body, and cultivate inner awareness. Keep any props you need — like a mat, blocks, or strap — in this space, so they're ready when you are.

>> **Be consistent:** If you start small but aim to move at least three days a week, you'll have an easier time being consistent than if you bite off more than you can chew at first. Start small and build on as you feel you can.

For more on staying motivated and setting goals, see Chapter 15.

Selecting Movements

Choosing the right movements is essential for building a somatic flow that aligns with your goals. Whether you're seeking flexibility, mindfulness, or general fitness, selecting movements that resonate with your intentions makes your practice more meaningful and effective. In this section, you learn how to tailor exercises to meet your unique goals, find balance among different types of movements, and refine your practice through self-assessment.

Selecting movements that align with your goals

Once you've clarified your goals, it's time to select movements that support them. By choosing exercises that align with your intentions, you'll create a somatic flow that's enjoyable and purposeful:

>> **For increased flexibility:** Focus on mindful stretching and yoga-inspired movements. Gentle, sustained stretches can help release tension and improve range of motion. Chapter 5 includes exercises for increasing flexibility.

>> **To enhance mindfulness:** Prioritize meditation, breathwork, and body scans. Slower, intentional movements help deepen your mind-body connection. Chapters 4 and 10 include exercises for this purpose.

>> **For general activity:** Include dynamic practices like Pilates or brisk walking. These exercises will get your body moving while building strength and endurance. Chapter 6 includes exercises for this purpose.

>> **To reduce anxiety or tension:** Try somatic exercises like gentle shaking or somatic dance. These movements help you "shake off" stress, calming your nervous system. Chapter 7 includes exercises for this purpose.

TIP

Don't overwhelm yourself with too many types of movement. Choose a few that appeal to you and focus on building a consistent practice around them.

Balancing different types of exercises

As you design your somatic flow, finding a balance between different types of movement is key. Too much of one exercise can lead to burnout or even strain. Blending vigorous movements with gentler, calming practices helps you stay energized and balanced:

>> **Balance active and passive exercises:** If your practice consists mostly of meditation, body scans, or passive modalities like Feldenkrais or Trager work (where someone else moves your body — turn to Chapter 11 to read more), consider adding more active movement. You'll start to recognize what your body is missing and what you may be doing too much of. As wonderful as a massage feels, at some point, you need to learn to loosen up your muscles and joints on your own.

>> **Consider your tendencies:** If I could do yoga all day, I would. But over time, I realized that my body was becoming hypermobile without enough stability and strength. This was one of the reasons I decided to train for a marathon; running introduced stability work and more grounding movements. Notice if you tend toward flexibility or stability exercises and find ways to create a balance that strengthens and supports your whole body.

>> **Mix up fiery and calming practices:** If you do somatic dance every day, you might find yourself overheating or burning out. Try balancing it with something gentler, like Yin yoga. For example, maybe you do somatic dance twice a week, Yin yoga twice a week, and go for a long, mindful walk once a week. This way, you're giving your body stimulation and relaxation.

TIP

Pay attention to your body's signals over time. Balancing your movements doesn't mean you need to force anything. As you become more in tune, you'll sense what feels "just right" for you.

Incorporating feedback and self-assessment

Taking time for regular feedback and self-assessment is essential as you progress in your somatic journey. Use different methods to track your experiences and changes. This monitoring helps you notice the subtle shifts in your body and mind, so you can refine your practice along the way:

>> **Adapt your flow as needed:** Use your self-assessments to adjust your practice. Prioritize movements that release tension or help you feel more connected. If certain exercises don't seem to work, feel free to try new ones. Since your body and mind are always evolving, let your practice adapt to meet you where you are.

>> **Celebrate your progress:** Somatic practice isn't about numbers or hitting measurable milestones. Instead, you'll start to notice shifts like holding less tension in your shoulders, dropping into a relaxed state more easily, or breathing deeper. You may feel taller or find yourself moving with more ease. Recognize and enjoy these changes as signs of growth in your practice.

>> **Check in with body scans:** Personally, I love body scans. They're a simple but powerful way to connect with how you're feeling physically and mentally. Schedule a body scan once a week or once a month, choosing a specific day and time, and make sure to stick with it. After each scan, jot down a few notes: How do you feel? Where are you tense? What do you want to release? How busy is your mind? By recording these insights, you'll start to establish a "baseline" to compare against over time. Turn to Chapter 6 for the full rundown on how to do a body scan.

REMEMBER

Somatic work isn't about pushing yourself to extremes. Instead, focus on learning, listening, and responding to your body's natural rhythms. These small, steady adjustments create meaningful change over time.

Sequencing for Success

Creating an effective sequence is essential for building a somatic flow that feels natural, enjoyable, and sustainable. Start small and grow from there, listening to your body's cues as you go. Also, establish some basic habits early on to create a strong foundation upon which to build:

>> **Begin with grounding:** Always start your sequence by grounding yourself. Whether you're standing, sitting, or lying down, connect to the Earth beneath you. Use your breath to help slow down and center yourself before moving. Consider a short grounding technique, like a breathing exercise or meditation, to set the stage.

>> **Build consistency over time:** Aim to practice somatic sequences several times a week to let your intuition and creativity grow. Developing a regular routine helps your body integrate the movements more fully and makes somatic flow feel like a natural part of your day.

>> **Ease into movement:** Begin with smaller, gentler movements, giving your body a chance to warm up. For instance, you might start with seated Cat-Cow stretches or gentle spinal rotations before moving into larger motions like Upward and Downward Dog. Don't rush; let each movement flow naturally and allow your body to settle into the sequence.

Creating a logical and effective sequence

Designing a logical sequence allows you to move smoothly through each part of your body while maintaining balance and connection. By following a general structure, you'll keep your flow focused and effective.

Start with a few sequencing basics:

>> **Focus on flexion and extension:** Begin by working with either the front or the back of your body, depending on what needs the most attention. For instance, if you tend to have forward head posture, starting with core (front) exercises may help. If you have more of a sway back, you may want to focus on exercises that engage your back muscles.

>> **Move from center to periphery:** Start with movements that engage the spine, such as flexion and extension exercises like Arch and Flatten, shown in Figure 12-3. Then, progress to exercises for the sides of your body (for example, side curls). Gradually work your way outwards to include the arms, shoulders, hips, legs, and finally, the head and neck.

>> **Use gentle rotations and finish with walking:** After working the spine and limbs, try some gentle twisting or rotation movements. Finish by practicing mindful walking, using your newfound awareness to notice how your body feels and moves as you walk.

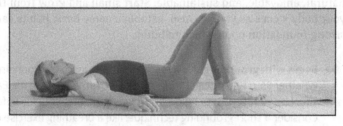

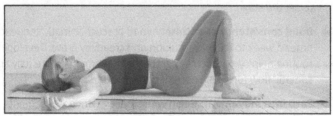

FIGURE 12-3:
The Arch and Flatten extension exercise engages your spine.

Photograph by Guen Egan

If you're beginning with flexion and extension, the Arch and Flatten with Rolling Head sequence is great to try. It works well as a stand-alone practice, a warm-up, or a cool-down. Use it to introduce gentle movement before a Pilates session or a yoga flow:

1. **Start on your back with your feet flat on the floor, hip-width apart.**

Feel the Earth beneath you and take a moment to ground yourself. Place your hands on your stomach, following the rhythm of your breath.

2. **Breathe into your stomach and let your tailbone rest on the floor as you gently arch your lower back.**

On your exhale, let your lower back melt into the floor, tilting your tailbone slightly upward.

3. **Slowly increase the movement by rocking your pelvis back and forth, allowing your head to respond naturally to the motion.**

As you roll your hips forward, let your chin move toward your chest; as you roll back, let your head gently rock back. Repeat for 2-3 minutes.

4. **Lengthen your legs on the floor, noticing how your lower back and neck feel.**

5. **Consider closing with a body scan or short meditation to end the practice on a calm note.**

Sequencing doesn't have to follow a strict formula. As you experiment, you'll get a feel for what feels right and can adjust based on what your body is asking for each day.

Ensuring smooth transitions between movements

To create smooth transitions between movements, think of your transitions as part of the flow, not just a way to get from one movement to the next, by following these guidelines:

>> **Moving in a natural sequence:** If you're working on your shoulders, it makes sense to then move down through your arms and hands. After working with your upper body, shift focus to your legs and feet. You wouldn't suddenly jump from your shoulders to your feet! Moving from one area to the next allows you to keep a sense of connection and flow.

>> **Staying connected to your breath:** Use each inhale and exhale to guide you as you move. If you start from the center of your body and move outward,

you'll feel the natural flow from one area to the next. This connection with your breath will help you sense how to move fluidly without forcing anything.

>> **Transitioning gradually when changing positions:** If you're lying down, don't rush to standing. Ease your way up. Try coming into a Child's Pose, shown in Figure 12-4, then move to all fours, and step one foot forward before eventually standing upright. When you make smooth, gradual transitions, you keep your body connected to the flow, without disrupting your focus.

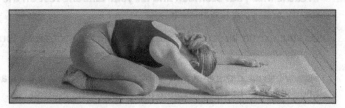

Photograph by Guen Egan

REMEMBER

Everything in your body is connected. Take your time to "connect the dots" as you move through each area. The more awareness you bring to your transitions, the more fluid and connected your practice will feel.

Using flows as warm-ups, cool-downs, or stand-alone practices

You can use somatic flows as warm-ups, cool-downs, or even as their own complete practice. Some exercises, like the Arch and Flatten, work beautifully as a stand-alone sequence or as a gentle warm-up or cool-down for more intensive movement.

There's a great quote from Mel Siff, author of *Facts and Fallacies of Fitness*, that says, "Programming your brain is more important than strength training and aerobics. Central nervous system programming must never be neglected at all stages of training." Somatic movement does exactly this — it trains your brain. You're programming your nervous system to pay close attention to your body and how it moves. It's a deep dive into how everything connects, which prepares you for any type of movement.

Here are some somatic exercises that work well as warm-ups or as stand-alone practices:

>> **Arch and Curl:** Lie on your back with your knees bent and feet flat on the mat. Start by arching your lower back and then returning to neutral. Engage your abdominals and lift your head, curling toward your knees. Think of this as a mindful, slow-motion crunch. You'll activate your core and release tension in your back. See Figure 12-5.

>> **Back Lift:** Lie on your stomach with your head turned to the right. Rest your left arm by your side, bend your right arm, and let the elbow point out. Start by lifting just the right elbow to feel the rear deltoid engage, then lower. Next, lift your head and neck, keeping your head turned. Finally, try lifting your head, neck, and left leg together to activate your back muscles. Repeat on the opposite side. See Figure 12-6.

>> **Cross Lateral Arch and Curl:** With your hands behind your head and knees bent, bring your right knee toward your chest and your left elbow in an arch toward the right knee. Lower, then switch sides. This isn't about crunching your abs; it's about connecting the movement and noticing how your spine, chest, and core work together.

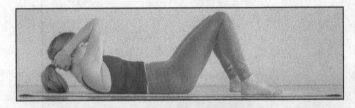

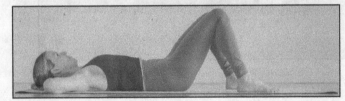

FIGURE 12-5:
The Arch and Curl activates your core and releases tension in your back.

Photograph by Guen Egan

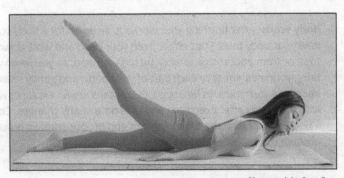

FIGURE 12-6:
The Back Lift activates your back muscles.

Photograph by Guen Egan

>> **Steeple Movement:** Lie on your back with your legs crossed and arms in the air. Slowly turn your arms to one side while letting your legs drop in the opposite direction. This movement wakes up your obliques, releases tension, and improves your torso's ability to twist. See Figure 12-7.

>> **Walking Exercise (or "Windshield Wipers"):** Lie on your back with your feet wider than hip-width. Let your knees drop to one side to feel the internal rotation in your opposite leg. Repeat several times on each side. This simple movement helps relax the pelvis and prepares your body for natural movements like walking or running.

>> **Washrag Exercise:** Lie on your back with your knees bent and arms out to the sides. Inhale, then exhale as you let your knees fall to one side, bringing them back to center, and then letting them fall to the other side. Continue moving side to side, then add a gentle twist with your upper body by alternating the palms up and down. This exercise releases stress, improves breathing, and helps your body move more freely.

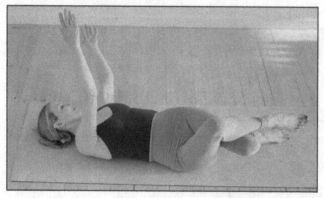

FIGURE 12-7:
The Steeple Movement wakes up your obliques.

Photograph by Guen Egan

After your workout, try these practices to help your body relax, release tension, and seal in the benefits of your movement session:

>> **Body scans:** After finishing your workout, lie down for a body scan to notice how your body feels. Start either from your head and work down to your toes, or from your toes and work up to your head. As you lie on your back, bring your awareness to each part of your body, and gently relax each area, imagining your muscles letting go. Body scans are an excellent way to check in with your body after exercising and take note of any changes. Consider doing a body scan both at the beginning and end of your somatic practice to observe the shifts before and afterward.

>> **Conscious breathing:** Spend some time noticing your breath to stay connected after your movement. Sit or lie in a comfortable position, placing one hand on your stomach and the other on your chest. Observe the rise and fall of your chest and abdomen as you breathe. This conscious breathing practice helps you maintain a sense of connectedness and appreciation for your body's effort. By breathing mindfully, you seal in the practice and show gratitude for the time spent.

>> **Gentle yoga postures:** Cool down with these soothing yoga poses, which help your body transition from activity to rest:

- **Cat-Cow:** Start on your hands and knees. Inhale as you arch your spine (Cow), and exhale as you round your spine (Cat). Alternatively, you can do Cat-Cow seated in a cross-legged position. See Chapter 7 for more about the Cat-Cow.

- **Happy Baby:** Lie on your back, hug your knees toward your chest, then take hold of each foot with your hands, pulling your knees toward your armpits. Rock gently from side to side, breathing deeply. See Figure 12-8.

- **Supine Goddess Pose:** Lie on your back with the soles of your feet together and knees open to the sides. Breathe deeply and relax in this position for one to two minutes. See Figure 12-9.

FIGURE 12-8:
The Happy Baby helps your body relax.

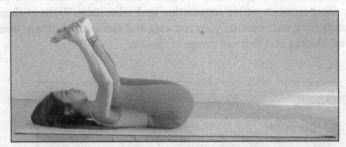

Photograph by Guen Egan

FIGURE 12-9:
The Supine Goddess Pose.

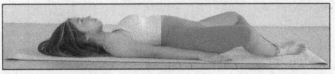

Photograph by Guen Egan

- **Supine Twist:** Lie on your back, cross one leg over to the opposite side, and reach the same arm out, turning your head toward it. Hold for five to eight breaths, then switch sides. See Figure 12-10.

» **Pandiculation:** This movement, often accompanied by yawning, stretches and contracts your muscles, waking up your sensory-motor system and sending feedback to your brain. Pandiculation helps release muscle tension and prevents chronic tightness. This natural reflex — like when a dog or cat stretches after sleeping — helps reset your muscle tension and improve circulation. Try these variations:

  - Sitting or standing, lift your shoulders, contract them, and let them drop.
  - Lift your arms up to the sky, let out a big yawn, and stretch from side to side.
  - Take your arms behind your back, arch your chest up to the sky, and yawn deeply.
  - Try a Downward-Facing Dog stretch. Start on your hands and knees, then lift your hips up and back, pressing your hands firmly into the floor. For more, you can have a partner push your hips into the stretch; see Figure 12-11.

TIP

Pandiculation works well both before and after a workout, helping your muscles release through active contraction and relaxation. Without these yawning-and-stretching movements, your muscles and fascia can tighten, leading to structural imbalances and reduced range of motion.

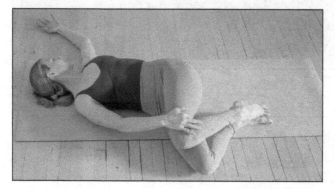

FIGURE 12-10:
The Supine Twist.

Photograph by Guen Egan

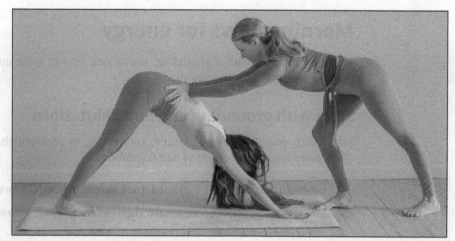

Photograph by Guen Egan

FIGURE 12-11:
The Downward-
Facing
Dog stretch.

Adapting Flows for Different Times of the Day

You can always adapt somatic movements to fit your energy throughout the day. Some people are morning people, while others are night owls. You may like to wake up and get moving right away or you may feel more energized toward the midafternoon or early evening.

TIP

Get to know yourself and what you prefer and adapt your movement to meet you where you're at.

I personally love to move in the morning. However, morning exercises have their challenges. Your brain may be more awake, but your body needs time to catch up. Start slowly in the morning and use breath and grounding exercise to prepare your body for larger movements. Ease into the exercises in the morning.

In the afternoon, your body is now more open and has been moving more; but your brain may be fried at this point. Focus on exercises that help you stay focused and that release and relax your mind so you can drop into your body. Use restorative postures to unwind from a long day. Maybe try some somatic dance since your body feels nice and alive and your brain doesn't need to do much thinking.

REMEMBER

The time of day that you do your somatics practice is up to you. If you're up for it, try a morning practice and a short evening practice to release the tension you built up throughout the day.

Morning flows for energy

Kickstart your day with a grounding, energizing flow to wake up your body and prepare your mind for the day ahead.

Start with grounding and Sun Salutations

Stand with your feet firmly planted, connecting to your breath and the Earth. Then move into three rounds of Sun Salutations:

1. Inhale to lift your arms overhead, then exhale as you fold forward.

2. Step back into plank on an inhale, then exhale to lower yourself to the ground.

3. Inhale as you lift your chest into Cobra or Upward-Facing Dog, and exhale back into Downward-Facing Dog. Hold for five breaths.

4. Step forward on an inhale, fold into a forward bend on an exhale, then inhale to lift your arms overhead. Exhale to return your arms to your sides.

5. Finish with the Tree Pose on each side to build focus and energy for the day.

Figure 12-12 shows the process, step by step.

Add a somatic flow with Cat-Cow and joint movements

Warm up your spine with Cat-Cow movements, then move into circular movements on all fours. Afterward, stand up and "shake it off," releasing any lingering tension or negative energy. Follow up with gentle movements for each joint — roll your neck, shoulders, and hips, bend and extend your knees, and finish by rolling out each ankle.

Try a Pilates-inspired workout

Lie on your back to engage your core. Begin with "the Hundreds" by lifting your head and neck, extending your arms by your sides, and pumping your arms up and down five times on an inhale and five times on an exhale, repeating ten times (for a total of 100 pumps; see Figure 12-13). Follow with some slow roll-ups, then lie back for a few Articulating Bridges, shown in Figure 12-14. End with conscious breathing to set your intentions for the day.

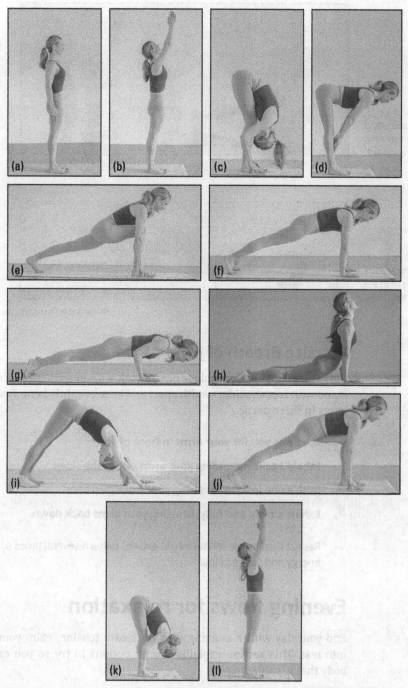

FIGURE 12-12:
The steps for the
Sun Salutation.

Photographs by Guen Egan

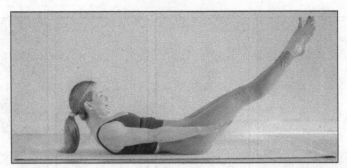

FIGURE 12-13:
The Hundreds is
a common
Pilates move.

Photograph by Guen Egan

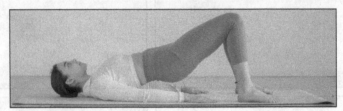

FIGURE 12-14:
The Articulating
Bridge releases
tightness.

Photograph by Guen Egan

Practice Breath of Joy

This energizing flow combines breathwork with movement to elevate your mood. Stand with feet shoulder–width apart and knees slightly bent. Imagine filling your lungs in three parts:

1. **Inhale as you lift your arms in front of you.**

2. **Inhale again, extending your arms out to the sides.**

3. **Inhale one last time, raising your arms overhead.**

4. **Exhale slowly and fully, bringing your arms back down.**

   Repeat this "inhale-inhale-inhale-exhale" pattern several times to boost your energy and sense of joy.

Evening flows for relaxation

End your day with a relaxing flow to release tension, calm your mind, and ease into rest. This section explains several options to try so you can signal to your body that it's time to rest.

Restorative Yin yoga sequences

Yin yoga includes many gentle, restorative sequences. Here are some you can try:

» **Constructive Rest Pose:** Lie on your back with knees bent and feet wider than hip-width, letting your knees fall toward each other. Stay here for three minutes.

» **Banana Pose:** Lie with your legs extended. Cross one ankle over the other and reach both arms overhead toward the same side, creating a banana shape. Hold for three minutes, then switch sides. See Figure 12-15.

» **Half Butterfly:** Sit up, drawing one leg in with your knee bent to the side, foot against the inner thigh of the opposite leg. Fold over the straight leg for three minutes, then switch sides. See Figure 12-16.

» **Sleeping Swan:** From a seated position, sweep one leg behind you so your front knee is bent and the back leg is extended. Lean your torso forward over the front leg and stay for three minutes. Repeat on the other side.

» **Finish with Legs-Up-The-Wall (the *Savasana*):** End with a few minutes of Legs-Up-The-Wall or lying in Savasana, allowing your body to fully relax. See Figure 12-17.

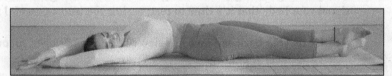

FIGURE 12-15:
The Banana Pose.

Photograph by Guen Egan

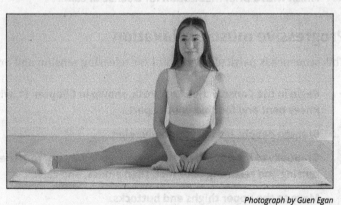

FIGURE 12-16:
The Half
Butterfly Pose.

Photograph by Guen Egan

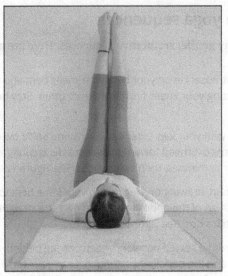

FIGURE 12-17:
Finish with your
Legs-Up-The-Wall.

Photograph by Guen Egan

Gentle evening flows with articulating bridges and twists

Incorporating these gentle evening flows and breathing exercises regularly helps signal your body that it's time to rest, easing you into a peaceful night's sleep.

1. Lie on your back and do a few slow Articulating Bridges, followed by Windshield Wiper Legs.

2. Move into gentle Supine Twists and a Reclining Goddess Pose.

3. Finish with a brief meditation for a sense of calm.

Progressive muscle relaxation

This sequence is particularly helpful for releasing tension and preparing for bed:

1. Begin in the Constructive Rest Pose, shown in Chapter 11, with your knees bent and feet hip-width apart.

2. Breathe deeply, letting your body relax.

3. Gradually extend your legs, then work your way up from the feet, tensing and releasing your feet, then ankles, and calves.

4. Move to the upper thighs and buttocks.

5. Continue with the middle back and abdomen.

6. **Finish with the arms, shoulders, hands, and facial muscles, releasing each area fully.**

7. **End with mindful breathing using any calming breathing technique to wind down, such as 4-7-8 breathing or *Viloma* breathwork.**

REMEMBER

4-7-8 breathing is when you inhale for a count of four, hold for seven, and exhale for eight. *Viloma* breathwork is when you practice a three-part breath in a Restorative yoga posture such as a Reclined Goddess or Supported Bridge Pose.

Adapting Flows for Special Needs and Preferences

Somatics is all about discovering what works best for you and honoring your body's rhythms and requirements. You can adapt somatic flows to meet your unique needs, goals, and preferences by

>> **Adjusting flows based on your goals and life stage:** As your needs change over time, tailor your practice accordingly:

- If you're an athlete, focus on somatic movements that aid recovery, release muscle tension, and enhance mobility.

- If you're healing from an injury, prioritize gentle, rehabilitative exercises that support pain management and gradual strengthening.

- If you're going through menopause or experiencing other hormonal changes, incorporate cortisol-lowering somatic exercises to help manage stress and promote relaxation.

>> **Customizing the duration and intensity of your practice:** Start small, aiming for 15 to 20 minutes a day, and build from there as your practice becomes more intuitive. Somatic movement is a learning process where you become the expert in your own body, so give yourself time to explore and adjust based on how you feel.

>> **Listening and responding to your body's feedback:** Notice the effects of each movement and make adjustments accordingly. No one knows your needs better than you. If a movement feels too intense, feel free to modify it or try something different. Consistency is key, so find ways to make your practice sustainable and enjoyable.

Integrating Somatic Flows into Your Daily Life

You can easily integrate somatic flows into your daily routine. Somatic movement isn't limited to formal practice sessions — you can weave it into everyday moments to stay connected with your body and mind.

>> **Incorporate movement breaks:** Mid-morning, do some simple chair yoga or stretches to release any tension that's built up. Take a few moments to reset your posture, stretch your shoulders, and breathe deeply.

>> **Practice mindful breathing during daily tasks:** While making your coffee or tea, take a few intentional breaths. Engage in mindful eating by using the 5-4-3-2-1 technique — noticing five things you can see, four things you can feel, three things you can hear, two things you can smell, and one thing you can taste.

>> **Replace afternoon slumps with movement:** Instead of reaching for caffeine or a snack, try an energizing meditation or some gentle stretches. Reconnect with your body and refresh your energy naturally.

>> **Start your morning with gentle movement:** When you wake up, stretch out any stiffness with a few simple movements. Reach your arms overhead, take a few side bends, and yawn to release tension. As you get out of bed, feel your feet on the floor and take a few deep breaths to ground yourself.

>> **Take a mindful walk:** When walking to work, dropping off kids, walking your dog, or even just heading to the mailbox, turn your walk into a mindful experience. Pay attention to the sensation of each step and the rhythm of your breathing. This small act can help you stay present and grounded.

>> **Unwind with somatic movement at the end of the day:** Before making dinner or winding down, do a few gentle yoga poses or breathwork exercises to release the day's accumulated tension. Finish your day with some calming breathwork, a body scan, or progressive muscle relaxation.

REMEMBER

By integrating somatic flows into small, daily moments, you maintain a deeper connection with your body and mind. This practice allows you to experience the benefits of somatic movement in a natural and consistent way, even on the busiest days.

5
Living a Somatic Lifestyle

Incorporating somatics to address body pain, improve flexibility, and enhance balance and coordination.

Combining cardio, strength training, and somatic exercises to improve your fitness.

Learning how to make somatic exercise a lifelong commitment.

IN THIS CHAPTER

» **Helping your hips**

» **Soothing your shoulders**

» **Being good to your back**

» **Easing foot and ankle pain**

» **Comforting your chronic pain**

» **Improving your overall mobility**

Chapter **13**

Addressing Specific Needs with Somatic Exercises

I n this chapter, I tackle the not-so-fun reality that sometimes, life *is* a pain — literally. Trust me, I get it; you're not alone in feeling those mysterious aches, stiffness, and stubborn tension that seem to show up at the worst possible moments. Maybe your neck is stiff from staring at screens all day, or your back is giving you grief for no apparent reason. Whatever your body's complaint, know that you're among friends here — and I'm here to help you find relief.

Think of this chapter as your go-to guide for saying goodbye to those daily discomforts. Here, you explore simple, effective somatic exercises that can make a real difference. These aren't high-intensity moves meant to push you to the limit; they're gentle, mindful movements that help you reconnect with your body and listen to what it needs. Whether it's a quick stretch for shoulder relief or a calming breathwork routine to ease anxiety, each technique is designed to help you feel better, one small step at a time.

So, take a deep breath and get ready to meet your body where it is. This chapter is packed with practical, approachable exercises to address specific areas like hips, back, shoulders, and more. Let's work together to bring comfort, mobility, and a bit of ease back into your daily life — because when you feel better, everything else feels a little bit easier too.

TIP

To identify the source of your pain and discomfort, consider the type of pain and its location. Ask yourself, "Does it get worse with movement? What's my range of motion? Are both sides the same?" As you perform the exercises in this chapter, be sure to stop and notice your emotions. Somatic exercises often bring up emotional responses. As you work out, notice if any particular emotions (for example, frustration, joy, calmness) arise and connect them to physical sensations in your body.

ADAPT MOVEMENTS TO INDIVIDUAL NEEDS

Everyone has specific areas or issues that may need more attention than others. You know your body best, so always listen to it. While it's important to focus on your body as a whole, give a little extra attention to areas that need additional support. For example, if you experience tightness in your hips or lower back, incorporate targeted stretches or mobility exercises for those areas. Remember, somatic movement is all about customizing to your individual needs for optimal mobility and comfort.

Many of these exercises you may have seen elsewhere or performed at the gym or with a physical therapist or in a class. To make them somatic is bringing your conscious awareness to the body and its sensations during each exercise. Slow down the pace, pay attention to the specific muscles involved and how your body feels as you move. Stay connected to your breath and tune into sensations, muscle engagement and any discomfort or tension you feel. Stay curious instead of pushing through. You can begin each exercise or pose with a body scan or check in mid-way or after each exercise too. Be aware of your energy and how it flows, slow down your transitions, and use your focus and visualization as you move through each phase of each exercise or posture. Stay present and every time your mind wanders gently bring it back.

You may find that certain movements bring up different emotional responses. For example, an intense physical effort might stir feelings of empowerment or frustration. A deep hip-opening pose may bring up sadness or stuck energy. Acknowledge these feelings without judgment, letting them flow naturally.

Relieving Hip Pain

Hip pain often results from inactivity, misalignment, overuse, or the natural wear and tear of aging. By keeping you mindful, strong, and flexible, somatic exercises offer powerful tools for managing and relieving hip pain. In this section, you uncover common causes of hip pain, practice gentle stretches to boost hip flexibility, and strengthen your hips for better stability.

TIP

If you're just getting started, review the foundational somatic stretches in Chapter 5, which introduces gentle movements that can prepare you for more targeted hip work.

Understanding common causes of hip pain

Hip pain can arise from several sources:

>> **Bursitis:** Repetitive activities that overwork or irritate the hip joint often cause this inflammation of the bursae, the fluid-filled sacs between tissues.

>> **Muscle or tendon strain:** Activities that strain the muscles, tendons, and ligaments supporting the hips lead to this type of pain.

>> **Osteoarthritis:** Aging or wear and tear on the hip joint causes the cartilage to deteriorate, leading to pain.

>> **Tendinitis:** Overuse often triggers this condition, which inflames or irritates the tendons.

TIP

In many cases, you can manage hip pain by keeping your hip joint strong through exercise and mobile with flexibility moves. Somatic strength work and stretching are ideal for addressing hip pain because they allow you to stay mindful throughout the movements and avoid overdoing it. Somatic exercises teach you to listen to your body and work within your own range of motion and skill level. You can build up to many of these poses and exercises, and always modify as needed.

You can also incorporate breathwork, meditation, and visualization to help manage pain or discomfort. Think of the hips as the basement of the house. You may store a lot down there that you don't realize. Somatic stretches let you "clean house" in the hips, while somatic strengthening moves help you build an even stronger foundation.

REMEMBER

Maintaining good posture, covered in Chapter 8, can help prevent hip pain by promoting proper alignment in your hips and lower back.

Gentle stretches for hip flexibility

I teach specific hip-opening yoga classes, and they are my favorite. I love hip openers and find that everyone can benefit from them. Most gentle hip openers can work wonders for your mobility. Keeping your hips flexible can prevent and alleviate pain.

WARNING

Always listen to your body, and if you're new to stretching, consider consulting your doctor first. Be sure to recognize when discomfort becomes pain and stop anything that is causing you true pain!

The poses in this section can be performed lying down (in the *supine* position). Work up to those you can do while seated, and finally, hip stretches you do while standing. Start off slowly with stretches you can do in the supine position:

» **Supine Figure Four:** Lie on your back with your knees bent. Cross your right ankle over your left knee, lift both legs, and gently pull your left thigh toward you. As shown in Figure 13-1, this position targets the outer hip area and releases tension in your lower back. Hold for five to eight breaths, then switch sides.

» **Supine Cow Face Pose:** Lying on your back, bring your legs to a tabletop position. Cross your right leg over your left leg at the upper thighs. Hold the tops of your outer ankles and gently bring the legs toward you. After five to eight breaths, switch sides. Figure 13-2 illustrates this pose, which helps release tension in the inner hip.

» **Supine Inner Hip Opener:** Lying on your back, place the right ankle above the left knee, letting the right knee open to the side. Drop both legs to the left so the right foot touches the floor, braced by the left knee. Gently press the right knee away from you. Hold for five to eight breaths, then switch sides. Figure 13-3 demonstrates this gentle opener.

FIGURE 13-1:
Supine Figure Four stretch, focusing on the outer hip area and lower back release.

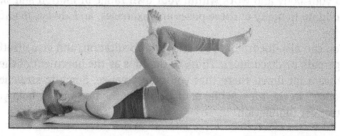

Photograph by Guen Egan

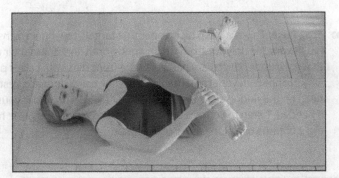

FIGURE 13-2: Supine Cow Face Pose, targeting inner hip flexibility.

Photograph by Guen Egan

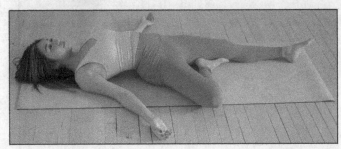

FIGURE 13-3: Supine Inner Hip Opener, promoting gentle inner hip release.

Photograph by Guen Egan

» **Happy Baby Pose:** Lying on your back, hug both knees to your chest, then pull on the outer ankles as you lift your feet toward the ceiling and draw the knees toward your armpits. Try to lengthen your tailbone into the mat. Hold for five to eight breaths. Check out this pose in Chapter 12 (Figure 12-8).

» **Goddess Pose:** Lie down on your back with your feet together and your knees open to the sides. Hold for five to eight breaths or up to three minutes. Goddess Pose feels especially good with support under your knees. Check out this pose in Chapter 12 (Figure 12-9).

» **Pigeon Pose:** From Downward-Facing Dog or on all fours, slide your right shin forward between your hands, positioning it as parallel to the front of the mat as possible without shifting to the outer hip. Keep your back leg long and aim the of the back leg toward the floor so that it stays internally rotated. Place a block or blanket under your front hip for support. Walk your hands forward and take five to eight breaths, then switch sides. You can check out this pose in Chapter 8 (Figure 8-5).

» **Frog Pose:** This is a deep hip opener that targets the inner thighs, groin, and hip flexors. Lie on your stomach and bring both legs out to their own sides so that your upper thighs are parallel to the front mat, with calves perpendicular. Stay propped on your forearms or walk your hands forward, resting your head on the floor (see Figure 13-4). Use extra cushion under your inner knees if needed. Listen to your breath, as this can be an intense pose; hold for five to eight breaths or as long as it's comfortable.

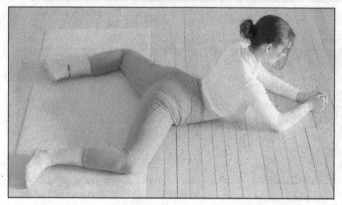

FIGURE 13-4:
The Frog Pose, a powerful inner thigh stretch.

Photograph by Guen Egan

TIP

For deeper awareness and body connection in each pose, review the somatic breathing techniques in Chapter 4. Coordinating breath with movement enhances stability and ease during stretches. Single-tasking can help you make each movement somatic. Focus solely on the task at hand. When you find your mind tip toeing away, gently bring it back to the sensations and the movement.

Seated poses

These exercises take you through seated positions to help you cultivate stable, strong hips:

» **Seated Figure Four:** Sitting upright, bend your knees and place your feet on the floor. Cross your right ankle above your left knee, letting the right knee open to the side. Bring your hands close behind your back and lift out of your lower back. Breathe into the outer hip for five to eight breaths, then switch sides (see Figure 13-5).

» **Ankle to Knee Pose:** Sitting tall, bend your right leg so your shin is parallel to the front of the mat. Place your left ankle on your right knee, letting your left knee fall on top of your right foot. Walk your hands forward and fold over your legs (see Figure 13-6). If this is too intense, you can stick with Seated Figure Four. After five to eight deep breaths, switch sides.

» **Half Hero Pose:** Sit up tall with your legs extended straight in front of you. Bend your right knee and bring the top of your right foot to the outside of your right hip. You can stay here, recline back to your elbows, or lie down fully. This stretch (see Figure 13-7) deeply targets the front of your hip and thigh. Hold for five to eight breaths, then repeat on the other side.

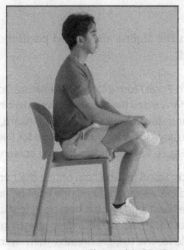

FIGURE 13-5:
Seated Figure Four, targeting the outer hip in a seated position.

Photograph by Guen Egan

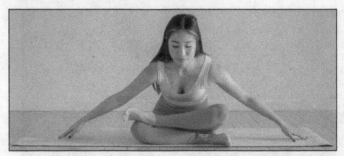

FIGURE 13-6:
Ankle to Knee Pose, providing a deeper hip stretch for both hips simultaneously.

Photograph by Guen Egan

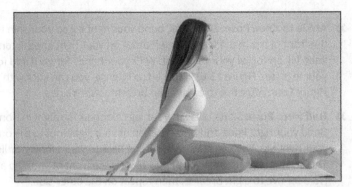

Photograph by Guen Egan

FIGURE 13-7:
Half Hero Pose,
lengthening the
hip flexors and
quadriceps.

Standing stretches

When you're comfortable with the supine and seated positions, these standing exercises take things up a notch:

» **Lizard Pose:** I love the Lizard Pose! From a Downward-Facing Dog or on all fours, lunge your right foot forward to the outside of your right hand. Slide your back leg farther back and start to walk your hands forward, lowering your elbows to the floor or using blocks for support. Hold for five to eight breaths, then switch sides. Figure 13-8 illustrates this hip-opening posture.

» **Standing Hip Flexor Stretch:** Stand tall and hold onto a chair or place your hand on the wall if you need extra support. Bend one knee behind you and catch the foot with the same hand, bringing the heel close to your hip while aligning your knees (see Figure 13-9). You'll feel a deep stretch in the front of the thigh and hip flexor. Hold for five to eight breaths, then switch sides.

FIGURE 13-8:
Lizard Pose, an
intense hip
opener that
targets the inner
thigh and
hip flexors.

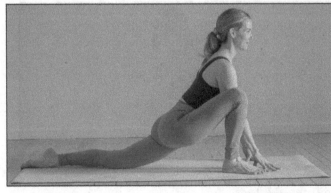

Photograph by Guen Egan

>> **Yogi Squat:** Stand with your feet slightly wider than hip-width and your toes turned slightly out. Lower your hips into a deep squat. You can press your elbows against your inner thighs or knees as you bring your hands into a prayer position (see Figure 13-10). If this deep squat is too intense, place a tall block under your hips or use the Happy Baby Pose as an alternative.

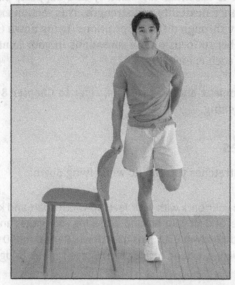

FIGURE 13-9: Standing Hip Flexor Stretch, targeting the hip flexors and quadriceps.

Photograph by Guen Egan

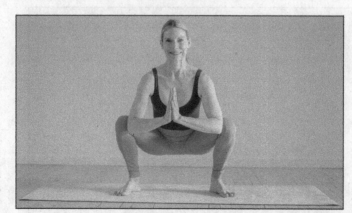

FIGURE 13-10: The Yogi Squat, a versatile movement for hip flexibility and stability.

Photograph by Guen Egan

In addition to gaining flexibility in your hips, building strength in your hips is essential to long-term mobility and health. Somatic movement is all about finding balance — developing strength and flexibility while managing effort and ease.

Strengthening exercises for hip stability

Building hip strength is essential for stability and support, particularly when you're working to balance flexibility and strength. This section explores exercises that target hip stability through different positions: Lying down (supine), sitting, and standing. Remember to focus on the sensations in your joints, muscles, and bones as you perform each exercise.

TIP

For foundational alignment and posture tips, refer to Chapter 8 to support safe and effective strengthening.

Supine exercises

Start off slowly with stretches you can do while lying down:

>> **Hip Bridge:** Lie on your back with your feet hip-width apart and knees bent. Press into your feet and lift your hips up, engaging your glutes and core. Hold briefly at the top, then lower your hips back down. Repeat for 10 to 12 reps. For an added challenge, extend one leg for a Single-Leg Hip Bridge, as shown in Figure 13-11.

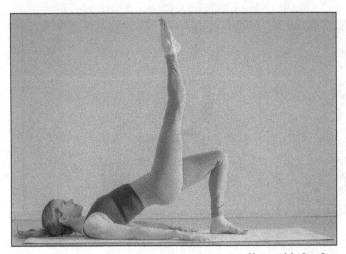

FIGURE 13-11:
Single-Leg Hip Bridge, building strength in the hips and glutes.

Photograph by Guen Egan

>> **Side-Lying Leg Work:** Lie on your side, propped up on one elbow, with your legs slightly in front of your hips. Lift the top leg up and down about 12 inches, then practice internal and external rotations, and finally, lift the leg higher, then lower. Aim for eight to ten reps of each movement, then switch sides. This sequence strengthens hip muscles while promoting mobility. Side-Lying Leg Work offers benefits similar to other hip openers, but here the focus is on strengthening through controlled movements rather than passive stretching.

Standing exercises

When you're comfortable with the supine and seated positions, these exercises take things up a notch:

>> **Goddess Squat:** Stand with feet wide and toes turned out. With your hands in prayer at your chest, squat down until your thighs are parallel to the floor, or as low as you can comfortably go. You can also hold on to a chair. Keep your back upright, as shown in Figure 13-12. Hold this pose for 30 to 60 seconds, then stand. Repeat two to three times.

>> **Warrior I, II, and III:** Each Warrior pose works different areas of the hip and lower body strength:

● **Warrior I:** Step one foot back and turn the outer heel down. Bend your front knee over your ankle and lift your arms overhead, pressing your palms together, as shown in Figure 13-13. Hold for five to eight breaths, then switch sides.

● **Warrior II:** In a wide stance, turn one foot forward and bend that knee, extending your arms out to the sides. Align your front knee and open your hips. Hold for five to eight breaths, then switch sides. Figure 13-14 shows the correct stance.

● **Warrior III:** Stand on one leg and extend your other leg back behind you, bringing your torso parallel to the floor. Your arms can extend back, forward, or to the sides, as shown in Figure 13-15. Hold for five to eight breaths, then switch sides.

These are just a few ideas for hip strengthening through yoga and Pilates. You can also strengthen your hips by taking mindful walks and moving through a full range of motion.

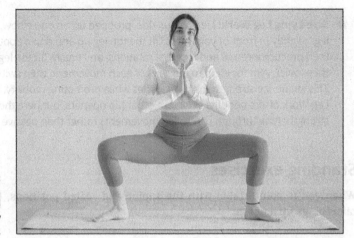

FIGURE 13-12:
Goddess Squat,
a powerful
lower-body
strengthener.

Photograph by Guen Egan

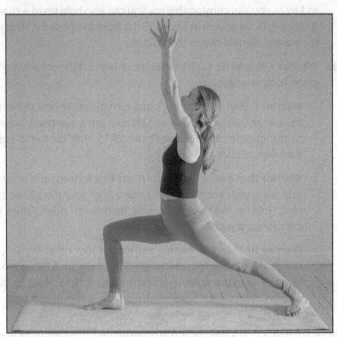

FIGURE 13-13:
Warrior I,
strengthening
the hips, legs,
and core.

Photograph by Guen Egan

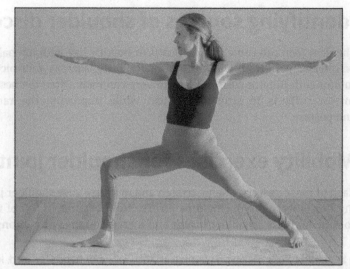

FIGURE 13-14:
Warrior II, a strengthening posture that stabilizes the hips and knees.

Photograph by Guen Egan

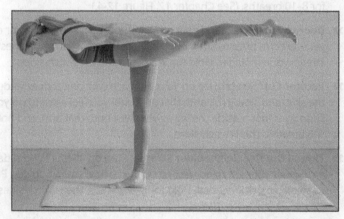

FIGURE 13-15:
Warrior III, an advanced balancing posture that strengthens the hips and glutes.

Photograph by Guen Egan

Easing Shoulder Pain

Sometimes you may feel like you must hold the weight of the world on your shoulders. From balancing your work, your family, your personal life, your health, and so much more, it can feel like a lot of pressure. Releasing tension from your shoulders not only helps on a physical level but also on an emotional level.

Identifying sources of shoulder discomfort

Shoulder pain can come from arthritis or bursitis like with hip pain. It could also be referred pain from another part of the body, such as your biceps, triceps, or rotator cuff. Rotator cuff injuries are very common. Often the best treatment for rotator cuffs is to strengthen them while improving the range of motion and posture.

Mobility exercises for shoulder joints

Each of these exercises helps stretch and mobilize your shoulder joints, promoting flexibility and reducing tension. Try to incorporate a few of these into your routine for better shoulder health and increased range of motion:

>> **Child's Pose:** Begin on your knees and walk your hands forward, letting your upper body relax toward the floor. For a deeper stretch, turn your palms up to the ceiling and bend your elbows, placing your hands on your back. Hold for 8–10 breaths. (See Chapter 12, Figure 12-4.)

>> **Doorway Stretch:** Stand near a wall or doorway, and bend your elbow so your forearm presses straight up against the wall. Turn your chest away to stretch your shoulder. Hold for 5–8 breaths, then switch sides.

>> **Rotator Cuff Stretch:** Lie on your stomach with one arm extended out to the side, and slowly roll onto that arm until you feel a stretch in your shoulder. Drop your foot outside the leg as you twist onto that arm, and hold for 5–8 breaths. Then switch sides.

>> **Thread the Needle Shoulder Stretch:** Start on all fours and slide your right arm under your left hand, resting on the back of your shoulder. Place your head on a block if needed. Hold for 5–8 breaths, then switch sides.

Strengthening routines for shoulder muscles

Building shoulder strength not only enhances your stability but also helps protect your shoulders from injury. You can do these effective bodyweight exercises anywhere to strengthen your shoulder muscles:

>> **Downward-Facing Dog:** Begin on all fours, tuck your toes, and lift your hips up and back. Press firmly into your hands, externally rotating your upper arms, and feel your shoulders glide up the back. Hold for five to eight breaths. See Figure 12-11 in Chapter 12.

>> **Plank:** Start on all fours and walk your feet back to come into a plank. Hold for eight to ten breaths. To modify, drop your knees to the floor or lower onto your forearms for a forearm plank.

>> **Pushups:** From a plank or modified plank with your knees on the floor, bend your elbows and lower your chest toward the floor, then press back up. Perform these with control, ensuring your shoulders don't round forward.

>> **Side Plank:** From a plank, stack your hips and feet as you shift onto your right hand and raise your left arm toward the ceiling. Hold for eight to ten breaths, then switch sides. You can also do this on your forearm.

>> **Upward-Facing Dog:** From a plank, lower your hips as you lift your chest, coming onto the tops of your feet. Keep your hips lifted off the floor and use your upper body, core, and legs to hold the position for 30 seconds. See Figure 13-16.

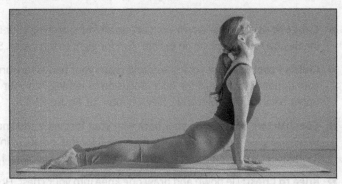

FIGURE 13-16: The Upward-Facing Dog.

Photograph by Guen Egan

Stay connected to your body and your breath as you practice these shoulder-strengthening exercises.

REMEMBER

Understanding and Alleviating Back Pain

Back pain affects millions, often resulting from weak core muscles, tightness, poor posture, stress, and inactivity. Lifestyle factors such as excess weight, prolonged sitting, and unhealthy habits can worsen the issue, and stress or injuries may trigger or aggravate pain. Fortunately, you can make small but powerful adjustments to reduce discomfort. Incorporating activities like stretching, improving posture, and balancing movement with rest can bring relief and help prevent recurring pain. When you understand how to support your back through these habits, you're on the path to long-term comfort and a healthier lifestyle.

WARNING

Some postures can exacerbate back pain if you have acute pain or specific issues/injuries. Always consult with your doctor first and pay close attention to how each move makes you feel. If you ever have a sharp or shooting pain, back off and eliminate that exercise.

Use the power of the pause and notice how your body feels in the moment. Do a mini body scan and tune into sensations of tightness or fatigue. Slow down your transitions and pause for a moment of stillness or meditation so you can reset your body awareness each time.

Stretches for lower and upper back

These stretches can alleviate back pain and reduce tension and stress:

>> **Cat-Cow:** As a familiar warm-up, start on all fours, arching your back on an inhale and rounding it on an exhale. Aim for eight to ten cycles. See Chapter 7.

>> **Child's Pose:** Begin on your knees and reach your hands forward, sinking your upper body toward the floor. Focus on breathing into your lower and upper back for 60-90 seconds. (See Chapter 12, Figure 12-4.)

>> **Constructive Rest:** Lie on your back with your feet wide and knees together to release your lower back. This pose is ideal for immediate pain relief — use it whenever you need a gentle lower back reset. (See Chapter 11, Figure 11-1.)

>> **Knee to Chest:** Lie down and draw one knee into your chest. Hold for 30 to 60 seconds, then switch sides. This simple, effective stretch complements the Supine Figure Four exercise for a deeper lower back release.

>> **Shoulder Rolls:** Sit tall and roll your shoulders up and back ten times, then reverse the direction. This exercise for upper back tension is also found in the shoulder mobility section, where it's recommended as a great warm-up.

Core strengthening for back support

In addition to stretching your back muscles, it's important to strengthen the core muscles that support your back and spine. The *transverse abdominals* are the deepest layer of your core, and you should focus on these when protecting and strengthening your back. Pilates is especially effective in this case, because it targets these deep core muscles through controlled, mindful movement.

In these postures, be sure to keep a neutral hip position, which is crucial for strengthening the deep core and for supporting the back and spine. For more on Pilates principles and techniques, see Chapter 5. These Pilates-inspired exercises work your core and help stabilize your back:

>> **Bird Dog:** Start on all fours, engaging your core. Stretch one arm forward and the opposite leg back, keeping your hips stable and abdominals engaged. Return to all fours, then switch sides. This exercise helps build core stability by challenging your balance and alignment. (See Figure 8-8 in Chapter 8.)

>> **Dead Bug:** Similar to the Bird Dog but done on your back, this exercise stabilizes your core while allowing you to stay in a neutral spine position. Lie on your back, lift your knees to a tabletop position, and extend your arms toward the ceiling. Lengthen your left arm backward as you reach your right leg forward without letting your torso move (see Figure 13-17). Return to center and repeat on the other side. Focus on keeping your core engaged, moving only one arm and the opposite leg at a time. Try six to eight reps for optimal core engagement and back support.

>> **Standing Knee Lifts:** Doing core work in a standing position can show you how your abdominals support you upright. Stand with your feet hip-width apart, arms overhead with palms facing each other. Lift one knee at a time toward your chest, using your core to drive the movement. Stay tall and steady, using your breath. Aim for 10 to 12 reps per side.

>> **Toe Taps:** Lie on your back and find a neutral pelvis (hips neither tucked nor arched). Tap one foot to the floor, then lift it back up using your abdominals. Keep alternating your legs and aim to move from the hip rather than bending at the knee. Do 10 to 12 reps.

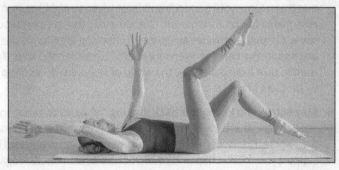

FIGURE 13-17: The Dead Bug helps strengthen your core and back.

Photograph by Guen Egan

Tips for maintaining a healthy back

Maintaining a healthy back requires daily attention to movement, posture, and self-care practices. By incorporating these simple habits, you can protect your back, reduce pain, and support long-term comfort:

» **Consider regular massages or sessions with a Feldenkrais or Alexander Technique practitioner:** For a deeper understanding of these methods, refer to Chapter 11. Chapter 6 also explores bodywork approaches that alleviate discomfort and improve range of motion.

» **Drink enough water to maintain the fluidity of your joints and the elasticity of your soft tissues:** Eating a healthy diet helps you maintain a healthy weight, which reduces strain on your back. You may also want to increase your calcium and vitamin D intake to maintain strong bones and prevent osteoporosis.

» **Improve your posture when standing, sitting, or walking:** Chapter 8 provides postural exercises and tips to support a healthy back alignment in various positions.

» **Lift with care and mindfulness:** When you pick something up from the floor, bend your knees into a squat, keep your back long, and engage your core. Avoid rounding your spine or putting too much strain on your back.

» **Practice meditation to relieve stress and anxiety:** Reducing mental stress can help you avoid holding tension in your back and spine, as back pain can often be a physical manifestation of pressure and stress. For stress-relief practices, flip to Chapter 10, which covers relaxation techniques that help reduce physical and mental tension.

» **Sleep well and make sure you're using supportive pillows and a good mattress:** Since you're spending at least seven to eight hours in bed, it's essential to be comfortable and sleep in a way that supports your back and spine. Chapter 9 provides guidance on choosing ergonomic sleep positions and supportive bedding to ensure restful, back-friendly sleep. If you really want to take a deep dive into the world of sleep, check out *Sleep For Dummies* by Dr. Clete Kushida!

» **Stay active and keep your back moving:** While it's common to think you need to rest your back when it hurts, lack of movement often makes back pain worse. Exercises that strengthen your core, arms, and legs can better support your back. Chapter 5 covers Pilates fundamentals. Yoga is also beneficial, as it stretches and strengthens your back, and Chapter 7 covers specific yoga poses for back health.

Managing Knee Pain

Knee pain can be debilitating. Years ago, I blew out my ACL while skiing. Thank goodness for my yoga and strength practice — I was able to rehabilitate it on my own. I didn't even realize until a recent MRI that my ACL was completely gone, and I was supporting my knee through the strength of the surrounding muscles, ligaments, and tendons. I'll always have to be a bit careful with my right knee and mindful of my movement. I credit my yoga and meditation practice with helping me manage the pain, and I'm also grateful for my Pilates practice, which keeps my core strong and reduces stress on my knees when I'm doing certain exercises and activities, especially running.

Causes of knee pain

Knee pain can have many causes and include injuries (like my torn anterior cruciate ligament), sprains, strains, cartilage tears (very common), and even broken bones. Repetitive stress can also cause knee pain as well as any overuse from running, jumping or kneeling for too long. Some medical conditions such as arthritis or lupus can contribute to knee pain. Iliotibial band syndrome as well as bursitis can also cause knee pain.

Stretches and exercises for knee relief

Here are some stretches and exercises that can help relieve knee pain:

>> **Knee Stretch:** Lie on your back and bend one knee toward your chest. Hold behind your thigh and gently pull the leg toward your head. After 30 to 60 seconds, switch sides.

>> **Triangle Pose:** This yoga posture helps build awareness around lifting and supporting the knee joint. Step into a wide stance, turn your right foot out 90 degrees, and turn your left foot in about 75 degrees. With both legs straight, hinge over your right leg and place your right hand on a block outside your calf or on your shin. Look up to your top hand and take five to eight breaths. Then, come to standing and switch sides.

REMEMBER

Tight hips can contribute to knee pain, so be mindful when stretching your hips. Make sure you're opening from the hip itself and not twisting or putting stress on the knee. The hip joint is a ball-and-socket joint, giving it a wide range of motion, whereas the knee joint is a hinge joint that only moves front to back. Avoid putting pressure on the inner or outer knee when doing poses like Pigeon or Ankle to Knee. If you experience knee pain, you may want to skip poses that place strain on your knee.

TIP

Whenever you're on all fours or kneeling, be sure to use a blanket, towel, or extra cushion under your knees for added support.

Strengthening surrounding muscles

Strengthening the muscles around your knees can improve knee stability and mobility, helping to protect your knee joint. Try these exercises to build support for and relieve strain on your knees:

» **Bridges:** Strengthen the glutes, hamstrings, core, and lower back to take pressure off the knees. Lie on your back with feet hip-width apart, lift your hips up off the mat, and hold for 30 seconds. Lower back down and repeat eight to ten times.

» **Calf Raises:** Strengthen the muscles in your calves, which support your knees and help reduce knee pain. Stand while holding on to a chair or wall, then lift onto the balls of your feet and lower back down. Aim for 20 reps, or try ten reps on each leg if you want to attempt single-leg calf raises.

» **Lateral Steps:** Loop a small resistance band around your ankles. Step out to the side, then bring your feet back to hip-width distance. Continue stepping to one side, then reverse direction, leading with the other leg. This exercise strengthens the outer thighs and glutes, helping the knees track properly.

» **Lunges:** Various lunges and warrior poses can strengthen the muscles around the knee. For a high lunge, step one foot back until the front thigh is parallel to the floor. Ensure the front knee doesn't move past the toes. Engage your core and stretch through the back thigh. Hold for 30 to 60 seconds, then switch sides. Repeat three to five times on each leg.

» **Seated Knee Extension:** This exercise mimics the knee extension machine at the gym and strengthens the quadriceps. Sit in a chair and loop a resistance band around your foot (or use an ankle weight). Extend your leg straight out, then bend it back to the floor. Repeat 10 to 12 times on each leg. This exercise can be beneficial for symptoms of medial meniscal tears, MCL sprains, and bursitis.

» **Step-Ups:** Practicing Step-Ups can make climbing stairs and moving around easier and safer on your knees. Find a short bench or step, place one foot on it, and bring the other foot up to meet it. Step down with the same foot first, followed by the opposite foot. Alternate starting legs for 20 reps total.

» **Wall Squats:** This exercise strengthens the quadriceps, which support the knees. Stand with your back against a wall (or use a stability ball for added core work), feet hip-width apart, and slide down until your thighs are parallel to the floor. Make sure your knees don't go past your toes. Hold for 30 to 60 seconds, and repeat two to three times.

Preventive measures for knee health

Preventing knee injuries and managing knee pain requires proactive care and mindful habits. By incorporating these strategies into your routine, you can protect your knees and support long-term joint health:

>> **Avoid sudden changes in activity levels:** Gradually increase or decrease exercise intensity and duration. For example, if you're new to running, start with run/walk intervals, gradually increasing the running periods and mileage over time.

>> **Cross-train with a mix of impact and non-impact exercises:** Incorporate both high- and low-impact activities to balance stress on your knees. Focus on strengthening your core, glutes, and quads to reduce force on the knee joints.

>> **Maintain good posture:** Slouching can contribute to knee pain. Keep good posture during daily activities to prevent strain.

>> **Maintain a healthy weight and a joint-friendly diet:** Keep a healthy weight to minimize strain on your knees. Eat a balanced diet rich in fruits, vegetables, nuts, fish, lean protein, complex carbohydrates, and healthy fats to support joint health.

>> **Turn with the balls of your feet:** When changing directions, pivot on the balls of your feet rather than twisting at your knees to avoid unnecessary stress on the knee joints.

>> **Wear supportive shoes:** Choose shoes with good cushioning to absorb impact and reduce pressure on your knees.

>> **Warm up before exercising:** Prepare your muscles and joints by warming up with low-impact movements. Walk before you run, march in place before lifting weights, or do any activity that gets the blood flowing to your leg muscles. Warming up helps ensure your knees are ready for exercise.

Addressing Neck Pain

Neck pain is a common issue that can disrupt your daily activities, reduce mobility, and even lead to headaches or tension in the shoulders and upper back. By understanding and addressing the common triggers of neck pain, you can take proactive steps to prevent discomfort and support a healthier neck.

Common neck pain triggers

Many daily habits and lifestyle factors can contribute to neck pain, but understanding these common triggers is the first step toward finding relief. By identifying and addressing the causes, you can reduce neck strain and improve overall comfort:

» **Allowing your head to fall forward:** Letting your head drop forward, whether during seated activities or while walking, places strain on the neck and upper spine.

» **Enduring stress and anxiety:** High levels of stress or anxiety can cause tension in your neck, shoulders, and upper back, leading to chronic neck pain.

» **Having poor posture:** Slouching or rounding your shoulders can strain the muscles in your neck, especially when sitting for extended periods.

» **Lifting heavy objects:** Lifting incorrectly or with poor body mechanics can strain the neck muscles, particularly if you're lifting with your head and shoulders out of alignment.

» **Looking at small screens:** Frequent use of phones or other small screens can lead to "tech neck" from constantly looking down.

» **Sleeping in a bad position:** Sleeping without adequate neck support or in an awkward position can lead to stiffness and pain upon waking.

» **Using computers for extended periods:** Sitting at a computer for long hours often leads to a forward head position and rounded shoulders, putting stress on your neck.

Gentle neck stretches and exercises

The good news is that you can decrease neck pain and start living with more ease in your head, neck, and shoulders. Physical tightness in your head and neck often leads to more tension and anxiety, so consistent stretching can be especially beneficial. Performing daily neck stretches and exercises can help combat forward head syndrome, improve your posture, and even reduce stress levels:

» **Head to Side:** Sit up tall and drop your right ear toward your right shoulder. You can place your right arm over your head to deepen the stretch, but avoid pulling on your neck — just let it relax to the side. After five to eight breaths, switch sides.

>> **Head to Chest:** From a neutral position, let your head drop straight down toward your chest. You can place your hands behind your head for a gentle assist or simply let gravity work. Keep your chest lifted and let the back of your neck relax. Hold for five to eight breaths.

>> **Head to Ceiling:** From center, lift your chin up and gently drop your head back. You can brush your hands up along the front of your neck for an added soothing effect. Hold for five to eight breaths.

Techniques to reduce tension and improve mobility

Incorporating gentle neck exercises into your daily routine can help increase mobility and reduce tension, making it easier to maintain a relaxed and pain-free neck:

>> **Chin Tucks:** Chin Tucks are excellent for preventing forward head syndrome and strengthening the neck muscles. Standing or sitting, gently move your head forward (without tipping down), then pull your head straight back, tucking your chin as if making a "chicken head" motion. Repeat for six to eight reps.

>> **Forward and Backward Tilts:** Move your head up and down by tilting it forward and then backward. Complete six to eight reps for a full range of motion.

>> **Head Circles:** Slowly circle your head around in a clockwise direction, then reverse to counterclockwise. Continue circling in both directions for 30 to 60 seconds. Stop in the center and notice how your neck feels.

>> **Shoulder Rolls:** Sit or stand tall and roll your shoulders forward, up, back, and down. Repeat six to eight times, then reverse the direction for another six to eight reps. Releasing tension in the shoulders can help free up the neck.

>> **Shoulder Shrugs:** Shoulder Shrugs help reduce tension in your upper back and shoulders, which can relieve neck strain. Sitting or standing, lift your shoulders up toward your ears, then let them drop down. Repeat eight to ten times.

>> **Side to Sides:** From a neutral position, gently turn your head from side to side, gradually increasing your range of motion. Aim for 30 to 60 seconds.

Ergonomic adjustments to prevent neck strain

Making a few ergonomic adjustments to your workspace can go a long way in preventing neck strain. By improving your posture and optimizing your setup, you can reduce the risk of stiffness and pain during long periods of sitting:

» **Adjust your chair:** Ensure your chair supports your lower back, and keep your feet flat on the floor with your legs parallel to the ground.

» **Align your keyboard:** Position your keyboard so your arms can rest comfortably by your sides, with your elbows bent at a 90-degree angle.

» **Consider ergonomic accessories:** An ergonomic headrest, a speaker or headset for phone use, and a high-quality chair can provide additional support. If you use a laptop, consider adding an external keyboard and mouse for better positioning.

» **Position your monitor:** Set your monitor so the top of the screen is just below eye level and about an arm's length away from your face. This distance helps prevent eye strain and reduces the need to lean forward.

» **Practice good posture:** Sit with your shoulders relaxed, spine long, and chin parallel to the floor. Take periodic stretch breaks to avoid slouching. A quick stretch, like clasping your hands behind your back and lifting your chest, can help reset your posture.

» **Take frequent breaks:** Aim to stand up or take short stretch breaks every hour. Even two to three minutes of movement can help prevent stiffness and discomfort.

Handling Foot and Ankle Pain

The Chinese proverb "Death begins in the feet" highlights the importance of caring for your feet as the foundation of your body. Healthy feet are essential for stability, mobility, and overall wellness. Neglecting them can lead to a range of issues that may impact your quality of life and physical abilities.

Understanding foot and ankle issues

Foot and ankle issues can arise from injuries, aging, or other factors. Common problems include sprains, strains, fractures, arthritis, flat feet, bunions, neuromas, calluses, plantar fasciitis, and ankle instability. Mobility and strength are crucial for maintaining healthy feet and ankles. Building strength in the muscles around these joints, along with regular stretching and mobility exercises, can prevent pain and reduce the risk of injury.

Exercises to strengthen feet and ankles

Strong feet and ankles can help prevent sprains, improve balance, and support better posture. Here are some effective exercises to strengthen and stretch these areas:

>> **Ankle Flexion:** While seated in a chair, extend one leg out straight and flex your toes back toward you. Hold for 20 seconds, then release. Repeat six to eight times on each side.

>> **Heel Raises (Calf Raises):** Stand with or without support, then lift up onto the balls of your feet and lower your heels back down. Aim for 20 reps. To further challenge your balance, try single-leg raises by lifting one foot at a time and completing ten reps per side.

>> **Marble Pickup:** Sit on the floor or in a chair and use your toes to pick up marbles and place them in a cup or bowl. This exercise helps improve toe dexterity and strengthens the small muscles in your feet.

>> **Resistance Band Exercise:** Loop a resistance band around a sturdy object (like a chair or table leg), then place the band around the top of your foot. Pull back with your toes to stretch the band, hold for a few seconds, and slowly release. Repeat on the other side.

Flexibility routines for better mobility

Improving mobility in your feet and ankles can help reduce injuries, support joint health, and enhance both athletic performance and daily activities. Try incorporating these exercises regularly:

>> **Alphabet Tracing:** Trace each letter of the alphabet with your feet. Start with one foot and trace each letter as a capital letter; halfway through, switch feet to complete the alphabet. This exercise improves ankle mobility and coordination.

>> **Ankle Circles:** Rotate your ankles in a circular motion, clockwise and counterclockwise. This exercise improves flexibility and reduces tension in the ankles.

» **Arch Raises:** Lift just the arch by contracting the muscles in your foot. Try lifting one arch at a time or both at the same time. This exercise helps strengthen the intrinsic muscles of the foot, which can aid in balance and stability.

» **Ball Roll:** Roll a golf ball, lacrosse ball, or even a pickle ball under the sole of your foot, focusing on releasing tight areas. Roll each foot for about a minute or two, especially at night for relaxation and relief.

» **Towel Scrunch:** Place a small towel on the floor and use only your toes to scrunch it toward you. Repeat a few times with each foot to build strength in the toes and arches.

» **Toe Raises:** Lift your heels off the ground while spreading your toes as you lift and lower. Focus on spreading your toes wide as you lift for added mobility.

» **Toe Spreading:** Stand tall and try to spread all your toes as wide as possible. Relax, then repeat eight to ten times. This exercise enhances toe dexterity.

Improving mobility and flexibility in your feet and ankles supports overall joint health and makes daily activities and athletic movements easier.

Coping with Chronic Conditions

Somatic movement can be a valuable tool for managing chronic conditions by increasing body awareness, enhancing sensations, and helping you identify areas of tension and pain. Through mindful movement and a better understanding of your body's signals, you can develop strategies to manage discomfort and find ways to release stress and anxiety associated with coping with chronic pain or other persistent conditions.

Somatic movement assists with chronic conditions in several key ways:

» **Emotional processing and coping skills:** Somatic practices provide a safe space to process emotions and develop resilience. Chapter 11 includes additional techniques for emotional resilience through mindfulness and movement.

» **Increased body awareness:** By tuning into your body, you can better recognize patterns of tension or areas of discomfort. See Chapter 2 for some foundational exercises.

>> **Mindful movement:** Moving with intention helps you avoid aggravating sensitive areas and can create a greater sense of ease. For mindful movement practices, refer to Chapter 11.

>> **Stress reduction:** Somatic practices help calm the nervous system, making it easier to manage the emotional and physical toll of chronic pain. Chapter 10 explores meditation techniques that complement somatic movement for stress relief.

REMEMBER

The Alexander Technique, Feldenkrais Method, and mindfulness meditation are all excellent options for managing chronic conditions, as each method can be tailored to address specific challenges you're facing. For more details on these methods, see Chapters 6 and 11, which cover these approaches and their applications to chronic pain and other conditions.

Somatic exercises for arthritis relief

Somatic exercises can help release chronic muscle tension that compresses the joints, allowing you to retrain your posture and movement patterns that may be straining these areas. By releasing tight muscles, you create space around the joints, easing discomfort and improving mobility. As you become comfortable with these exercises, consider incorporating light strengthening routines or weight-bearing activities like yoga and Pilates. Becoming more mindful of your choices around nutrition and stress management can also contribute to osteoarthritis relief.

TIP

Tai Chi is an excellent practice for arthritis, as it combines mindfulness with gentle movement that doesn't stress the joints. The focus on body awareness supports range-of-motion exercises that gently mobilize affected joints. Mindful breathing and gentle stretching around specific joints are also highly effective. Modified yoga postures, such as chair yoga, can be particularly beneficial for those with arthritis. For more about Tai Chi, check out *T'ai Chi For Dummies* by Therese Iknoian.

Here are some other somatic exercises you can incorporate for arthritis relief:

>> **Ankle Circles:** Rotate your ankles in circles, clockwise and counterclockwise, to improve mobility.

>> **Cat-Cow Pose (Modified Yoga):** Start on all fours, arching your back on an inhale and rounding it on an exhale.

>> **Gentle Neck Rolls:** Slowly roll your head in each direction, being mindful of your range of motion and any joint sensitivity.

» **Hip Circles:** Move your hips in large circles, both clockwise and counter-clockwise, to mobilize your hip joints.

» **Knee Flexion and Extension:** Carefully bend and straighten both knees, focusing on smooth movements and keeping the knees aligned over the ankles. This exercise promotes joint mobility without strain.

» **Modified Tree Pose (Yoga):** Place one foot against the opposite inner ankle, letting the knee open out to the side. Press your hands together in prayer position, focusing on lengthening through the standing leg and engaging your core for balance. See Figure 13-18.

» **Shoulder Shrugs:** Lift and lower your shoulders to release tension and mobilize the shoulder joints.

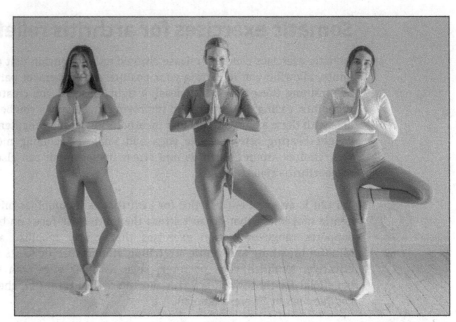

FIGURE 13-18:
The Modified
Tree Pose.

Photograph by Guen Egan

By regularly incorporating these gentle movements, you can alleviate arthritis pain and improve overall joint mobility. Remember to move mindfully, staying within a comfortable range of motion to avoid any strain.

Managing fibromyalgia symptoms with movement

When you practice somatic movement and exercise regularly, you can better deal with your fibromyalgia symptoms. *Fibromyalgia* is an autoimmune disease that causes musculoskeletal pain accompanied by fatigue, sleep, memory, and mood issues. Somatic movement helps reduce pain and fatigue, improves sleep, and can increase your sense of control and awareness.

Tai Chi can be very beneficial at reducing fibromyalgia symptoms and may even be better than aerobic exercise. Yoga is good for improving pain and reducing fatigue as well as boosting your mood. Stretching and strengthening exercises can help you overcome the pain and feel better in your body as well as give you move energy.

Adapting exercises for chronic fatigue syndrome

If you or someone you know is suffering from chronic fatigue syndrome, start slowly and begin with short, achievable activities, such as a short walk around the block or some gentle stretches in the evening. Make sure to choose the right activities. Yoga, Tai Chi, walking, and light weight training or Pilates are best.

Make sure to pace yourself and listen to your body. Somatic movement is the greatest in this case in that it really helps you listen in and breathe and not overdo it. Monitor how you feel each day and take note of your progress. Stay focused on functional strength and what you need to live happily and fully in your body while dealing with CFS.

Techniques for living with chronic pain

Managing chronic pain requires a holistic approach, incorporating various techniques that address physical and emotional well-being. Regular exercise, breathwork, mindfulness practices, and relaxation techniques can all help reduce pain and improve quality of life.

Setting goals, maintaining a balanced diet, and connecting with others are also essential components of chronic pain management. Journaling can be a powerful tool as well; writing down your feelings can help release emotions that may be tied to the pain or holding you back. You can also use your journal to reflect on the positives in your life, building gratitude even amid discomfort.

REMEMBER

Human touch is another valuable element in managing pain. Techniques like Feldenkrais, Rolfing, the Alexander Technique, and massage can provide physical relief and emotional support, making a dramatic difference in how you feel. For more on these and other somatic practices that include physical touch, see Chapters 6 and 11. For more on relieving pain using somatics, see Chapter 5.

Improving Overall Mobility

The good news is that there are many ways to work on and improve your mobility:

» **Stretching** can improve your mobility and flexibility, especially with stretches like the 90/90 stretch (a seated hip stretch where each leg forms a 90-degree angle) or the kneeling Hip Flexor Stretch (a lunge position stretch targeting the hip flexors).

» **Strength training** can also help your mobility as you build muscle. By using free weights, machines, or your own body weight, you're moving your joints through ranges of motion and improving your mobility.

» **Cardiovascular activities** — from running to dance to walking — can also help improve your mobility, as you're moving your joints through various ranges of motion. Think of a swimmer doing a full stroke or a golfer going through a full swing.

» **Yoga, Tai Chi, and Pilates** all improve mobility, overall balance, and core strength.

» **Foam rolling** can help increase mobility and relieve stiffness. Hip circles, lateral walks, lateral lunges to balance, forward lunges to balance, and deep squats are all examples of moves that will increase your mobility.

Combining different exercises for full-body mobility

To improve full-body mobility, try combining a variety of exercises and practices:

» **Foam rolling with Pilates:** Use a foam roller to release tight muscles, then follow up with Pilates exercises to improve flexibility and core strength.

» **Lunges and Warrior poses:** These yoga-inspired movements target the legs, hips, and core while enhancing balance and mobility.

>> **Squats:** Perform squats to build lower-body strength and mobility. Focus on a full range of motion for best results.

>> **Strength training with dynamic stretching:** Combine weightlifting or resistance exercises with dynamic stretches to improve mobility and flexibility while building muscle.

>> **Sun Salutations:** A yoga sequence that flows through poses targeting the whole body, improving flexibility, strength, and coordination. See Figure 12-12 in Chapter 12.

>> **Yoga and Pilates combinations:** Blend these two practices to enhance both mobility and core strength, as each focuses on body alignment and flexibility.

TIP

Most somatic workouts incorporate full-body movements, and combining exercises from different practices can create a well-rounded routine. Yoga and Pilates, in particular, align beautifully with mobility training, as they emphasize flexibility, core strength, and mindfulness.

Long-term strategies for maintaining mobility

Maintaining mobility requires consistent effort and should be a priority in your daily routine. To support lasting flexibility and mobility, follow these guidelines:

>> **Eat a healthy diet:** A balanced diet supports muscle recovery and joint health, contributing to long-term mobility.

>> **Get quality sleep:** Restful sleep is essential for recovery, especially when you're engaging in regular physical activity.

>> **Incorporate stretching and mobility exercises:** Add stretching and mobility moves to your workouts daily, focusing on a full range of motion.

>> **Make small, consistent effort:** Concentrate on doing a little each day, and pay attention to your progress. Notice how great you feel, and let that be your motivation to keep prioritizing flexibility and mobility.

>> **Manage stress:** Consider incorporating meditation and mindfulness activities into your daily routine.

>> **Practice good posture and movement patterns:** Be mindful of your posture throughout the day and focus on healthy movement patterns that avoid strain.

>> **Stay hydrated:** Hydration supports joint lubrication and overall flexibility, making it an important part of any mobility routine.

IN THIS CHAPTER

» **Coordinating cardio and somatic exercise**

» **Seeing how somatic movement can blend with strength training**

» **Warming up and cooling down somatically**

» **Designing your dream fitness plan**

» **Adjusting movements for all abilities**

» **Feeling proud of your progress**

Chapter **14**

Incorporating Somatic Exercises into Your Fitness Routine

I magine feeling completely connected to your body during every workout, understanding its cues, and moving with purpose and ease. That's what somatic exercises bring to your fitness routine — a unique blend of mindfulness and movement designed to enhance your well-being and deepen your mind-body connection.

In this chapter, you learn how to seamlessly integrate somatic practices into your existing fitness plan, whether you're running, lifting weights, or unwinding with yoga. You discover how to tailor your exercises to your fitness level, boost endurance, and prevent injuries — all while enjoying the journey. Somatic techniques aren't just about physical fitness; they're about building awareness of how you move, breathe, and recover, allowing you to thrive mentally and physically.

You also explore practical ways to incorporate somatic elements into every part of your routine — from warming up and cooling down to using props like resistance bands or foam rollers for deeper muscle activation. With these techniques, you optimize your performance while nurturing your body, ensuring it stays strong and balanced for the long haul. Somatic practices create a space for reflection and growth, empowering you to move with intention and confidence in every aspect of your fitness journey.

Combining Cardio and Somatic Exercises

Integrating cardio with somatic exercises creates a well-rounded routine that keeps you tuned into your body while moving. When you start, begin slowly and focus on practicing regularly. Pay attention to how your body feels as you move, and keep things slow and steady, gradually increasing intensity. To start, the cardio activities in Table 14-1 blend beautifully with somatic awareness.

TABLE 14-1 **Cardio Activities That Blend Well with Somatic Exercises**

Activity	Description	Making It Somatic	For More
Dancing	A fantastic way to connect with your body while getting your heart rate up. Moving to music can make you feel alive and in tune with yourself. This activity engages both mind and body, encouraging self-expression and releasing stress.	Tune into your body's internal sensations and let them guide you. The focus shifts from trying to "do" the movement in a particular way, or for an external audience, to becoming fully present with what's happening inside you.	Chapter 5 covers dancing as somatic movement.
Diaphragmatic breathing	Starting each day with diaphragmatic breathing can reduce stress while engaging your entire cardiovascular system. This practice also prepares you for physical activity by increasing oxygen flow.	Focus on the sensations of your breath. Place one hand on your stomach and feel the breath moving. It's about becoming aware of the sensations happening inside you, not just the act of breathing itself. Think of it like a mini check-in with your body — feel what's going on with each breath.	Chapter 4 covers diaphragmatic breathing in detail.
Cycling	Cycling is a low-impact exercise that gets your heart racing. When you're on a stationary bike, you can get lost in your how you feel without worrying about traffic.	Cycling becomes deeply somatic when you focus on how your body moves and stay mindful of your body's alignment and movement in space.	

Activity	Description	Making It Somatic	For More
Jumping rope	This can act as a "shake it off" exercise, helping you release physical and mental tension.	To make jumping rope somatic, you can approach it in a way that fully engages your body and your awareness of physical sensations, grounding the movement in your body and breath. The idea is to transform jumping rope from a purely mechanical activity to an embodied practice that connects your mind, body, and breath. Make the rope an extension of your body!	Chapter 2 talks more about "shake it off" exercises.
Walking	An accessible, effective, and endlessly versatile exercise. Start with a grounding exercise.	Somatic walking is about being fully present with the body's movements and sensations in the moment. When you walk somatically, you intentionally tune into the physical experience of each step.	Chapter 10 covers grounding, whereas Chapter 11 covers mindful walks.

TIP

Schedule time to mentally process what you release during these movements, as they can often have emotional as well as physical effects.

Improving Efficiency and Form

Somatic techniques help you recognize and correct habits that interfere with balanced movement and alignment, enabling you to move with better form and efficiency. The exercises outlined in Table 14-2 help improve your form and reduce unnecessary strain so you can naturally move more effectively.

Somatic stretching is focused on increasing body awareness and reconnecting the mind and body. The goal is to cultivate a deep sense of self-awareness in how your muscles and joints move and feel, with an emphasis on release and relaxation. Regular stretching, on the other hand, focuses primarily on improving flexibility, mobility, and muscle elongation. It may not emphasize body awareness to the same degree as somatic stretching, and the intention is often more physical rather than emotional or cognitive.

TABLE 14-2   **Somatic Exercises That Improve Form**

Discipline	Description	For More
Alexander Technique	This method focuses on recognizing habits that cause tension and poor form. By cultivating positive movement patterns, you move with less strain, increasing efficiency across all activities.	Chapter 11 guides you through how to do the Alexander Technique.
Breathwork	Deep breathing enhances core stability and oxygen delivery, helping you maintain better posture and relax your nervous system. With less tension, you conserve energy and sustain good form longer.	See Chapter 4 for more on different breathwork exercises to try.
Movement therapies	Practices such as yoga, Pilates, and Tai Chi integrate physical movement with emotional awareness, teaching you to breathe deeply and move intentionally. These therapies help you develop muscle memory for good form, which improves efficiency not only during exercise but in everyday life.	Chapter 5 explains these therapies in more detail.
Somatic stretching	Enhances posture, flexibility, range of motion, and balance. Tight muscles pull your spine out of alignment, so creating length and ease in your muscles helps improve overall function.	Gentle beginner stretches are described in Chapter 5. For stretches that target specific body parts, see Chapter 13.

Preventing Injury

Somatic movement helps prevent injury by teaching you to listen to your body and respond to its needs in the moment. This awareness allows you to recognize when you're pushing too far, adapt exercises to your current capacity, and build strength mindfully. Somatic exercises also help you identify signs of overuse and fatigue, so you can adjust and recover as needed.

Recognizing signs of overuse and fatigue

Signs of overuse and fatigue can include

>> **Emotional symptoms:** You may feel fatigued, exhausted, or low on energy throughout your day. Irritability, anger, moodiness, or depression can also signal overexertion.

>> **Health-related symptoms:** Getting sick more often, becoming more prone to infections, or experiencing increased blood pressure or heart rate may indicate overuse.

» **Performance issues:** You might find it hard to concentrate or focus, feel scattered or forgetful, or notice a decline in work or school performance. Struggling to organize your thoughts can also be a sign.

» **Physical symptoms:** Muscle pain, stiffness, or a general feeling of heaviness in your muscles may occur. Unusual weight changes, bloating, or constipation can also be physical indicators of overexertion.

» **Reduced motivation:** A loss of interest in activities you once enjoyed, coupled with decreased self-esteem, may indicate the need for rest.

» **Sleep issues:** Insomnia or waking up feeling tired and unrested are common signs of overdoing things.

Incorporating recovery practices

Recovery is a vital part of any fitness routine. Make sure to schedule regular rest days and find ways to unwind and de-stress that don't tax your body. As always, listen to what your body is telling you and respect those messages. Try these recovery practices:

» **Active recovery:** Include gentle movements like Yoga *Nidra* (see Chapter 7), mindful slow walks (Chapter 11 tells you more about these), or light stretching on your recovery days. These allow your body to stay active without strain.

» **Diet and hydration:** Stay hydrated and focus on eating nutrient-dense, high-quality foods with plenty of protein.

» **Massage and bodywork:** Try massages, warm baths, or bodywork therapies to release tension and support muscle recovery.

» **Mind-body practices:** Explore meditation, breathwork, or quiet time to help reduce stress and promote relaxation. See Chapter 10 for more on meditation.

» **Sleep and rest:** Prioritize good sleep habits and take breaks from high-intensity workouts when needed.

» **Temperature therapies:** Experiment with methods like cold plunges or saunas to soothe sore muscles.

WARNING

Always include proper warm-ups and cool-downs during exercise to prepare your body and allow it to relax afterward. Taking care of your body with recovery practices not only prevents injury but also supports long-term fitness and well-being.

Adding Somatic Elements to Strength Training

When you're strength training, you can incorporate somatic movements and exercises to enhance your workouts. These techniques help you become more mindful of your movements, improving both your physical and emotional connection to the exercises. By integrating somatic elements, you can increase awareness, reduce the risk of injury, and get more out of every rep.

Integrating somatic awareness

Integrate somatic awareness into your strength routines by slowing down and moving more consciously. This approach helps you maintain good form and control over your muscles. To deepen your awareness and make each movement more intentional, try to

>> **Engage in body scanning:** While working out, scan your body to connect your mind to your muscles, helping you focus on the physical and emotional effects of your exercise.

>> **Experiment with slower movements:** Try a pushup or squat, performing the movement at a slower pace while keeping proper form. This allows you to build greater control and awareness.

>> **Focus on your breathing:** Notice how exhaling during exertion can help you complete a few more reps or lift heavier weights. Use diaphragmatic breathing to bring more oxygen into your lungs, powering you through your workout.

>> **Practice good posture:** Use a mirror to check and adjust your posture before lifting or performing a move. This allows you to build greater control and awareness.

REMEMBER

By applying somatic movement and mindfulness to your strength training, you stay present in each movement, gaining more from your workouts without distractions.

Focusing on muscle activation and control

When lifting weights, focus on the muscles you want to activate and control your movements with proper form. Start with small, deliberate movements to build control as you engage specific muscle groups. Contract and release your muscles slowly, paying attention to their activation. Use touch to ensure you're targeting the correct muscles — for example, place your hand on your bicep during a one-arm curl or on your glutes during a squat to avoid overusing your quads.

Enhancing mind-muscle connection

When you enhance your mind-muscle connection, you get so much more out of your workout — physically and mentally. Focusing on your movements and your intentions with certain techniques helps you optimize your exercises and deepen your results:

>> **Explore bodyweight exercises:** Exercises like pull-ups provide a full range of motion and help you properly engage muscles. With bodyweight movements, there's no room to "cheat" — they naturally encourage proper form. Rather than focusing solely on strength or speed, a somatic pushup emphasizes tuning into your body, cultivating a deep awareness of each movement, and exploring the sensations you experience. Slow down, focus on your breath, feel the transitions, and reflect on how the movement makes you feel.

>> **Flex and relax targeted muscles:** Before starting your workout, flex and release the muscles you want to work on. This simple practice increases blood flow and prepares your body for movement.

>> **Incorporate mindfulness:** Stay present in each movement by using meditation, mantras, or visualization before your workout. Take a few moments to set your intention and focus on what you aim to achieve.

>> **Prepare with a warm-up:** Warming up improves muscle strength, power, and reaction time. It helps your muscles contract and relax faster, getting you ready for the movements ahead. You can do a "shake it off" somatic movement or some gentle arm swings or leg swings to get your blood pumping a bit.

>> **Use touch to guide activation:** Lightly touch the muscles you're engaging to ensure proper activation. You can also ask a friend or coach to assist by gently tapping the target area.

>> **Visualize your movements:** Picture the muscles you're working and imagine them contracting in your mind. Visualization improves focus and helps direct oxygen and blood flow to those muscles.

Whether you're in the gym or preparing for an activity, taking a few moments to mentally prepare will help you stay focused and get the most out of your workout.

Balancing strength and flexibility

You can balance your strength and flexibility by incorporating a variety of exercises throughout your week. Stretching improves flexibility, strength training builds muscle, balance exercises enhance coordination, yoga combines strength and flexibility, and dancing boosts coordination, strength, and mobility.

WARNING

A lack of balance, strength, or flexibility in one area can negatively impact the others, increasing your risk of injury and affecting overall well-being.

Combining strength exercises with stretching

Combining strength training with stretching offers numerous benefits, including building strength, improving flexibility, reducing the risk of injury, and increasing mobility. This approach allows you to move through a greater range of motion while supporting overall balance and performance:

» **Alternate training days:** Follow a strength-training day with a yoga or mobility-focused day to allow your muscles time to recover and improve flexibility. Alternate throughout the week.

» **Stretch between sets:** Incorporate stretches between strength-training sets to relax and elongate the muscles you're working, helping to reduce tension and maintain balance.

» **Warm up and cool down properly:** Use dynamic stretches during your warm-up to prepare your body for movement and target the areas you plan to work on. After your workout, perform static stretches to relax and lengthen the muscles you just used.

Addressing muscle imbalances

When one side of your body is stronger or more flexible than the other, this imbalance can affect your performance and increase your risk of injury. You can correct muscle imbalances with intentional exercises and mindful lifestyle adjustments:

» **Adopt somatic practices:** Use methods like the Alexander Technique, Feldenkrais, or Rolfing to create a personalized plan for identifying and correcting imbalances. (See Chapter 11 for more.)

» **Be mindful throughout your day:** Stay aware of how you move, sit, and stand to avoid reinforcing imbalances outside of your exercise routine.

>> **Evaluate external factors:** Check your shoes, sleeping position, and posture to uncover and address contributors to muscle imbalances.

>> **Use unilateral exercises:** Work one side of your body at a time with exercises like single-arm rows or one-legged squats. Unilateral movements help you identify which side is stronger or weaker so you can begin to balance them.

Using Somatic Exercises as a Warm-Up and Cool-Down

Somatic exercises can be highly beneficial for warming up and cooling down. These gentle, intentional movements help relax the fascia around your muscles, increase blood flow, and improve sensory awareness to your brain. Incorporating somatic exercises into your warm-up routine not only prepares your body for movement but also provides a mental check-in.

Warming up with somatic techniques

Every day, your body is in a different state depending on factors like sleep, nutrition, and previous activities. Warming up gives you a chance to connect with your body and notice how you feel in the moment. It also helps you release tension, regulate your nervous system, and foster a sense of relaxation and safety as you prepare to exercise.

Try incorporating the somatic warm-up techniques listed in Table 14-3 into your warm-up, which will allow you to ease into activity while increasing circulation, reducing muscle tension, and enhancing your mind-body connection.

TABLE 14-3 **Somatic Warm-Up Techniques**

Technique	Description	For More
Dynamic stretches	Prepare your body with controlled movements like high knees, squats, or lunges to get your heart rate up and blood flowing	See Chapter 13.
Gentle somatic movements	Try Cat-Cow stretches, hip circles, or "shaking it off" to loosen your muscles and wake up your core.	See Chapter 13.
Intentional movement	Perform the exercise you're about to do, but more slowly and mindfully, focusing on proper form.	See Chapters 2 and 5.

Preparing the body with gentle movements

The mind–body practice of somatic exercise uses gentle movements to release tension and build awareness of your body. These exercises help you feel prepared and relaxed as you transition into more intense activity:

» **Butterfly Hugs:** This movement fosters a sense of safety, confidence, and support as you move into your workout. Cross your arms over your chest, placing your hands on your shoulders or upper arms. Tap one hand on your shoulder or arm, then alternate with the other hand in a slow, rhythmic motion. Focus on slow, deep breathing as you continue tapping. This gentle, self-soothing technique helps regulate your nervous system, reduce stress, and promote a sense of safety and relaxation. Turn to Chapter 7 for more guidance on self-hugging.

» **Diaphragmatic breathing:** This technique calms your mind and body while improving oxygen flow, helping you ease into activity. See Chapter 4.

» **Progressive muscle relaxation:** Alternately contracting and releasing muscles decreases tension, preparing your body for smoother movements. See Chapter 7.

» **Seated Cat-Cow:** This seated movement guides your spine through flexion and extension, making it a great warm-up for any activity. Turn to Chapter 7 for the how-to guidance on this stretch.

» **Supine Spinal Twists:** Gentle spinal twists help open your spine and prepare your back for motion. See Chapter 5.

Activating key muscle groups

Muscle activation exercises are short, targeted movements designed to prepare your body for physical activity. These exercises increase blood flow to your muscles, relax overactive areas, and ensure the targeted muscles work efficiently.

» **Band pull-aparts:** Hold a resistance band at shoulder height and pull it open, stretching your arms wide, as shown in Figure 14-1. Relax and repeat 10 to 12 times.

» **Fire hydrants:** With a small resistance band around your knees, lift one leg open to the side while on all fours, as shown in Figure 14-2. Try ten reps on each side.

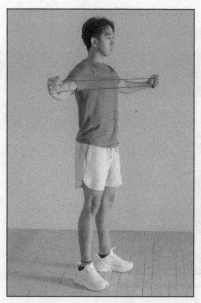

FIGURE 14-1:
Band pull-aparts help activate your shoulders.

Photograph by Guen Egan

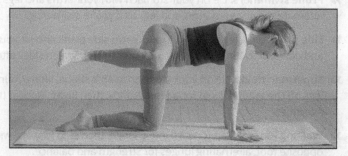

FIGURE 14-2:
Fire hydrants are great for activating your hips, knees, and legs.

Photograph by Guen Egan

>> **Monster walks:** As shown in Figure 14-3, loop a band around your ankles, bend your knees slightly, and step sideways while pressing against the band. Move forward and backward for balance.

>> **Plank march:** In a forearm plank, lift one leg straight behind you, alternating legs to engage your core and glutes.

>> **Plank with single-arm lift and hold:** From a plank position, lift one arm forward and hold, switching sides to challenge your core stability.

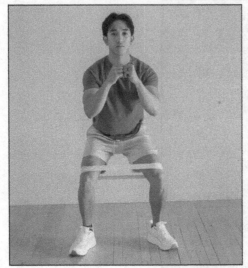

Photograph by Guen Egan

FIGURE 14-3: Monster walks are funny and fun!

>> **Prone swimmers:** Lie on your stomach with your arms and legs lifted. Alternate moving your arms and legs as if you're swimming.

>> **Side plank with leg raise:** Hold a forearm side plank and lift your top leg up and down, activating your core and outer thighs. Switch sides after ten reps.

>> **Superman holds:** Lie on your stomach in an X shape, lifting your arms and legs off the ground. Hold for a few seconds, then lower. Repeat three to five times.

>> **Walking lunges:** Step forward into a lunge, then step forward with the opposite foot, alternating lunges for strength and balance.

To deepen the experience of these somatic exercises, you can take it a step further by incorporating mindfulness and sensory awareness. Here's how:

1. **Pay attention.** Slow down, feel the ground, and pay attention to the mechanics.

2. **Practice body scans, starting at your feet and moving your way up.** Notice any tension you can release and only activate the muscles you are using.

3. **Connect your emotions to your body.** Feel the emotions in your body as you do these.

4. **Keep breathing and find your flow.**

5. **Be aware of your movement and make micro adjustments as needed.**

6. **Embrace fluidity.** Allow your movements to feel fluid and organic, rather than rigid or mechanical. This can help you stay more connected to the experience of each exercise.

Cooling down with somatic practices

At the end of your workout, somatic practices help your body recover while promoting relaxation. The techniques in Table 14-4 release tension, calm your nervous system, and leave you feeling restored.

TABLE 14-4 **Somatic Cool-Down Techniques**

Technique	Description	For More
Breathwork	Practice deep, diaphragmatic breathing to calm your body and reduce stress.	See Chapter 4.
Body scans	Check in with how your body feels after activity, focusing on areas of tension or fatigue.	See Chapter 6.
Progressive muscle relaxation	Contract and release muscles to gently ease into rest. Start with your toes and move up your body until you reach the top of your head	See Chapter 7.
Static stretches	Incorporate relaxing poses like Pigeon Pose, Seated Forward Folds, Ankle-to-Knee Supine Twists, and Supported Bridge Pose.	See Chapter 8.

REMEMBER

Throughout these practices, stay mindful and connected to your movements. Let your breath guide you and listen to what your body needs in the moment. By keeping your focus on intentional relaxation, you can create a space for recovery that leaves you feeling restored and ready for your next activity.

Reducing muscle soreness and tension

Somatic movement is an effective way to reduce muscle soreness and tension. By incorporating proper warm-ups and cool-downs into your routine, you prepare your muscles for activity and give them time to relax afterward, making soreness less likely. Somatic movements naturally calm the nervous system, which promotes healing and helps release tightness and discomfort.

To alleviate soreness, try swaying gently back and forth with your arms overhead. Move naturally with your breath, as if you're being rocked by the wind. This flowing motion helps release tension and improves blood circulation. You can practice this anytime you feel sore or include it at the end of every workout.

Try these other practices to reduce muscle soreness:

>> Child's Pose is another great way to rest, recover, and ease muscle tension throughout your body. For added relief, try heel drops by lifting and lowering your heels while focusing on the sensations in your lower back and feet.

>> Wave breathing is also helpful for releasing tension in your nervous system. It's similar to Cat-Cow but has a gentler, wave-like rhythm. Sit or stand comfortably, inhale as you arch your back, then exhale as you round your spine. Close your eyes and focus on the movement of your spine, letting it flow naturally with your breath.

>> Incorporating practices like yoga and meditation further supports muscle recovery. Meditation, in particular, helps you enter a deeply restorative state, promoting healing and relaxation throughout your body.

Creating a Balanced Workout Plan

A balanced workout plan is like a balanced diet — variety is essential. Focusing on only one type of movement can create imbalances or increase the risk of injury. Think of your routine like a plate:

>> **Your main activity** is your "main course," making up the biggest portion. Choose something you love and enjoy doing most frequently.

>> **A complementary activity** supports your main activity, like strength training to enhance yoga or Pilates to support posture and alignment.

>> **A fun or recovery activity** adds an element of relaxation or joy, such as hiking, swimming, dancing, or Restorative yoga.

For example, if yoga is your primary activity, you might do yoga three to four times a week. Add two to three strength-training sessions to supplement your practice, and include hiking or walking for fun and variety. Finally, include a daily relaxation practice to wind down and connect.

Integrating cardio, strength, and somatic exercises

A well-rounded routine combines cardio, strength, and somatic exercises, each offering unique benefits to your fitness and well-being. Cardio improves heart health and endurance, strength training builds muscle and bone density, and somatic exercises promote flexibility, alignment, and body awareness.

To build a balanced routine:

>> **Include a few days of cardio each week**, choosing activities you enjoy, such as walking, cycling, swimming, dancing, or rowing. If you're new to cardio, start with shorter sessions and gradually increase your duration and intensity.

>> **Aim for at least one day of strength work** using weights, Pilates, or bodyweight exercises like pushups or squats. Resistance bands or functional training moves are great alternatives for variety and accessibility.

>> **Incorporate mindful practices** like yoga, stretching, Feldenkrais, or restorative movements daily, either as part of your warm-up or cool-down, or as a stand-alone practice for recovery and relaxation.

Here's a sample weekly schedule to integrate all three:

>> **Monday/Wednesday/Friday:** Cardio activities such as brisk walking or swimming.

>> **Tuesday/Thursday:** Strength training using weights or bodyweight exercises.

>> **Daily:** Somatic exercises like stretching, yoga, or mindful body scans, either as a warm-up or cool-down.

By combining these components thoughtfully, you can create a routine that supports your physical fitness, reduces injury risk, and enhances your mind-body connection.

Scheduling rest and recovery days

Rest and recovery are just as important as movement, allowing your body to heal, rebuild, and recharge. Without adequate recovery, you risk injury, burnout, and diminishing returns from your workouts. Dedicate at least one day a week to full recovery. Sundays are a popular choice, but any day that works with your schedule is fine.

On recovery days, prioritize activities that support relaxation and restoration. Stretch, meditate, or engage in gentle somatic practices to release tension and reconnect with your body. If you prefer movement, consider active recovery options like a slow walk, Restorative yoga, or light foam rolling. These can promote circulation and help alleviate muscle soreness without overtaxing your body.

To maximize recovery, focus on:

>> **Hydration:** Drink plenty of water throughout the day to support muscle repair and reduce fatigue.

>> **Nutrition:** Fuel your recovery with nutrient-dense foods, including protein, healthy fats, and antioxidant-rich fruits and vegetables.

>> **Sleep:** Prioritize quality sleep, as it's during rest that your body heals and regenerates.

By taking time to rest, you'll improve your performance, prevent injuries, and set yourself up for long-term fitness success.

Modifying Exercises for Accessibility

Using props and modifications can make exercises more accessible, ensuring comfort and safety as you start slowly and progress at your own pace. These adjustments allow everyone, regardless of fitness level, to engage in movement that feels supportive and empowering.

>> **Chair yoga:** Chair yoga is a fantastic way to modify exercises for greater accessibility. Try seated Cat-Cow stretches, gentle twists, side bends, or poses like Modified Warrior II, Tree Pose (while holding the chair), or Downward Dog with your hands on the seat of the chair. You can also stretch your hamstrings by placing one leg on the chair seat.

>> **Pushup modifications:** Start with pushups against a wall. Stand about a foot away from a wall and place your hands on the wall at shoulder height. Bend your elbows out to the side bringing your chest toward the wall, then press back to starting position. Try these before transitioning to kneeling pushups or full pushups over time.

>> **Squat modifications:** If a full squat feels too challenging, try squatting onto a chair and standing back up.

>> **Strength training without weights:** Begin with bodyweight-only exercises, such as lunges or planks, before adding weights. You can also try lunges while holding onto a chair (see Figure 14-4).

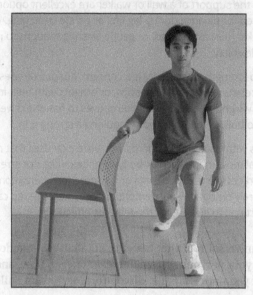

FIGURE 14-4:
Use a chair for balance while lunging.

>> **Using props for yoga and stretching:** Props like yoga blocks, straps, and towels can help you deepen stretches or modify yoga postures to suit your abilities.

Adapting movements for different abilities

Every body is unique, and adapting movements for different abilities ensures that exercise is accessible, empowering, and safe for everyone. Whether you're managing a disability, recovering from an injury, experiencing mobility challenges, using assistive devices, or navigating hearing or vision impairments, the key is to listen to your body and choose modifications that meet you where you are:

>> If you use a wheelchair, there are numerous seated exercise options to explore. Chair yoga is a great place to start, with movements like seated

twists, Cat-Cow stretches, or side bends. Resistance bands can add variety, enabling strength training for the upper body without requiring standing. You can also practice breathwork and mindfulness exercises from a seated position to build a strong mind-body connection.

» For those using canes, walkers, or other assistive devices, focus on stability and safety. Exercises like wall pushups, squats to a sturdy chair, or standing stretches with the support of a wall or walker are excellent options. A walker can also be used for balance during leg lifts or gentle stretching. When seated, you can try ankle rolls, arm circles, or gentle twisting motions to maintain mobility and flexibility.

» If reduced grip strength or dexterity is a concern, adapt exercises using tools like grip aids, resistance bands with loops, or weights with built-in handles. Ankle or wrist weights are also great alternatives to handheld weights, allowing you to build strength without requiring a strong grip.

» For individuals with vision impairments, prioritize exercises that require minimal spatial movement, such as bodyweight exercises or stretches, and use tactile markers like textured mats or furniture for orientation. For hearing impairments, rely on clear visual demonstrations, step-by-step captions, or written instructions to guide your movements effectively.

Breathwork is a universal tool that benefits all abilities. Practice diaphragmatic breathing to calm your nervous system, increase oxygen flow, and stay connected with your body. If you notice fatigue, discomfort, or tension building, slow down and take a break.

REMEMBER

Above all, honor your body's needs. Adaptations might mean reducing intensity, modifying posture, or seeking guidance from a professional experienced in adaptive fitness. Accessible fitness is about creating a movement practice that works for you — empowering, enjoyable, and aligned with your abilities, including any assistive devices you use in daily life.

Ensuring your safety and comfort

When trying new exercises, take it slow and prioritize safety. The most important thing is to feel comfortable with the movements and avoid injury. For example, when training for my first marathon, my goals were to finish the race and avoid injury. I focused on listening to my body, building up gradually, and staying within my limits.

Here are a few tips for staying safe and comfortable:

>> **Distinguish between discomfort and pain:** While stepping slightly out of your comfort zone can promote growth, sharp, shooting pain or burning sensations are warning signs to stop immediately.

>> **Monitor your breathing:** You should still be able to talk and stay present in your movements. If you find yourself holding your breath or feeling overly strained, take a step back.

>> **Prioritize recovery:** Schedule breaks and recovery days, stay hydrated, eat nourishing foods, and get quality sleep to help your body heal and rebuild.

TIP

Keeping your fitness routine enjoyable and varied is essential for long-term success. Choose activities that genuinely bring you joy, whether it's dancing, hiking, or practicing yoga. Switch up your workouts regularly to keep things fresh and prevent boredom — try a new class, explore outdoor activities, or incorporate playful movements like jumping rope or balancing challenges. When you look forward to your workouts, staying consistent feels less like a chore and more like self-care. Variety also helps work different muscle groups, reducing the risk of overuse injuries while keeping your body and mind engaged. Above all — and yes, it bears repeating — listen to what your body is telling you and work to stay connected in the moment.

Chapter **15**

Maintaining a Lifelong Somatic Practice

C ommitting to a lifelong somatic practice is like planting a garden that grows with you — sometimes flourishing wildly, sometimes needing a little pruning, but always full of potential. Whether you're just getting started or refining years of experience, somatic exercises are designed to adapt, evolve, and move with the rhythm of your life.

This chapter focuses on creating sustainable habits, adjusting your practice to different life stages, and overcoming challenges. You learn to set actionable goals, track progress, and keep your enthusiasm alive — even on those days when you'd rather stay under the covers (we've all been there). And don't worry — this isn't about perfection. It's about finding joy in the process and celebrating even the smallest victories. Let's dive in and explore how to keep this journey vibrant, fulfilling, and as delightful as your favorite playlist. You've got this!

Setting Goals and Staying Motivated

Maintaining motivation begins with setting clear and meaningful goals. Think of your goals as guideposts that keep you focused while leaving room for flexibility. Whether you aim to improve flexibility, manage stress, or enhance your overall well-being, breaking goals into daily, weekly, monthly, and annual targets makes the journey more manageable — and a lot more fun.

This process is a journey of self-discovery that allows you to deepen your connection to your body and mind. This section guides you in making somatic practices a consistent part of your life.

Establishing a daily routine

Your daily somatic practice is the foundation of your journey. By incorporating small, consistent actions into your routine, you create habits that stick.

TIP

Make your daily goals simple and easy to accomplish to help you build momentum and confidence. The practices don't have to take up much time, but can still make a big difference in how you feel throughout your day.

A daily routine can help keep you accountable and give you structure so you don't end up wondering where the time went by at the end of the day. Think of it as laying the groundwork for your somatic practice. Start by blocking out time for somatic practices. Target the times when you have the most energy or can create a quiet space for focus. Here's one way to set up your day:

>> **Morning check-in:** Start your day with a moment to set your intention. Take a deep breath, stretch gently, and think about what you want to achieve.

>> **Midday pause:** Schedule your somatic practice when your energy dips. A short breathing session, a quick mindful movement break, or a ten-minute meditation can refresh your focus.

>> **Evening reflection:** Before bed, revisit your day. Reflect on what worked well, notice how your body feels, and mentally release any tension.

Write down your routine to solidify your commitment, whether in a planner, a journal, or even a note-taking app. Lay it out like a to-do list or a daily schedule:

>> 7:00 AM: Five minutes of mindful breathing.

>> 12:30 PM: Ten minutes of yoga or somatic stretching.

>> 8:00 PM: Body-scan meditation before bed.

The key is to start small, choosing practices you can manage without overloading your day. Stick to this routine for a few weeks to build consistency. See if you notice a difference in your energy and awareness.

TIP

INCORPORATING SOMATIC PRACTICE INTO DAILY ACTIVITIES

If you find it hard to set aside dedicated time, you can blend somatic exercises into the activities you're already doing. You can enhance your practice without needing extra hours in your schedule by weaving mindfulness and movement into every-day moments:

- **At your desk:** Try gentle chair yoga poses, like Seated Twists or Shoulder Rolls, to release tension.

- **During chores:** Pay attention to how your body moves while washing dishes or vacuuming. Move deliberately, engaging your core and focusing on posture.

- **While brushing your teeth:** Do calf raises or balance on one leg to strengthen your ankles and core.

- **While walking:** Turn a regular walk into a mindful one by focusing on your breath and the sensation of your feet touching the ground.

Use transition moments in your day — like waiting for your coffee to brew or standing in line — to practice mindfulness or body awareness. Even a few seconds of somatic breathing or a subtle stretch can help you stay present and reduce stress.

These activities don't replace dedicated somatic practice, but they do complement it by keeping you tuned in to your body throughout the day. As a result, you'll find it easier to stay connected and consistent, even during busy times.

TIP

Use technology to help you stick to your plan. Set reminders on your phone or use a calendar app to schedule your practices just like appointments. For example, create recurring events labeled "Mindful Breathing" or "Somatic Stretch Break" at your chosen times. Many apps also offer guided meditations, movement sessions, or habit trackers to keep you motivated and on track.

Setting weekly milestones

Your weekly somatic practice builds on your daily habits and lets you take a broader view of your progress. Weekly goals allow you to

» Experiment with new techniques

» Reflect on what's working

» Set a rhythm that fits your lifestyle

TIP

Use your weekly milestones to reinforce your progress, explore fresh ways to enhance your practice, and build consistency. Adjust your goals as needed to keep things fun and achievable.

Weekly goals are like stepping stones toward bigger achievements. These milestones are a chance to push yourself a little further without feeling overwhelmed. They also help you see how, over time, even small efforts add up:

>> **Add a new somatic movement** to your practice, such as Tree Pose or Child's Pose (see Chapter 7 for the full how-to on different movements).

>> **Dedicate one day to reflection** by journaling your physical and emotional progress, identifying what's working and what could improve.

>> **Experiment with movement timing** by shifting your daily practice to a new part of the day and see how it impacts your energy or focus.

>> **Incorporate a mindful activity into your week**, like journaling, cooking a meal with full attention, or practicing mindful walking.

>> **Meditate for 10 minutes daily** and evaluate how it feels by week's end. For ideas and guidance on meditation, turn to Chapter 10.

Revisit your weekly plan at the end of each week. Reflect on what worked well, what didn't, and what changes you want to make for the upcoming week. This process of trial, error, and refinement keeps your practice personalized and effective.

Managing monthly check-ins

Monthly check-ins allow you to zoom out and assess the progress you've made from your daily and weekly practices. This is a chance to celebrate your wins, refine your goals, and set intentions for the month ahead. These moments of reflection ensure your somatic practice stays fresh and aligned with your needs.

As you go, you can always adjust. Nothing is set in stone. These are your goals, and as long as they suit your life and make you feel better overall, carry on!

REMEMBER

Consistency builds habits, but reflection builds growth. Use monthly check-ins to celebrate progress and course-correct where needed. Consider journaling your thoughts to capture your progress and uncover trends over time. Look at

>> **Consistency:** Did you stick to your daily and weekly goals? Why or why not?

>> **Mental well-being:** How do you feel after your exercises? Are they helping you to feel calmer, more centered, or better equipped to manage stress?

>> **Physical changes:** Have you noticed any improvements, such as in flexibility, posture, or balance?

Documenting these reflections gives you clarity about what's working and high-lights areas where you may want to shift your focus.

Reflect on progress and set new targets

Once you've assessed your month, it's time to refine your goals and set new targets. Use your reflections to inspire growth while keeping your goals realistic. For example:

>> **Build on your successes:** If you've consistently practiced one movement, challenge yourself by adding a new movement or increasing the duration of your sessions. Maybe you meditated every day for five minutes each day. Next month, you may want to increase to ten-minute sessions or add an additional five-minute meditation.

>> **Deepen your mindfulness:** If you've been practicing basic breathing techniques, consider trying more advanced options like coherent breathing, covered in Chapter 4.

>> **Expand your focus:** If you've worked on improving flexibility, add strength-building exercises to your routine, covered in Chapter 14.

Make adjustments

Your plans are not set in stone — think of them as flexible tools rather than rigid rules. Adjustments allow you to respond to how your body and mind feel, ensuring that your somatic practice remains enjoyable and supportive. If something isn't working, reflect on why and tweak it to fit your needs.

Try adjusting your goals by

>> **Modifying intensity:** If a movement feels too challenging, simplify it by reducing the range of motion or using props for support. For example, you might use a wall or chair for balance while practicing certain poses.

>> **Shortening duration:** If meditating for 15 minutes feels overwhelming, break it into two shorter sessions or reduce it to 10 minutes. Consistency is more important than length!

>> **Switching activities:** If a specific exercise doesn't resonate with you, swap it for something you enjoy more. For instance, replace a standing stretch with seated movements or try a different breathing technique.

>> **Tuning into your energy levels:** If you're feeling fatigued one week, focus on gentler practices like Restorative yoga or body scans instead of dynamic flows.

REMEMBER

Listen to your body as you adjust. It's okay to scale back when you feel tired or overextended, or try something new to stay engaged. Progress isn't always linear — it's about finding what works best for you at any given moment.

Setting annual goals

Your annual somatic check-in is a time to dream big, reflect deeply, and celebrate how far you've come. Long-term goals give your practice a sense of purpose and direction, while yearly reflections help you track the lasting benefits of your somatic journey. This is also a great opportunity to set intentions for the year ahead and adjust your focus.

Long-term goals give you something to work toward over the course of a year. These goals are often larger or more complex than daily or weekly ones and require consistent effort to achieve. Think of them as your North Star — they guide you forward, inspire you to stay committed, and remind you of the big picture. Your long-term goals reflect what excites and inspires you:

>> **Commit to a new somatic skill**, like mastering the Tree Pose or balancing in a handstand

>> **Focus on a lifestyle goal**, such as incorporating somatic awareness into a mindful 5K run/walk or practicing sobriety for a year

>> **Integrate new techniques** into your practice, such as somatic flow sequences (see Chapter 12) or advanced breathwork

TIP

To make your bigger goals achievable, break them into smaller, actionable steps by linking them to your daily, weekly, and monthly practices.

Keep in mind, long-term goals are about progress, not perfection. Celebrate the effort you're putting in and don't stress if your timeline shifts — life happens, and your goals can adjust to fit it. No matter what happens, the journey toward your long-term goal is just as important as achieving it. Think of each small win along the way as a reason to high-five yourself (or treat yourself to an extra cozy cup of tea).

Celebrating the year

The end of the year is your chance to pause, reflect, and celebrate how far you've come. Somatic practices are about more than physical improvements — they touch every part of your well-being, from your mental clarity to your emotional resilience. Taking the time to honor your journey helps you stay motivated and reconnect with your purpose.

Start your reflection by asking yourself these questions:

» **Have I noticed improvements in my physical health**, such as better posture, greater flexibility, or reduced pain?

» **Have I developed more emotional resilience**, with a steadier mood or better tools for managing stress?

» **Have I cultivated new habits** or skills that bring joy and meaning to my life?

TIP

Write down your thoughts or share them with a trusted friend or mentor. Acknowledging even the smallest wins can spark gratitude and inspire you to keep going.

Once you've reflected, it's time to celebrate! Try marking your progress by:

» **Hosting a mini celebration** by sharing your favorite somatic techniques with friends or family. Teach them a movement or mindfulness trick you've mastered this year.

» **Planning a somatic retreat for yourself**, whether it's an afternoon in nature, a workshop with an expert, a quiet day dedicated to journaling and body awareness, or something else that rejuvenates you.

» **Treating yourself to a somatics-related reward**, like a new yoga mat, meditation cushion, or class pass to deepen your practice.

REMEMBER

Celebrations don't have to be elaborate. Sometimes the best reward is taking a day to relax, reflect, and simply enjoy the progress you've made.

Finally, use your yearly reflection to set intentions for the next year. What do you want to build on? What new skills or practices excite you? Let your successes guide you as you step into another year of growth.

Making Adjustments for Age

Somatic practices grow and change with you, making them accessible at any stage of life. Whether you're maintaining flexibility during midlife or focusing on balance and mobility as a senior, adapting your practice ensures it continues to meet your needs.

REMEMBER

Your body is your best guide. Listen to it as you adjust for different life stages, and let your practice evolve naturally.

Addressing common middle age concerns

Midlife often brings busier schedules and changing physical needs. Somatic practices during this phase can help you stay strong, flexible, and mindful amid life's demands. They also offer a valuable opportunity to reclaim time for yourself in a hectic schedule, grounding you in the present moment.

Middle age often comes with unique challenges, including health, mental well-being, lifestyle shifts, and even financial worries. This is a critical time to take charge of your overall wellness and set yourself up for a vibrant, fulfilling life.

Physical health

During middle age, the risk for certain health conditions — such as heart disease, cancer, high cholesterol, weight gain, or muscular issues — can increase. Now is the perfect time to prioritize your health by adopting habits that support long-term well-being:

>> **Build muscle mass:** Incorporate strength training to maintain muscle tone and support your joints.

>> **Eat a balanced diet:** Focus on meals rich in fruits, vegetables, lean proteins, whole grains, and healthy fats.

>> **Get regular health screenings:** Stay proactive about your health by scheduling checkups and addressing concerns early.

>> **Include cardiovascular activity:** Do something that gets your heart rate up, like brisk walking, cycling, or dancing.

>> **Practice somatic movement regularly:** Gentle yet consistent movement helps maintain flexibility, reduce stress, and support overall fitness.

Taking small, consistent steps now can make a big difference in preventing future health issues.

Mental health

Your mental health is just as important as your physical health, and the two are closely interconnected. For some, middle age can bring emotional challenges, including signs of a midlife crisis, irritability, or depression. To support your mental well-being:

>> **Incorporate somatic exercises:** Meditation, breathwork, and hands-on therapies are powerful tools for reducing stress and increasing self-awareness.

>> **Prioritize self-compassion:** Be kind to yourself, practice gratitude, and embrace a positive mindset.

>> **Seek connection:** Engage in supportive communities or relationships, as touch and social interaction can be profoundly healing.

Somatic practices can help you process emotions, increase resilience, and foster a sense of calm and clarity.

Lifestyle changes

If you haven't already, middle age is an excellent time to reevaluate your daily habits and make meaningful lifestyle changes:

>> **Prioritize sleep:** Quality rest is essential for both physical and mental recovery.

>> **Reassess your diet:** Ensure you're fueling your body with nutritious foods that support energy and longevity.

>> **Stay active:** Regular movement not only keeps your body strong but also boosts mood and reduces stress.

Simple changes, made consistently, can lead to profound improvements in how you feel every day.

Tailor exercises to maintain flexibility and strength

As you age, it's natural to lose some muscle mass and flexibility if you aren't actively working to maintain them. According to findings by Harvard Medical School, adults can lose 4 to 6 pounds of muscle per decade starting in their 30s. Without consistent stretching or moving your joints through their full range of motion, flexibility and mobility can also decline.

The good news? Somatic movement can help you preserve — and even improve — muscle mass and flexibility. A balanced routine that incorporates strength training and flexibility exercises can make a significant difference.

Here are some strategies to tailor your practice:

>> **Balance your routine:** Incorporate at least two strength-training sessions per week or add weight-bearing activities like yoga and Pilates to your schedule.

>> **Be consistent:** Maintaining muscle mass doesn't require long workouts, but it does require dedication to regular, mindful movement that fits your lifestyle.

>> **Focus on flexibility and mobility:** Include mindful stretching, dance, or somatic flow sequences to keep your joints supple and maintain your range of motion.

If you're worried about "bulking up" from strength training, don't be! More muscle mass boosts your metabolism, making it easier to maintain a healthy weight while staying strong and resilient.

Stay mindful in midlife

Midlife often comes with a full plate — whether you're balancing career, family, or personal goals, your mindset plays a crucial role in helping you navigate it all. Staying mindful can help you feel grounded, focused, and better equipped to live the life you want.

Somatic exercises, such as meditation and breathwork, can dramatically improve your outlook and strengthen your relationship with yourself. Personally, I credit my well-being to my twice-daily meditation practice.

Try these simple ways to stay mindful throughout your day:

>> **Engage your senses:** Use your five senses to fully experience each moment — whether it's enjoying a meal, taking a walk, or spending time with loved ones.

>> **Incorporate mindful movement:** Stretch, open your body, and welcome the possibilities of the day ahead.

>> **Set mindful reminders:** Schedule a timer on your phone to pause every hour or so. Take a mindful moment to reflect on where your thoughts are and reconnect with the present.

>> **Start your day with gratitude:** When you wake up, take a few deep, full breaths. Acknowledge the gift of being alive and thank your body for all it does for you.

>> **Use your breath as an anchor:** Throughout the day, pause and take deep breaths to help you stay present and centered.

Mindfulness doesn't have to be time-consuming. Small, intentional moments throughout your day can make a big difference in how you feel and function.

Making senior adjustments

As you get older, somatic movement becomes an invaluable tool for maintaining joint lubrication, muscle strength, and mental alertness. Every senior's journey is unique, so it's important to modify exercises to match your current abilities. The key is to move safely and consistently, even if that means shorter sessions more frequently. Remember, sometimes less is more, especially when it allows you to maintain consistency.

Modify exercises for seniors

Seniors may need to make any number of tweaks to stay comfortable and safe:

>> **Adjust the range of motion:** If deep movements feel challenging, start with smaller motions. For example, try partial squats or use a chair to sit down and stand back up.

>> **Slow it down:** Adjust the speed and tempo of movements to suit your comfort level. Slower, deliberate movements can be just as effective as faster ones.

>> **Support your balance:** Hold onto a wall or chair during standing exercises until you feel steady.

>> **Use props:** Chairs, resistance bands, and blocks can make movements more accessible. For example, do pushups against a wall or a modified plank using a chair. Chair yoga is another excellent option for gentle strengthening and mobility.

Focus on balance, mobility, and gentle strengthening

For seniors, maintaining balance and mobility is crucial for preventing falls and staying active. Focus on:

>> **Balance-building exercises:** Practice standing on one foot with support nearby or gentle walking drills to improve stability (see Chapters 5 and 13).

>> **Gentle strength training:** Use light resistance bands or bodyweight exercises to strengthen key muscle groups without overexertion.

>> **Mobility-enhancing movements:** Perform wrist rolls, shoulder shrugs, or ankle rotations to maintain joint flexibility.

REMEMBER Always listen to your body and adjust the pace or intensity of your exercises to what feels comfortable. Gentle and consistent practice leads to long-term benefits.

These somatic exercises are excellent for building strength, improving mobility, and enhancing balance:

>> **Bird Dog:** From all fours, extend one arm forward and the opposite leg back. Hold for five seconds, then switch sides. This move strengthens the core, glutes, and lower back.

>> **Calf raises:** Stand near a wall or chair for support and lift your heels up and down. This keeps your feet and ankles mobile. Aim for 20 repetitions.

>> **Knees to chest:** Lie on your back and bring one knee into your chest at a time. This stretches the lower back and hips.

>> **Leg raises:** Lie on your side and lift your top leg, or lie on your stomach and lift one leg at a time to strengthen the lower back and improve posture.

>> **Sitting to standing:** Strengthen your lower body by sitting in a chair and standing back up. Repeat 10 to 12 times.

REMEMBER Consistency is key. Even small movements done regularly can lead to noticeable improvements in strength, mobility, and overall well-being.

Accommodating Different Abilities

Somatic practices are for everyone, regardless of physical ability or experience level. Somatic movement isn't about striving for perfection or fitting into someone else's mold — it's about learning to connect with your body on your terms. There's no "one-size-fits-all" approach here, and that's what makes it so empowering. With simple adaptations and the right mindset, your practice can be as unique as you are. Somatic exercises can meet you exactly where you are. This is your journey, and it's all about finding what feels good and right for your body.

The tennis legend Arthur Ashe said, "To achieve greatness, start where you are, use what you have, do what you can." You have a unique opportunity to craft the body, mind and spirit that you want. It is never too late to start. Starting where you are right here and right now is the most productive way to create lasting change.

REMEMBER

Somatic practices aren't about doing things perfectly — they're about connecting with your body in a way that feels right for you.

Starting where you are

Everyone's somatic journey begins from a different place. The key is to honor where you are today and create a practice that works for your unique abilities and circumstances.

Here's how to assess and adapt to your starting point:

» **Begin with gentle movements:** If you're new to somatics or have limited mobility, start with seated or lying-down exercises, such as spinal twists or gentle stretches (see Chapter 5).

» **Focus on consistency:** Building a regular practice, even if it's short, is more important than trying to do too much too quickly.

» **Listen to your body:** Pay attention to what feels good, what feels challenging, and what feels uncomfortable. Adjust your movements accordingly to avoid strain.

Remember, it's not about how much you do — it's about how mindful and present you are during each practice.

Assess your individual needs and capabilities

Understanding your current fitness level is the first step in tailoring your somatic practice to your unique needs. Take stock of key factors like body composition, endurance, bone density, flexibility, and posture. Tools like a DEXA scan can measure bone density, while BMI calculators or modern scales can provide detailed stats beyond weight. If you're curious about endurance, consider investing in a VO2 max reading or scheduling a postural assessment.

Once you've assessed your baseline, reflect on your goals. What do you want to achieve? How much time and energy can you dedicate to your practice? And most importantly, how can you ensure your safety and comfort while working toward those goals?

Health and fitness are often measured by flexibility, movement patterns, and muscular endurance. You can check these on your own or consult a fitness professional for more accurate assessments. Start with simple tests:

» **Flexibility:** Can you touch your toes while keeping your spine long? Can you hold opposite elbows behind your back?

>> **Mobility:** How easily can your joints move through their full range of motion?

>> **Strength and endurance**: How many pushups can you do? How long can you hold a plank?

Over time, as you continue to practice, you'll notice improvements in these areas. Tracking these changes can provide you motivation and show you how far you've come on your journey.

Customize your exercises for different levels

Once you understand your baseline, you can begin tailoring your workouts to focus on what your body needs most to feel its best. Everyone's starting point is unique, and customization is key to making progress in a safe and sustainable way.

After 30 years of yoga practice, my physical therapist told me something unexpected: "You're too flexible, and your joints need more stability." This revelation shifted my focus to strength training, which has become a critical part of my routine. As a woman approaching perimenopause, maintaining and building muscle is especially important for my health.

What works for me may not work for everyone. Someone younger who sits at a desk all day might benefit from more mobility training combined with light strength work. On the other hand, an older individual who experiences high levels of stress and limited movement might start with mindful walks, light resistance band training, or chair yoga.

The key is to meet yourself where you are and work with what you have. Assess your unique needs and customize your exercises accordingly, whether that means focusing on stability, flexibility, strength, or stress relief. By honoring your current level, you can build a practice that supports your growth and well-being.

One of the strengths of somatic practices is their adaptability. Almost any exercise can be modified to match your current abilities. Here's how:

>> **For beginners:** Simplify movements by reducing your range of motion or focusing on just one part of the body at a time.

>> **For intermediate practitioners:** Increase the duration or add dynamic elements to your practice, such as flowing between poses.

>> **For advanced practitioners:** Deepen your connection by holding poses longer or incorporating more challenging variations, like balancing poses.

For more examples of how to adapt somatic movements to your fitness level, see Chapter 14.

Progressing at your own pace

Forward is a pace. If you're dedicating time each week to your somatic movements, you're making progress. Not all changes are immediately visible — sometimes, they're felt instead. You might notice that your energy improves, you wake up feeling more rested, or your body moves with greater ease. Instead of relying solely on the mirror for feedback, pay attention to how you feel. Notice your mood, your breath, and your overall sense of well-being each day.

REMEMBER

You are your only competition. There's no need to compare yourself to anyone else; simply aim to be a little better than you were yesterday. Journaling can help you track your progress and focus on small wins, which are far more sustainable than dramatic changes.

Consistency is key, so make your practice manageable. Go slow, stay steady, and trust the process. As long as you're investing in yourself, progress is inevitable.

Set realistic and achievable goals

Once you've assessed your needs, the next step is to set realistic goals that inspire and motivate you without overwhelming you.

When you're goal-setting

>> **Adjust as needed:** Life happens! It's okay to modify your goals as circumstances change.

>> **Be specific:** Instead of saying, "I want to get stronger," try, "I want to practice chair poses three times a week to build leg strength."

>> **Start small:** Focus on goals you can achieve in the short term, like practicing mindful breathing for five minutes a day or adding a single stretch to your morning routine.

Progress gradually to avoid overexertion

Somatic practices emphasize gentle, mindful movement, making them especially valuable for gradual progression. Overexertion can lead to strain or burnout, so taking your exercises slow is key.

To ensure you are safely progressing:

>> **Balance effort and rest:** Alternate between active poses and restorative exercises to give your body time to recover.

>> **Increase intensity gradually:** Add small increments to your routine, like holding poses a few seconds longer each week or incorporating a new exercise every month.

>> **Listen to your body:** Pay attention to signals of discomfort or fatigue and scale back if needed.

REMEMBER

Consistency matters more than intensity. Slow and steady progress builds a strong foundation for long-term success.

Utilizing adaptive equipment

Adaptive equipment is a gateway to empowerment. Whether you're living with a disability, managing an injury, or simply seeking comfort in your practice, props like chairs, blocks, and resistance bands meet you exactly where you are. These tools can support you and show you how much is possible.

Use tools and props to enhance practice

You can make somatic exercises more accessible and enjoyable for yourself with different tools and props:

>> **Balance aids:** Items like wobble boards or stability cushions can enhance balance exercises for advanced practitioners or create extra support for beginners.

>> **Blocks:** Help reduce strain by bringing the ground closer.

>> **Bolsters:** Offer support during restorative poses, reducing pressure on joints and muscles.

>> **Chairs:** Perfect for seated poses or to provide balance support during standing exercises. Chair yoga is especially beneficial for those with limited mobility.

>> **Resistance bands:** Add gentle strengthening elements to your practice without requiring grip strength.

>> **Yoga straps:** Help with flexibility by providing extra reach during stretches.

Modify the exercises for accessibility

Modifications make somatic practices inclusive and adaptable for a wide range of abilities. Here are some ways to modify exercises:

>> **Adjust positions:** For standing poses, try seated variations. For example, replace a standing forward fold with a seated version using a chair.

>> **Reduce strain:** Use cushions, blocks, or rolled-up towels to support sensitive areas like knees or wrists.

>> **Shorten duration:** If an exercise feels too intense, reduce the time spent holding a pose or performing a movement.

Maintaining Consistency and Motivation

If you feel joyful when you move or feel down when you're not doing your exercises, you'll likely stay motivated and consistent. Action creates motivation, and the more you incorporate somatic exercises into your life, the more likely you are to keep going. I always notice how I feel off if I've skipped a few days of meditation. Realizing that I feel so much better when I make time for it keeps me dedicated.

Staying consistent with your somatic practice can feel like a challenge at times, especially when life gets busy. However, creating a supportive environment and inviting others into your journey can help you stay motivated and connected to your goals. This section offers practical ways to build consistency and keep your practice sustainable.

Creating a supportive environment

A supportive environment is the foundation for any consistent practice. Your surroundings can encourage you to show up daily, even when motivation wanes. When you have a supportive environment around you, you are more likely to stay motivated and consistent. Create a space in your home that is welcoming and exciting for you to want to move or practice in. Find a network of supportive people in your area who love to see you succeeding.

Set up a dedicated practice space

A space just for your somatic practice doesn't have to be elaborate — a small, intentional corner is enough. Here's how to make it work:

>> **Add personal touches:** Decorate your space with items that bring you peace, like a favorite candle, soft lighting, or a calming piece of art. Hang fun encouraging quotes on the wall.

>> **Choose a calm, clutter-free spot:** Whether it's a corner of your living room or a small section of your bedroom, pick a space where you feel comfortable and undistracted.

>> **Keep your tools handy:** Store your mat, props, or cushions within reach so you don't have to search for them before practice.

Encourage family and friends to join

Your friends and family will want to join when they see you thriving. Actions speak louder than words, and you'll be a living representation of health and well-being. They'll want to support you and join your journey as you support them.

If your actions alone don't spark their interest, try sharing your personal success stories. Tell them what makes you feel so good, how you started, why you started, and what keeps motivating you to show up. Sometimes, simply explaining the benefits can inspire others to get involved.

Here are some ways to make somatic practices a shared experience:

>> **Connect with your partner:** Explore partner yoga poses or unwind together with a restorative class before bed.

>> **Do fun things together:** Join a local yoga community and set a regular class date with a friend, or find an awesome studio in your area where you can do a Pilates duet together.

>> **Involve your children:** Try a guided meditation as a family or let them join in a playful somatic movement session.

Tracking your progress

Tracking your progress and setting clear goals can help you stay motivated and on track. By monitoring your improvement, you can celebrate small gains and identify areas to adjust or improve. Tracking also provides a tangible way to see how far you've come, which can be incredibly encouraging.

Start by establishing a baseline for where you're starting, whether it's your endurance, strength, or flexibility. Use tools like fitness journals, apps, or progress photos — not for aesthetic changes alone but to observe improvements in posture, mobility, or strength over time. For example, take photos to track how your posture aligns after a month of somatic exercises.

Try this check-in/check-out strategy:

>> **Check in:** Set aside time to evaluate how you feel before and after your workouts.

>> **Check out:** Reflect on what you've accomplished and areas you'd like to improve.

Keep a fitness journal

A fitness journal is a powerful tool for staying motivated and tracking your journey. Write in the present tense as if you're experiencing your workouts in real time. Include details like these:

>> The exercises you perform.

>> How you feel physically and emotionally during and after the session.

>> Any sensations, challenges, or breakthroughs you experience.

>> Motivational quotes or affirmations that inspire you.

Review your entries periodically to see how far you've come and to identify patterns in your fitness journey.

TIP

Keep your journal somewhere easily accessible, like your gym bag, desk, or bedside table. Writing immediately after your workout ensures that you capture all the details while they're fresh.

REMEMBER

You don't have to limit your journal to somatic exercises or workouts. Journaling can encompass your entire body-mind experience. Maybe some movement released emotions you want to explore on paper, or perhaps you'd like to journal immediately after a session to capture how you feel.

If you need more inspiration, consider using prompts to get started:

>> What do I want to accomplish today?

>> Which movements made me feel best?

>> How is my mood?

>> What am I grateful for?

>> What has my body done for me today?

Use apps and technology for feedback

Fitness apps and trackers can provide real-time feedback and deeper insights into your progress. Apps like Fitbit, Garmin, or Apple Watch can track your steps, heart rate, and calories burned, while apps like Strava or Runkeeper monitor cardio performance. For strength training, try Caliber, Ladder, or Shred.

Use apps and trackers to

>> **Monitor your performance:** Use real-time data to adjust your intensity and stay in your target zones.

>> **Receive feedback on form:** Some apps analyze your movement patterns and provide tips to improve technique and avoid injury.

>> **Set personalized goals:** Input your baseline data to get customized workout plans.

>> **Stay motivated with cues:** Many apps offer audio guidance, reminders, or badges to celebrate milestones.

>> **Track your recovery:** Check metrics like sleep quality and heart rate variability to ensure proper recovery.

>> **Learn new exercises and techniques:** Apps can give you fresh ways to approach movements you already know. Personally, I love hearing new cues for familiar moves — it helps me experience them in a deeper way.

REMEMBER

Using technology doesn't just track your progress — it helps boost your confidence, motivate change, and organize your goals. Whether you're learning something new or reflecting on how far you've come, apps and tools make your journey more rewarding and accessible.

Finding inspiration

Inspiration comes in so many forms. As you deepen your connection to yourself through somatic movement, you'll find inspiration in ways you may not have expected. Reading motivational books, journaling, observing art, or learning a new skill can spark new ideas. Even social media can inspire you with new exercises or uplifting quotes.

Look for inspiration in nature, while traveling, or when collaborating with others. Sometimes, simply getting enough sleep or refreshing your environment can shift your perspective and reignite your energy.

Join communities

A supportive community can be incredibly inspiring and motivating. I love retreats for this very reason — you meet a group of like-minded people who share your passions and interests. Whether you join a cycling club, a walking group, or a Tai Chi class, communities like these offer a sense of connection and support, making your journey feel less lonely.

Check out your local YMCA, yoga studio, Pilates studio, or movement gym to find a welcoming and warm environment. For example, when I first fell in love with yoga, I joined a local studio in the East Village in NYC. It not only introduced me to amazing friends but also opened my eyes to new ways of thinking. Having a community to share your growth with can help you feel more grounded and comfortable in your practice.

Attend workshops and classes

Workshops and classes are wonderful opportunities to deepen your knowledge, connect with others, and reignite your motivation. You can learn a lot so much and walk away with new techniques to explore.

Workshops often provide in-depth experiences that immerse you in your practice, while regular classes can fill in gaps, offer new insights, or keep you motivated when practicing at home feels difficult. Personally, I love combining a home practice with the occasional class to keep things fresh and balanced.

Learn from experts

Learning from experts can transform your practice. Whether it's a class, workshop, seminar, or retreat, studying with someone who has dedicated years to their craft can be inspiring and educational.

For example, I've learned something new every time I've worked with mentors or teachers in Pilates, yoga, meditation, Feldenkrais, or Alexander Technique (see Chapter 11). Experts offer deep insights and unique approaches to somatic work, which can help you make huge strides in your progress.

If possible, consider saving up for a private session with an experienced teacher. One-on-one attention allows them to assess where you are, tailor the experience to your needs, and guide you in ways that can significantly accelerate your growth.

Overcoming Common Challenges

Every journey comes with its hurdles, but challenges can also be opportunities for growth. Whether you're facing plateaus, setbacks, injuries, or just a tough day, remember that these moments are a natural part of the process. With resilience and the right tools, you can move through them and come out stronger on the other side.

Dealing with plateaus

As the saying goes, "Fall seven times, get up eight." When you hit a dip or stall in your growth, welcome it as a chance to reflect and reassess. Maybe your body is finding a new baseline before its next leap. Try not to get discouraged — get curious! Do you need to push yourself a little more? Shake up your routine? Or maybe address lifestyle factors that could be interfering with your progress? Plateaus are a natural part of growth, and they're temporary — they can remind us to adapt, grow, and rediscover what excites us. Setbacks set us up for success by teaching resilience.

REMEMBER

When you bounce back from a fall, you build strength and grit, which helps you evolve.

Recognize a plateau

If you notice you've stayed stagnant for several months, it may be a sign of a plateau. Ask yourself first: Do I need to keep growing? Perhaps you've reached a point in your flexibility, strength, or practice that feels satisfying to maintain.

Signs of a plateau include:

>> Declining performance or progress

>> Feeling unmotivated or uninspired by your practice

>> Lack of focus, energy, or enthusiasm

>> Repeating the same mistakes without improvement

TIP

Your journal can be a helpful tool for spotting plateaus and identifying potential causes. Use it to track your energy, progress, and mindset.

Overcome stagnation

To break through a plateau:

>> **Focus on recovery:** Prioritize sleep, nutrition, and stress management to support your body's needs.

>> **Invest in learning:** Take a class, hire a personal trainer, or explore online courses. Fresh perspectives can energize your practice.

>> **Mix things up:** Try new exercises, routines, or activities to keep things interesting.

>> **Seek community:** Join a group or connect with others to share ideas and find motivation.

Staying motivated during setbacks

Setbacks can be frustrating, but they're also opportunities to learn more about yourself. Setbacks build resilience and grit. Remember: "You grow through what you go through." Look for ways to celebrate your progress, even in small ways, and remind yourself of the times you've overcome obstacles in the past. You're tougher than you realize!

To stay motivated:

>> Practice self-care and celebrate small wins along the way.

>> Seek support and feedback from friends, mentors, or a support group.

>> Set new goals or refresh old ones to focus your energy.

>> Use affirmations to keep a positive mindset. Hang them where you'll see them often — on your mirror, your desk, or even your phone background.

Cope with injuries and illness

Injuries and illnesses can be disheartening, but they're also opportunities to pause, reflect, and grow. If you suddenly get sick or hurt, the first thing to do is pause your regular routine. Then:

>> **Celebrate small wins:** Keep a journal to track victories, no matter how small, and remind yourself of your progress.

>> **Maintain a positive outlook:** Use mantras like "Safe, healed, whole" or "Every day, in every way, I'm getting better and better" to focus your mind on healing.

>> **Practice self-compassion:** Allow yourself the time and space to heal without judgment.

>> **Seek support:** Lean on family, friends, or support groups to help you manage stress. You don't have to go through this alone.

Relaxation is key to healing — try meditating, journaling, listening to music, or other calming activities to reduce stress and anxiety. Depending on your condition, gentle movement, like a short walk or a few stretches, can improve your mood and circulation.

Maintain a positive mindset

A positive mindset can make all the difference, especially during challenging times. To stay optimistic and focused, try to:

>> **Focus on self-care:** Develop a morning routine that sets the tone for your day and engage in activities that bring you joy.

>> **Practice gratitude:** Write down three things you're grateful for each day, or try a gratitude meditation.

>> **Surround yourself with positivity:** Spend time with upbeat people and avoid negativity when possible.

>> **Use affirmations and mantras:** Encourage yourself with phrases like, "I am resilient," or, "I'm growing stronger every day."

Challenges are part of the journey. Embrace humor, stay curious, and keep moving forward. You're capable of more than you think, and each step — no matter how small — brings you closer to your goals.

6

The Part of Tens

The Part of Tens

IN THIS PART . . .

Debunking the common misconceptions about somatic exercises.

Enhancing your somatic experience with quick tips.

Chapter **16**

Ten Common Misconceptions About Somatic Exercises

S omatic exercises are for everyone — not just those with pain or injuries. They invite you to listen to your body, tune into its sensations, and connect with your emotions. Despite the benefits, somatic movement is often misunderstood. This chapter busts the most common myths about somatic exercises, giving you clear and actionable insights so you can approach this practice with confidence and curiosity.

Somatics Is Only for People with Injuries or Chronic Pain

While somatic exercises are incredibly effective for easing pain and supporting recovery, the benefits of somatic exercise extend far beyond that. Everyone can benefit from somatic exercises. This form of exercise is accessible to people of all fitness levels — even those without pain issues and even for elite athletes. They can help you improve your posture, flexibility, overall movement quality, and quality of life.

Whether you're an elite athlete or someone new to mindful movement, somatic exercises can improve your posture, flexibility, coordination, and overall quality of life.

You can use somatic exercises to focus on subtle, intentional movements, which help you regulate your nervous system and release tension. You also become more aware of how your muscles contract and extend, helping you prevent injuries before they happen. It's like a built-in body awareness system that strengthens you from the inside out.

REMEMBER

Somatic movement isn't about limitations; it's about possibilities. It meets you where you are and grows with you, helping you become stronger and more balanced, one movement at a time.

You Need to Be Flexible

Flexibility is one of the benefits you gain from somatic exercises, but you don't need to be flexible to begin. I often have students come to me and say they can't do yoga because they aren't flexible. I think that's like saying, "I can't lift weights because I'm not strong." You practice yoga and somatic movement to become flexible; you lift weights to become strong. The beauty of somatic movements is that they meet you where you're at. You can tailor them to your level. You have to start somewhere, and flexibility is a practice like anything else. Some people may be naturally more flexible than others, but everyone can benefit from flexibility training. Whether you're feeling stiff or already have a yoga-like range of motion, somatic exercises guide you gently toward greater mobility. The beauty of this practice lies in its adaptability. You work within your current range, gradually expanding it without pushing or forcing.

Flexibility is a gift you give your body. Somatic exercises help you work within your own range of motion and gradually increase your mobility. Through slow, deliberate movements, you release tension and develop awareness, which allows you to gain flexibility over time. You feel comfortable as you grow because you don't push yourself too hard or force anything. Instead, somatic movement lets you ease into your body and open carefully and naturally.

They're Just Stretches

Somatic exercises aren't just stretches. What sets them apart is their focus on breath and total body awareness. These are mindful movements that emphasize the internal experience of your body. Instead of concentrating on how your body looks, you tune into how it feels, moving with intention and listening to your inner guide.

While somatic movements often involve stretching, they go deeper by addressing root issues and unlocking your potential. This approach creates long-lasting changes. I've worked with athletes who used to stretch for sports. When they started practicing yoga and connecting their breath to the muscles they were opening, it transformed their experience. One wrestler I taught recognized many of the moves from his pre-tournament stretches but had never used his breath to deepen them. That small change made all the difference.

Somatic exercises are gentle, slow, and intentional. They focus on what feels good and relaxing, rather than pushing you past the point of pain or discomfort. Growing up as a dancer, I had teachers who encouraged us to stretch far beyond what was safe. In contrast, somatic movements combine stretching with breathwork, awareness, visualization, and insight. This intentional approach supports your health, well-being, and deeper connection to yourself.

REMEMBER

Somatic movement does so much more than traditional stretching. It relieves stress, regulates your nervous system, eases muscle tension, enhances mind-body awareness, and helps you process emotional issues.

Many somatic exercises mirror natural, everyday movements — like reaching when you stand up, side-bending when you get out of bed, or making circles with your feet after removing your shoes. They also include practices like body scans, freeform dance, full-body stretching, yoga, Tai Chi, Pilates, and mindful strength exercises. When you explore somatic movement, you open the door to a world of options, each designed to help you live your best life.

They Don't Build Strength or Fitness

Somatic exercises don't aim to build strength or fitness directly, but they focus on improving your mind-body connection — and this makes you stronger and fitter in everything you do.

One of the biggest myths about yoga is that people don't expect it to deliver such an incredible full-body workout. I still remember my very first yoga class. I was sweating buckets, and it wasn't even in a heated room! Yoga challenges your entire body with poses that demand strength, stamina, and focus. Other somatic practices, like Pilates, also build strength, endurance, and fitness in unique ways.

TIP

When you tune into how your body feels as you move, you strengthen your intuition and deepen your connection to yourself. This awareness carries over into everything else you do. When you lift weights or do any other type of workout, you release tension more easily and channel your energy more effectively. Somatic movement also builds mobility, balance, and coordination — key components of aerobic capacity and strength. You can even recover from common musculoskeletal issues while getting stronger.

Practices like yoga, dance, Tai Chi, and Pilates reveal strength you might not even realize you have. I've never met a "weak" dancer. Their strength, balance, and body awareness always amaze me. Even adding a little somatic dance movement to your week can boost your strength, flexibility, and overall fitness.

When you hold a plank, balance in Tree Pose, or engage your core during Pilates, you actively build strength. Somatic movement makes strength training more intentional.

REMEMBER

Somatics is also about building flexible brains. Neuroplasticity tells us that people can train their brains to be more flexible. Somatics can help you build physical flexibility of course, but it can also build flexibility in your brain, which can change your behavior and how you relate to others.

You Need Special Equipment

You don't need special equipment to practice somatic exercises! These gentle, mindful movements work anywhere — no fancy gear, specific clothing, or shoes required. For the most basic warm-ups, all you need is

>> A comfortable place to sit or lie down.

>> A yoga mat or large towel (optional but helpful).

>> Your body, breath, and a willingness to move.

That's it! The simplest movements often deliver the most profound changes. Start with what you have and build from there. As you grow more familiar with your practice, you might choose to invest in small props, but every exercise works perfectly with just your body. You can explore a wide range of movements without any tools:

>> Body scans and breathing exercises (see Chapter 4 for detailed breathwork techniques)

>> Bodyweight strength exercises like planks, pushups, and core movements

>> Guided visualizations and progressive muscle relaxation

>> A good pair of comfortable, supportive shoes is all you need for mindful walking

>> Pilates and yoga (for more on these practices, turn to Chapter 5)

>> Tai Chi and other martial arts (for an introduction, head over to Chapter 6)

They're Too Easy to Be Useful

Somatic movements may appear simple at first glance, but they require a tremendous amount of awareness. In a world filled with distractions, tuning into your body on such a deep level presents a unique challenge. While you may not be lifting the heaviest weights or running the fastest, somatic exercises teach you to:

>> Align your body for proper form when lifting weights or performing other physical activities.

>> Improve mobility and flexibility in your joints, which enhances balance and coordination and supports healthy backs, hips, and shoulders.

>> Walk and run with good posture, naturally increasing your cardiovascular endurance while avoiding injuries.

For me, somatic movement is tougher than anything else I've ever done. It often involves unlearning or repatterning lifelong habits, which can feel daunting. Listening to your body on such a deep level can make you feel vulnerable. It requires you to let your guard down and remove the walls you've built over time. Opening yourself up like this can be intimidating but also deeply transformative.

Somatic movement challenges the outdated "no pain, no gain" mindset. You don't need to push your body to its limits to see results. Instead, holistic movement nurtures your entire body, giving it the love and understanding it truly needs. This approach reduces the risk of overdoing it or ending up sidelined by injuries. Even professional athletes use somatic exercises to improve performance and manage stress. These practices:

>> Increase body awareness, which allows for more efficient and effort-less movement.

>> Reduce muscle tension, easing both physical strain and mental stress.

>> Retrain reactions to stress, helping athletes perform better under pressure.

TIP

Staying present is one of life's hardest skills. Practicing somatic exercises helps you learn to return to the here and now whenever your mind starts to wander.

Keep in mind, too, that somatic exercises range from beginner-friendly to advanced. For example, you might start with slow toe taps in Pilates but eventually progress to a full teaser V-sit. Nothing about Pilates is "easy" — I've personally become stronger in countless ways thanks to my yoga and Pilates practice. I credit these exercises for improving my posture, core strength, and flexibility.

You Need a Class or Teacher to Practice

You don't need a class or a teacher to practice somatic movements. The goal is to look inward and start paying attention to your body, and you can do that on your own. Once you learn some basic moves, you're free to experiment, adjust, and discover what works best for you.

Classes or teachers can enhance your experience if you want to explore deeper techniques or gain new insights (see Chapter 3 for tips on finding the right guide), but they aren't required. This book offers step-by-step instructions and plenty of exercises to help you get started right away. Somatic movement is about trusting yourself and connecting with your body, and that's something you can do anywhere, anytime, without anyone else.

They Aren't Scientifically Proven

Somatic exercises have a long history. Yoga dates back 5,000 years, Tai Chi has been practiced for thousands of years, and Joseph Pilates introduced his method in the early 1900s. These practices wouldn't have remained so popular if they didn't work.

Modern science supports aspects of somatic movement, especially meditation and mindfulness. Research shows that meditation improves mental health, enhances sleep, reduces pain, lowers blood pressure, sharpens focus and memory, and fosters emotional resilience. It also increases compassion and *interoceptive awareness* — your ability to sense what's happening inside your body — and supports better decision-making. Somatic exercises incorporate these elements of mindfulness and meditation by combining movement with breath and focused awareness. Instead of avoiding sensations, you embrace and fully experience them.

REMEMBER

While not every somatic practice has conclusive scientific proof, evidence suggests that these exercises help relieve pain, reduce tension, and promote easier movement. They offer gentle, low-risk options for improving body awareness and emotional well-being. In a world filled with stress and distractions, it never hurts to get more in tune with your body and emotions.

They Aren't Different from Yoga

Yoga is one type of somatic movement, but if yoga doesn't resonate with you, plenty of other options exist. Practices like Pilates, the Alexander Technique, Feldenkrais, Tai Chi, and dance may share some similarities with yoga, but they are distinct in their methods and goals. When I first started teaching yoga in the 90s, I was often asked to substitute for Pilates classes. That curiosity led me to pursue a Pilates certification, and I discovered how different it is from yoga.

Other forms of somatic movement, such as mindful walking, shaking-it-off exercises, body scans, and meditation are also unique from yoga. While yoga classes can be taught in a somatic way, some styles focus more on achieving specific poses (asanas) and breathing techniques.

REMEMBER

Somatic movement emphasizes reprogramming the brain-muscle connection, while yoga often prioritizes postures and breathwork to reach particular poses. Somatic practices tend to be slower and more deliberate. That said, yoga and somatic movement complement each other beautifully, and the experience largely depends on the teaching style.

For instance, a Bikram yoga class may focus on building stamina and holding postures in a heated room, leaving less time for introspection. In contrast, a mindful Yin yoga session gives you the space to tune inward, listen to your body, and address emotions as they arise.

Yoga and somatic movement share the need for mindfulness, and yoga combined with meditation can further enhance your somatic practice. Together, they create a well-rounded approach to connecting with your body and mind.

Awareness Is Enough

Somatic awareness is an essential first step, but it's not enough to create real transformation. Awareness gives you the insight to recognize your patterns, but change happens when you turn that insight into action. This is where many people mistakenly think somatic exercises are too easy or not challenging enough to produce real results.

REMEMBER

The combination of awareness and mindful movement is what drives lasting change. When you slow down and move with intention, you begin to understand how your body works and what it needs to function at its best. True growth lies on the other side of discomfort. This doesn't mean pushing through pain — somatic exercises aim to release patterns that create pain — but it can feel uncomfortable to let go of old habits and embrace new ones.

Somatic practices help you acknowledge what holds you back, both mentally and physically. By becoming more aware, you can take deliberate, mindful action, creating a ripple effect of positive change. Awareness leads to action, and action sparks motivation. As you integrate these steps into your life, you'll feel inspired to keep evolving and uncovering your full potential.

Chapter **17**

Ten Tips for Enhancing Your Somatic Experience

S omatic exercises offer incredible opportunities to connect with your body, mind, and emotions, but like any meaningful endeavor, it's natural to face challenges along the way. That's why I'm so excited to share these tips with you! They're designed to help you stay motivated, build consistency, and truly enjoy the process. Think of them as your guideposts for making somatic movement a rewarding and sustainable part of your life.

Create a Schedule

The most important thing you can do is make time for yourself, and the best way to do that is by creating a schedule. At the start of each week, look at your calendar and block out time for your somatic exercises. Be specific — mark the days, times, and exactly what you plan to do.

For example, your schedule might look like this:

> » **Monday:** Yoga, 10–11 a.m., after the kids leave for school and before a mid-morning break.

>> **Tuesday:** Pilates, 11:30 a.m., during lunch.

>> **Wednesday:** Yoga, 10–11 a.m.

>> **Thursday:** Mindful walk with a friend, 8:45 a.m., after-school drop-off.

>> **Friday:** Yoga and Pilates blend, 9 a.m.

>> **Saturday:** Rest day.

>> **Sunday:** Yoga, 6:30 a.m., before the kids wake up.

>> **Daily:** Meditation at 5:45 a.m. and 2 p.m.

A schedule gives you a framework to stay organized and committed. It removes the stress of trying to squeeze in a session at the last minute — because let's face it, that rarely works. By planning ahead, you ensure that you prioritize yourself. For more detailed tips on scheduling your practice, see Chapter 3.

Give yourself the time you deserve to feel your best. Establishing a routine isn't just good for your physical health — it's an investment in your mental well-being too.

Track Your Progress

Just as you schedule your workouts, make sure to track your progress. Seeing how far you've come and how far you can go is so exciting and rewarding. The sky's the limit, and you have a lifetime of learning and getting to know yourself better. Track every small win at the end of the day and look back on each week and each month and then at the end of the year. You'll be amazed at how much you've grown and transformed. Your progress can be emotional, physical, and mental.

Tracking helps you stay focused and motivated while keeping you aligned with your goals. It allows you to identify areas that need more attention and helps you celebrate every win, no matter how small. For instance, while tracking my emotional state and handstand practice, I noticed I had neglected hydration. Once I started tracking my water intake and nutrition, I saw how much they influenced my overall progress.

Adjusting your goals is part of the journey, and tracking gives you the information you need to make smart changes. It also keeps you accountable to your actions. You can't blame outside circumstances when you have a clear record of what's supporting or derailing you. For example, if you missed a few days of movement, tracking can help you pinpoint why. Were you distracted by social media or other avoidable activities? By reviewing your progress, you can spot patterns, redirect your energy, and refocus on what matters.

REMEMBER

Tracking boosts your chances of success. The more you monitor your progress, the more motivated and accountable you become. It's a chance to check in on the effectiveness of your plans, your consistency, and whether your goals remain realistic. With this data, you can adjust your approach, tackle one goal at a time, and reward yourself as you move forward.

Do It with a Buddy

One of the best ways to stay accountable and enhance your somatic experience is to move with a buddy. It's no surprise that dog owners walk more than non-dog owners — having a companion makes it easier to stay motivated. A dog can be a great walking partner, but having a human buddy offers even more benefits.

A workout buddy keeps you accountable. When someone else is counting on you, it's harder to skip a session. You're less likely to make excuses when you know a friend is waiting for you. A buddy also provides encouragement and motivation, helping you push through moments when you feel like giving up.

TIP

Share your somatic journey with a buddy to make the experience more enjoyable. You can discuss sensations, process emotions, or simply connect on a deeper level. I've noticed how much people open up during one-on-one yoga sessions — having a trusted friend can offer the same kind of insight and connection.

A buddy also supports your safety and progress. They can spot you during exercises, help improve your form, and keep you injury-free.

Use Apps and Other Helpful Technology

Apps and technology can be great tools to support your somatic journey. Many apps offer somatic movement classes tailored to different interests. If you love Pilates, there are countless apps and YouTube videos to explore. You can also find apps for yoga, Tai Chi, mindful strength training, guided walks, meditations, and more.

TIP

Pilates Anytime and Yoga Anytime have extensive libraries of classes, while Alo Moves features options like breathwork, meditation, yoga, Pilates, and strength workouts. Tonal, a smart strength-training system, adapts to your body and feels like somatic strength training in action.

If you're a fan of tracking data, there are plenty of tech gadgets available to provide feedback on your health. Wearables like heart rate monitors, tracking watches, and glucose monitors offer insights into your well-being. While I personally prefer to journal and track progress based on how I feel, some people love the precision of data.

For example, the Oura ring tracks sleep, fitness, menstrual cycles, stress, and even signs of illness or burnout. It uses biometric sensors to monitor metrics like heart rate and skin temperature. Fitbit devices track activity, sleep, heart rate, and workouts while offering reminders to move. An Apple Watch does all of this while doubling as a communication tool.

Although some of these gadgets can be pricey, many apps offer free trials, so you can test them before committing. Plus, most smartphones already include basic fitness trackers to log steps or support meditation apps. Even simple tools like these can enhance your journey and keep you motivated.

Celebrate Small Achievements

Don't forget to celebrate your wins along the way. Recognizing even the smallest achievements helps you stay motivated and reminds you of the progress you're making. Showing up for yourself — even for just five minutes a day — is worth celebrating. Those small moments add up to big transformations over time.

Celebrate the everyday joys, too — laughter, love, fresh air, and movement. Recently, I found myself laughing so hard at something silly my boys said in the car that my stomach hurt. Those belly laughs reminded me how much happiness comes from the little things. Write down a list of small treats that make you feel good, like a warm bath, a smoothie, or even a new pair of cozy socks. Pick one each day to pair with your somatic practice to double the benefits.

You can use tools like badges, stickers, or charts to track your progress. My son practices Spanish on Duolingo, and he's on a streak because he loves earning daily rewards. You can create a colorful chart or mark milestones in your phone to keep yourself motivated.

Keep an attitude of gratitude and find joy in everyday tasks, like sipping tea, watering your plants, or unloading the dishwasher. Mindfulness in the little things makes it easier to appreciate your wins, no matter how small.

Work at Your Own Pace

Moving at your own pace means choosing a speed that feels right for you and letting go of comparisons. Comparison truly is the thief of joy — focus on your journey, not anyone else's.

Set realistic goals that align with your values and break them into smaller, manageable steps. Start slowly and choose somatic movements you enjoy, as you're more likely to stick with them. This isn't about quick fixes; it's about long-term growth. Celebrate your successes, no matter how small, because even the slowest pace is still forward progress. Listen to your body, take breaks when needed, and trust that you're exactly where you need to be.

REMEMBER

It's easy to feel like others are moving ahead faster, but everyone has their own challenges. Even if your progress feels like an inch at a time, it's still progress. Growth isn't always linear, and some days you may feel stuck. Those moments of frustration are part of the process. Call out those feelings, reframe your mindset, and be patient with yourself. Somatic movement lets you embrace the process, continually discovering and building a better relationship with yourself.

Find Ways to Incorporate Somatics into Other Activities

You can integrate somatic movement into nearly any activity. By weaving grounding exercises, body scans, and mindful techniques into your day, you deepen your connection to your body and enhance whatever you're doing. For more on incorporating somatic movement into everyday life, hop over to Chapter 4.

TIP

Grounding exercises help you stay present and feel more stable. Use them at any time — while at work, before a workout, first thing in the morning, or as you wind down at night. Ground yourself during conversations or moments of anxiety to feel calmer and more centered (see Chapter 10 for more on grounding techniques).

Body scans are another simple but powerful tool. Check in with your body during movement sessions, at the end of a yoga class, or even while sitting in traffic. A quick scan helps you tune into your body's sensations, letting you notice and release tension (explore body-scan techniques in Chapter 6).

Breathing exercises signal safety to your brain and body. Use them to calm down during workouts, meditation, or daily activities like showering or working.

Whether you start your day with intentional breaths or use them to wind down at night, this practice is invaluable. See Chapter 4 for guidance on breathwork.

Somatic movement also complements other physical activities like strength training, running, dancing, and hiking. Pay attention to how your body feels as you move. Let it give you feedback and use that information to guide your transformation. Whether you're lifting weights, hitting the trails, or jogging, somatic awareness helps you connect deeply with your body, enhancing both your performance and your enjoyment.

See a Professional

Working with an expert can greatly enhance your somatic journey. An expert can help you break through plateaus, deepen your practice, and give you personalized techniques to use at home. I love working with professionals when I feel stuck in my own practice — they always help me find new insights and move forward.

When you hire a professional, you can share your goals and personal history to create a tailored plan. They help you stay on track, monitor your progress, and guide you to the next level. Experts also provide unique cues, metaphors, and alignment tips to help you connect more deeply with your body and understand how it works. Under their guidance, you can tap into sensations, release tension, and feel safe exploring your range of motion.

Professionals often use hands-on techniques to help you go deeper, whether through physical adjustments, alignment assists, or massage. For example, when my yoga or Pilates teacher uses touch to guide me, it helps me activate the right muscles and feel where I need to focus. If you're carrying physical tension, a Rolfing expert or Feldenkrais practitioner can help you release stored tension and improve movement patterns.

Seeing a professional also helps you stay mindful and engaged. At home, it's easy to get distracted, but a private session eliminates outside noise and lets you focus entirely on yourself. Trained coaches can guide you through breathing, meditation, and movement with clarity and intention.

Finally, working with an expert allows you to process the "issues in your tissues." While not all professionals are therapists, they can help you relax, breathe into sensations, and feel supported in your journey. Knowing that you're not alone — and that others are also learning and growing — makes the experience even more valuable. Professionals draw from their experience with a variety of clients, ensuring your sessions are customized to meet your unique needs. If you need help finding a professional, turn to Chapter 3.

Share Your Experience

Sharing your somatic journey with others enhances your practice in countless ways. It reinforces what you're learning, gets you excited about your progress, and inspires others to explore their own journeys. The more you share, the more connected and motivated you'll feel.

TIP

When you share, be specific. Help others visualize your experience by describing how your body feels before, during, and after a session. For example: "Yesterday, I took a Pilates class to strengthen my core and discovered how to connect my glutes to my abs for better control. It was fascinating. Have you ever tried Pilates?" Being detailed reminds you why you're doing this work and spreads your enthusiasm. Use descriptive language to share the emotions and sensations you experience. Highlight your wins — learning crow pose or meditating for a week straight — and let others celebrate with you. Sharing success motivates both you and those around you.

Acknowledge challenges, too. Somatic movement isn't always easy, and it's okay to admit when something felt uncomfortable. Sharing how you worked through frustrations makes your journey relatable and inspiring. As you practice being open, you'll grow emotionally and learn to sit with sensations that arise.

REMEMBER

Avoid giving advice — no one likes being told what to do. Instead, lead by example. When my boys see me meditating daily, they get curious and eventually join in. Your consistency and commitment will naturally inspire others.

Be Open to Surprises

As you practice somatic exercises, notice and be aware of any unexpected changes, such as how you interact with your family, friends, and workmates. You might notice that you digest food better, react to stress in a different way, or sleep better. Be more curious about the people and things around you. Notice how/if your life changes color. Notice not only how you reach the goals you set up, but also other side-benefits.

Share Your Experience

Sharing your somatic journey with others enhances your practice in countless ways. It reinforces what you're learning, gets you excited about your progress, and inspires others to explore their own journeys. The more you share, the more connected and motivated you'll feel.

When you share, be specific. Help others visualize your experience by describing how your body feels before, during, and after a session. For example: "Yesterday, I took a Pilates class to strengthen my core and discovered how to control my glutes for my abs for better control. It was fascinating. Have you ever tried Pilates?" Being detailed reminds you why you're doing this work, and spreads your enthusiasm. Use descriptive language to share the emotions and sensations you experience. Highlight your wins — learning crow pose or meditating for a week straight — and let others celebrate with you. Sharing success motivates both you and those around you.

Acknowledge challenges, too. Somatic movement isn't always easy, and it's okay to admit when something felt uncomfortable. Sharing how you worked through frustrations makes your journey relatable and inspiring. As you practice being open, you'll grow emotionally and learn to sit with sensations that arise.

Avoid giving advice — no one likes being told what to do. Instead, lead by example. When my boys see me meditating daily, they get curious and eventually join in. Your consistency and commitment will naturally inspire others.

Be Open to Surprises

As you practice somatic exercises, notice and be aware of any unexpected changes, such as how you interact with your family, friends, and workmates. You might notice that you eat and feel better, react to stress in a different way, or sleep better. Be more curious about the people and things around you. Before long, if your life changes color. Notice not only how you reach the goals you set up, but also other side-benefits.

Index

Numbers

4-7-8 breathing, 69–70, 180–181

A

accessibility, modifying exercises for, 332–333
achievements, celebrating, 354
age, making adjustments for, 323–328
  middle age, 324–327
  seniors, 327–328
Aikido, 96
Alexander, Frederick Matthias, 13, 218
Alexander Technique (AT)
  creation of, 13
  incorporating into daily routine, 220–222
  managing chronic conditions using, 291
  physical relief and emotional support from, 294
  for posture and movement efficiency, 219
  practitioners of, 282
  principles of, 218–219
  similarities between yoga and, 350
Alo Moves app, 353
Alphabet Tracing exercise, 289
alternate nostril breathing, 65–68
anger, expressing with somatic exercises, 23–25
ankles, 288–290
  issues with, 288–289
  mobility exercises for, 289–290

strengthening exercises for, 289
Ankle-to-Knee Pose, 271, 283
anxiety, 20–21, 245
  grounding and, 203
  meditation and, 192
  sleep-related, 171, 185–186
Apple Watch, 336, 354
apps, 336, 353–354. *See also specific apps*
Arch and Curl exercise, 84–85, 251
arch raises, 290
Arm and Leg Waves exercise, 235
arm lifts, 227
arthritis, 291–292
Articulating Bridge exercise, 176–177, 260
Ashe, Arthur, 328
AT. *See* Alexander Technique
autogenic inhibition, 119
awareness. *See* relaxation and awareness
Awareness Through Movement (ATM), 225

B

back, 279–282
  core strengthening for support of, 280–281
  healthy, maintaining, 282
  stretches for lower and upper back, 280
Back Lift exercise, 251
Bainbridge Cohen, Bonnie, 222
balance, improving
  Body-Mind Centering, 224

for seniors, 327–328
for stability, 91–93
Standing Awareness exercise, 104–105
using strength training, 93–94
ball roll exercise, 290
Banana Pose exercise, 177–178, 259
baseline concept, 233
benefits of somatic exercises
  alleviating chronic pain, 28–29
  deepening emotional balance, 20
  easing anxiety, 20–21
  enhancing self-awareness, 18–19
  expressing anger, 23–25
  fostering relaxation, 30–32
  healing trauma, 32–33
  increasing flexibility and mobility, 29–30
  interoception, 80
  managing stress, 22–23
  overview, 13–14
  supporting healthy relationship with food, 25–27
BESS (Body, Effort, Shape, and Space), 228–229
Biles, Simone, 18
Bird Dog exercise, 159, 281, 328
blocks, 332
BMC. *See* Body-Mind Centering
Body, Effort, Shape, and Space (BESS), 228–229
body mapping
  benefits of, 109–110
  techniques for, 110–112

About the Author

Kristin McGee is a nationally recognized yoga and Pilates teacher, speaker, *mompreneur*, and author. With over three decades of experience in the fitness and wellness space, she has had a continuous roster of high profile celebrities, pioneered the launch of Peloton's yoga and Pilates program, and recently branched out on her own to launch Kristin McGee Movement. You can check out her website at www.kristinmcgee.com.

Dedication

To my three boys, who inspire me daily to keep growing, learning, and becoming the best version of myself. Your love and energy fuel my journey every day.

And to my mom, dad, and entire family — thank you for your unwavering support and encouragement. Your belief in me means the world.

To all those who seek balance, joy, and growth — whether on the mat, in life, or in the heart. May this book inspire you to embrace each breath, each challenge, and each moment with compassion and courage.

Author's Acknowledgments

A special thank you to all of my students and to Tracy Boggier, who encouraged me to step into this project.

Thanks also go to the exceptional staff at Wiley. A special thank you to Kezia Endsley, Sarah Sypniewski, Penny Stuart, and Saikarthick Kumarasamy, for their patience and countless hours making this book happen.

Publisher's Acknowledgments

Acquisitions Editor: Tracy Boggier

Senior Project/Copy Editor: Kezia Endsley

Technical Reviewer: Staffan Elgelid

Production Editor: Saikarthick Kumarasamy

Cover Image: Courtesy of Guisela Corado